Bipolar Disorder in Older Age Patients

Susan W. Lehmann · Brent P. Forester
Editors

Bipolar Disorder in Older Age Patients

Springer

Editors
Susan W. Lehmann
Department of Psychiatry and Behavioral Sciences, Division of Geriatric Psychiatry and Neuropsychiatry
The Johns Hopkins University School of Medicine
Baltimore, MD
USA

Brent P. Forester
Division of Geriatric Psychiatry
McLean Hospital
Belmont, MA
USA

and

Behavioral Health, Population Health Management
Partners Healthcare
Boston, MA
USA

and

Harvard Medical School
Boston, MA
USA

ISBN 978-3-319-48910-0 ISBN 978-3-319-48912-4 (eBook)
DOI 10.1007/978-3-319-48912-4

Library of Congress Control Number: 2016955929

Printed on acid-free paper

This Springer imprint is published by Springer Nature
The registered company is Springer International Publishing AG
The registered company address is: Gewerbestrasse 11, 6330 Cham, Switzerland

We dedicate this book to our patients and their families who have inspired us and taught us countless lessons about the impact of bipolar disorder on their lives.

Susan W. Lehmann, MD
Brent P. Forester, MD, M.Sc.

Preface

Over sixty years ago, Sir Martin Roth described a case series of patients over the age of 60 who were hospitalized for a psychiatric condition. He observed that patients with mania, who constituted 6% of all individuals with affective disorder, tended to have a worse outcome than other patients with depressive disorders and were discharged less often [1]. Roth was the first to distinguish a different clinical course and prognosis of elders with affective disorders compared to elders with dementia or paranoid disorders.

During the past six decades since Roth first published his findings, older age bipolar disorder has been relatively understudied compared with unipolar depression. Yet, older individuals with bipolar disorder continue to present clinical challenges. Over the next 20 years, the population of individuals over age 60 is expected to increase dramatically, due to the combined effects of increase in life expectancy and longevity as a result of advances in general health care, and the demographic influx of the baby boomer generation into older age brackets. Along with the rapid aging of the population are projections for significantly increased numbers of older individuals with mental health needs, including bipolar disorder [2].

Bipolar disorder occurs in individuals across the lifespan, from childhood through old age. At all ages, bipolar disorder can be difficult to diagnose and to treat. While depressive disorders are frequently managed by non-psychiatric healthcare clinicians, bipolar disorder—with its complexities of clinical presentation, comorbid substance use disorders, and varying affective states—often requires the specific expertise of a psychiatrist. In older age, issues of diagnosis and clinical management are compounded by the presence of comorbid medical disorders commonly occurring with aging. Changes in physiology (especially renal, hepatic, and cardiac function), concomitant medications, and concerns about cognitive impairment further complicate clinical decision-making for the psychiatrist caring for the older patient with bipolar disorder. Moreover, older age bipolar disorder causes significant psychiatric and social morbidity, including high use of outpatient and inpatient psychiatric resources [3]. Effective care of the older patient with bipolar disorder must also include advanced knowledge about best practices regarding optimum modes of psychotherapy, psychosocial support, and treatment care settings.

Fortunately, in recent years, there has been increased interest in understanding the clinical features, biological underpinnings, and best approaches to management for individuals with older age bipolar disorder. This book brings together experts in older age bipolar disorder, presenting current knowledge in these areas and highlighting future research directions. The scope of the book is broad, encompassing epidemiology, the clinical assessment and diagnosis of the older patient who may have bipolar disorder, the neurobiology of older age bipolar disorder, and the principles of clinical management. In addition, there are chapters on substance use disorders and cognitive impairment in bipolar disorder. Other chapters focus on lithium, neuromodulation, psychotherapy, complementary and alternative medicine and its relevance for older age bipolar disorder, and a review of treatment care settings. Each chapter includes at least one clinical patient "Vignette" with "Learning Points," which illustrates principles described in the chapter, and each chapter concludes with a summary list of "Clinical Pearls" for the clinician.

This book is aimed for the general psychiatrist caring for older adults with bipolar disorder. Throughout the book, we highlight aspects which are especially unique or important to the care of the older patient with bipolar disorder. As our co-authors frequently note, there still is much more to learn about older age bipolar disorder. Additional research is needed to better understand the neurobiology of the disorder, the relationship between older age bipolar disorder, cognitive impairment and risk for major neurocognitive disorder, optimum pharmacotherapy, and best practices for older patients with both bipolar disorder and substance use disorders. Collaboration across research centers will be required to collect consistent neurobiological and clinical data that will lead to a better understanding of the trajectory of bipolar disorder into older age and relevant neurobiological and psychosocial markers to guide the development of more specific and effective interventions.

We have benefited greatly from the collaboration and support of wonderful colleagues who are leaders in the field of old-age psychiatry and older age bipolar disorder and who have contributed so generously of their expertise and time to this book. We are especially indebted to the excellent editing guidance provided by Elizabeth Corra from Springer. We believe that this book will help the general and geriatric psychiatrist more effectively provide evidence-based and thoughtful psychiatric care to improve the quality of life and daily functioning of older adults with bipolar disorder.

Finally, we are indebted to our families. Brent thanks his wife, Kim, son Rylan, and daughter Sasha, for their endless support, patience, and good humor. Susan thanks her husband, Richard, for his unflagging support and encouragement, which make all things possible.

Baltimore, MD, USA — Susan W. Lehmann
Belmont, MA, USA; Boston, MA, USA — Brent P. Forester

References

1. Roth M. The natural history of mental disorder in old age. J Ment Sci. 1955;101:281–91.
2. Bartels SJ, Naslund JA. The underside of the silver tsunami—older adults and mental health care. NEJM. 2013;368:493–6.
3. Bartels SJ, Forester B, Miles KM, Joyce T. Mental health service use by elderly patients with bipolar disorder and unipolar major depression. Am J Geriatr Psychiatry. 2000 Spring;8 (2):160–6.

Contents

Contributors

Olusola Ajilore Psychiatric Institute, University of Illinois at Chicago, Chicago, IL, USA

Rayan K. Al Jurdi Department of Psychiatry and Behavioral Sciences, Baylon College of Medicine, Houston, TX, USA

Chaya Bhuvaneswaran West Newton, MA, USA

Danielle Carns Adler School of Professional Psychology, Chicago, IL, USA

Megan Y.S. Chan Department of Psychological Medicine, Tan Tock Seng Hospital, Singapore, Singapore

Peijun Chen Department of Psychiatry, Louis Stokes Cleveland VA Medical Center, Cleveland, OH, USA

Colin Depp Department of Psychiatry, University of California at San Diego, La Jolla, CA, USA

Annemiek Dols Department of Old Age Psychiatry, VU Medical Center, GGZinGeest, Amsterdam, The Netherlands

Eulogio Eclarinal Ambulatory Clinic, Neuropsychiatric Institute, University of Illinois at Chicago, Chicago, IL, USA

Rachel C. Edelman Department of Psychiatry, University of California at San Diego, La Jolla, CA, USA; Santa Monica, CA, USA

Oliver M. Glass Department of Psychiatry and Behavioral Medicine, East Carolina University, Greenville, NC, USA

Rita Hargrave Oakland, CA, USA

Adriana P. Hermida Department of Psychiatry and Behavioral Sciences, Emory University School of Medicine, Atlanta, GA, USA

Dimitris N. Kiosses Westchester Division, Department of Psychiatry, New York Presbyterian Hospital-Weill Cornell Medicine, White Plains, NY, USA

Susan W. Lehmann Department of Psychiatry and Behavioral Sciences, Johns Hopkins University School of Medicine, Baltimore, MD, USA

Nicole Leistikow Department of Psychiatry and Behavioral Sciences, Johns Hopkins University School of Medicine, Baltimore, MD, USA

Maria Cristina Poscablo-Stein Department of Psychiatry and Behavioral Sciences, Emory University School of Medicine, Atlanta, GA, USA

Soham Rej Division of Geriatric Psychiatry, Department of Psychiatry, Institute for Community and Family Psychiatry, Jewish General Hospital, Montreal, QC, Canada

Martha Sajatovic Department of Psychiatry, School of Medicine, Case Western Reserve University, Cleveland, OH, USA

E. Sherwood Brown Department of Psychiatry, The University of Texas Southwestern Medical Center, Dallas, TX, USA

Kenneth Shulman Department of Psychiatry, Sunnybrook Health Sciences Centre, Toronto, ON, Canada

Sara Weisenbach Department of Psychiatry, University of Utah School of Medicine, Salt Lake City, UT, USA

Lindsey C. Wright New York, NY, USA

Robert C. Young Westchester Division, Department of Psychiatry, New York Presbyterian Hospital-Weill Cornell Medicine, White Plains, NY, USA

Epidemiology of Older Age Bipolar Disorder

1

Nicole Leistikow and Susan W. Lehmann

1.1 Introduction

Worldwide population reports project significant increases in the population of older adults over the next 40 years [1]. Greater numbers of older adults and their longer life expectancy due to healthcare advances will result in greater numbers of older adults living with bipolar disorder. Older adults with bipolar disorder (OABD) utilize more healthcare services than similar-aged healthy peers, yet remain less well-studied than younger age groups [2–4]. Consequently, the identification of and care for elders with bipolar disorder represent a growing public health need [5], giving greater urgency to understanding the prevalence, clinical presentation, and course of OABD.

1.2 Definition

Researchers have defined OABD in different ways, contributing to methodological complexity. While there is no clear consensus regarding when "older age" begins, most studies have defined OABD as starting between age 50 and 60 [1, 4, 6–8]. However, it is important to recognize that older adults with OABD may comprise 3 or even 4 distinct groups of individuals: (1) persons living longer with bipolar

N. Leistikow (✉) · S.W. Lehmann
Department of Psychiatry and Behavioral Sciences, Johns Hopkins University School of Medicine, 600 North Wolfe Street, Meyer 4-181, Baltimore, MD 21287, USA
e-mail: leistikow@jhmi.edu

S.W. Lehmann
e-mail: slehman@jhmi.edu

S.W. Lehmann and B.P. Forester (eds.), *Bipolar Disorder in Older Age Patients*,
DOI 10.1007/978-3-319-48912-4_1

Table 1.1 Defining older age bipolar disorder

An adult >age 50 with	Early-onset bipolar disorder	=	Older age bipolar disorder
	Early-onset depressive disorder with new-onset mania		
	New-onset mania in individual with no prior mood illness (in the absence of a specific medical trigger, but may be associated with brain injury, silent stroke or cerebrovascular risk factors)		
	Secondary mania (temporally and directly linked to a specific medical trigger) followed by symptoms consistent with bipolar disorder		

disorder that began in the first half of their life, (2) those with a preexisting depressive disorder that started early in adulthood and converts to bipolar disorder in later life, (3) those without previous episodes of depressive illness who present with new-onset mania in later life, and (4) those individuals with "secondary mania" who acquire bipolar disorder, or a psychiatric condition appearing similar to bipolar disorder, as a direct result of other medical causes (Table 1.1). The definitions of early- versus late-onset and secondary bipolar illnesses will be discussed below in the next section.

1.3 Limitations

One of the major challenges in studying bipolar disorder in older age is that it is less common in older than in younger individuals. An important limitation to the majority of studies to date is small sample size. The largest research samples of individuals with bipolar disorder have had populations in the low thousands [9, 10], with the majority of studies looking at sample sizes in the low hundreds or less [5]. Because searching within inpatient populations is a convenient way to locate subjects with a relatively rare disorder, the majority of studies on late-life bipolar illness focus on this group. However, this approach skews samples toward those individuals with more severe illness, and thus, findings may not be relevant for individuals with milder symptoms and those who require only outpatient care [5, 11]. Additionally, there is a lack of longitudinal studies in this area, resulting in a paucity of information about the long-term course of older age bipolar disorder. Further, retrospective collection of historical details, such as an individual's age of onset and clinical presentation, is subject to recall bias or error. Lack of prospective data may also contribute to a selection bias of individuals who survive into later life.

In general, the studies we cite are from US samples unless indicated. Different countries have varying demographic proportions between old and young, different medical and mental health systems in place, and different social services available which may affect age of onset proportions and prevalence rates in inpatient versus outpatient populations as well as health services utilization.

1.4 Prevalence in the Community

Overall, the prevalence rates of individuals living in the community with bipolar illness decrease with age [1, 12, 13]. Whereas bipolar disorder is present in 1.4 % of individuals aged 18–44, prevalence rates decrease to 0.1–0.5 % in people aged 65 and older [11, 14]. When individuals with both bipolar type 1 and bipolar type 2 disorders are considered, prevalence of OABD has been reported to be 1 % of individuals over the age of 60 [15]. It remains unclear whether this is a historic effect, related to diagnosis and identification of older patients, a cohort effect related to a lower level of disease among adults born earlier, a result of increased mortality among individuals with early-onset bipolar disorder (EOBD), or a combination of factors [16].

1.5 Prevalence in Treatment Settings

However, in contradistinction to low prevalence rates among older people living independently in the community, late-life bipolar disorder is more common in treatment settings. Since the landmark Epidemiologic Catchment Area study (ECA) in the 1980s, which found bipolar illness in 9.7 % of chronically institutionalized adults in prisons or nursing homes, researchers have recognized that the illness is overrepresented in care settings, and this discrepancy increases as people age [14, 17, 18]. For instance, a recent survey of 2600 New York City senior living facility residents found a bipolar disorder prevalence rate of 7.8 % [19]. In addition, a large study of all veterans in a national database found that fully one-quarter of those receiving either outpatient or inpatient treatment through the Veterans Administration for a bipolar diagnosis were aged 60 or older [20].

On inpatient psychiatric units, there seems to be relatively equal rates of younger and older adults with bipolar illness, close to 10 % for each, despite the declining prevalence of bipolar disorder in older age [5, 12, 15]. An early study of patients with late-onset bipolar disorder (LOBD) found that they accounted for 9.3 % of geriatric affective disorder admissions over a 2-year period [21]. One recent review article calculated the prevalence of mania in adults over the age of 50 who were being treated in a hospital for any mental illness to be 6.0 %, with one-third of those having first-time late-onset mania [11]. Rates of bipolar illness among those presenting to psychiatric emergency rooms are higher than in inpatient settings. A study of 2419 adult visitors to a Seattle psychiatric crisis unit found that 14 % of these patients had bipolar disorder [22]. Another study that focused on psychiatric emergency department visitors older than age 60 found that 17 % had bipolar disorder [23].

Therefore, although the prevalence of bipolar disorder decreases with advancing age, individuals with OABD represent a sizable proportion of the bipolar community, with a need for acute psychiatric services as well as day hospital treatment and case management that is equal to or greater than their younger cohort [2, 5, 13, 20].

1.6 Age of Onset

The clinical heterogeneity of older individuals with bipolar disorder is an ongoing area of research. As a group, older adults with bipolar illness share qualities of aging, including greater medical comorbidity, increased risk for polypharmacy, and physiologic reduction in renal function. However, research over many years has identified two distinct types of bipolar disorder among older adults, each with varying courses: EOBD and LOBD.

When this phenomenon was initially observed, there was interest in distinguishing between these two groups. However, it has been challenging to assemble large sample populations, and most studies have had modest numbers and inconsistent findings, making conclusions hard to draw. Some trends have been observed but with uncertain clinical significance. Over the past decade, researchers have placed less emphasis on distinguishing between early- and late-onset illnesses. It remains to be seen whether larger studies may reveal important clinical distinctions between these two groups. However, generalizing about the nature of bipolar disorder in later life, without taking into account these possible subtypes, runs the risk of conflating age-related versus disease-specific effects.

1.6.1 Bimodal Distribution

Defining the age at onset of bipolar disorder has posed significant challenges for researchers and there continues to be no clear consensus about how this should be done. Does one use the age at first mental health contact, the age at first psychiatric hospitalization, or the first time the patient experienced significant mood symptoms causing impairment in functioning? Does onset of bipolar disorder begin at the first depression or the first mania? If manias present first, the task of determining age of onset is relatively straightforward. However, for as many as 25 % of individuals who eventually meet DSM 5 diagnostic criteria for bipolar disorder, the first psychiatric treatment or hospitalization for any mood disorder will be for major depression, sometimes years to decades prior to the emergence of mania, delaying a correct diagnosis [7, 13, 24–27].

Despite these challenges, multiple studies of bipolar disorder have found a bimodal distribution of age of onset, with two major groups: a larger group experiencing onset of manic symptoms before age 30 and a smaller group with onset after age 40 [1, 7, 10, 24, 25, 28–32]. Some studies have defined an additional group with early onset in childhood or adolescence [33–36]. For the most part, two groups of individuals have been described: those with early-onset and late-onset disease.

1.6.2 Cutpoints and Proportionality of Early- Versus Late-Onset Bipolar Disorder in the Treatment Population

It is important to recognize that although an estimated 90 % of patients who will develop bipolar illness over their life span are diagnosed by the age of 50, first mental health contact occurs after age 60 for a significant minority of 8–9 % [24, 25, 28]. Although the findings are not unequivocal, research suggests that those who experience bipolar disease onset later in life may have different demographic profiles, risk factors, clinical presentation, and disease course. Future research may delineate whether they have distinct etiologies.

Various studies not only differ in the definition of "age of onset" for their subject population, but also use different cutpoints to distinguish early- and late-onset groups, challenging comparisons across studies. Researchers have utilized different approaches to determine which age cutpoint to use. Some studies have attempted to calculate a mathematically likely age dividing line based on the statistical distribution of their sample, while other studies have used arbitrary or convenience cutpoints. Using a cutpoint at age 40, one study found the proportion of early- and late-onset bipolar patients in a community sample in England to be 78 and 22 %, respectively [25]. Using a cutpoint at age 50, a study looking at both inpatients and outpatients diagnosed with bipolar I disorder, found that of those over 60, about one-third had experienced late onset of their illness [37]. Using a later cutpoint at age 60, a large Veterans Administration study of both inpatients and outpatients found that at least 9 % of individuals over 60 with bipolar disorder had just been diagnosed with that disorder in the prior year [20]. Using a lower cutpoint at age 45, a small study of inpatients hospitalized with mania found the proportion of patients with late versus early onset to be roughly equal [7]. Using a cutpoint at age 47 based on first psychiatric hospitalization, a midsize retrospective study of inpatients with bipolar disorder found that only 6.3 % had LOBD [29]. There remains a wide variation in the proportion of OABD that current studies ascribe to early- versus late-onset disease. The International Society for Bipolar Disorders Task Force on Older Age Bipolar Disorder noted that while age 50 may be a reasonable cutpoint to distinguish EOBD from LOBD, this is an area requiring further study, and a lower cutpoint of age 40 may be warranted if supported by future research [1].

1.7 Demographic Distinctions

Individuals who present with bipolar illness at a later age tend to be skewed demographically in three ways. One distinction is that while male to female gender ratios are fairly even among younger adults with EOBD, women predominate in many late-onset bipolar samples [9, 21, 25, 27, 35, 38]. It remains unclear whether this indicates a survival cohort, a bias in users of medical services, or a correlation between female gender and vulnerability to late-onset disease. A large study of both inpatients and outpatients in Denmark saw no statistically significant gender difference among older patients with bipolar disorder [10], similar to results from an inpatient study in Scotland that took population gender rates into account [39] and a small study of outpatients in England [30]. One finding that has been consistent across studies is that individuals presenting with bipolar illness later in life are less likely than early-onset patients to have a family history of bipolar illness [21, 24–26, 31], raising the question of alternative pathways to disease.

Finally, bipolar illness impacts close relationships [40]. Two studies found that those with later onset of illness were more likely to be married or living with someone in their older age than those with earlier onset of disease [32, 35]. One of the few prospective examinations of age of onset in bipolar illness found that 52 % of those who first became ill after age 30 were married at the time of the study compared to 27 % of those who experienced illness before age 21 and 40 % of those first ill before age 30 [33]. Another small study found that those with later onset reported more social support and perceived their social support to be more adequate compared with those who had earlier onset of bipolar disease [26]. These results suggest that social support may be a casualty of the disease striking before or during the age when people often find and consolidate partnerships and also has ramifications for prognosis and service utilization as patients age.

1.8 Heterogeneous Etiologies—Including Cerebrovascular Risk Factors and Secondary Mania

The bimodal distribution of age of onset, demographic differences, and possible distinctions in natural course of disease all beg the question, "Could LOBD be secondary to or exacerbated by cerebrovascular disease or any other focal neurobiological insult?" There seems to be clear evidence that cerebrovascular disease is frequently associated with LOBD, but not through one definitive pathway, and little characterization of predisposing factors. Furthermore, there is evidence for both new-onset mania in the setting of cerebrovascular risk and secondary mania triggered by a proximate medical cause.

The hypothesis that cerebrovascular insult may initiate onset of bipolar disorder later in life comes from rare observations of new-onset mania following brain injury. Mania-inducing strokes represent <1 % of all strokes but seem to predominate in the right frontal or temporal region [41–45]. There are no prospective studies following these patients over the long term; what evidence there is suggests that a proportion have resolution of their manic symptoms after one episode of mania and others go on to have bipolar disorder with recurring episodes of mood disturbance [44].

In addition to strokes causing mania, there is a growing literature suggesting a role for silent cerebral infarctions in late-onset bipolar illness. These are brain lesions seen on imaging but not known to be linked temporally to symptoms. An early small study found that 65 % of patients with LOBD had silent brain infarcts compared to 25 % of patients with early onset of either depression or bipolar disorder [46]. A more recent small study found that 92 % of patients with LOBD (compared to 53 % of those with EOBD) had visible brain infarctions on imaging, the majority of which, 62 %, were silent [47]. A small study of patients with their first episode of mania after age 65 found that 71 % had a comorbid neurologic disorder, twice as many compared to their age cohort with earlier onset bipolar illness [48].

More broadly, the link between LOBD and general cerebrovascular risk has been examined by many studies, with inconclusive results. An early study found that elderly patients with bipolar illness had significantly more cortical atrophy and poorer scores on cognitive tests than age-matched controls but did not find differences between those with early- versus late-onset illness [24]. However, a later study found that those with LOBD had significantly more cerebrovascular abnormalities [32]. Another small study that rigorously matched late-onset and early-onset patients by race, sex, and age found that the late-onset group had significantly more vascular risk factors and disease than those who were their same age but had disease onset earlier in life [29]. A small study in England found that among an older group of outpatients, those whose bipolar disorder occurred later had a significantly higher stroke risk compared to those who had earlier onset [30]. A large prospective Danish registry study of more than 200,000 patients found that having dementia, a disease of diverse etiologies but always related to structural brain disease, significantly increased the risk of developing mania or bipolar disorder [49].

In fact, the relationship between brain ischemia and bipolar illness may be more complex. Cerebrovascular disease may be a cause of LOBD, but early-onset bipolar illness itself, or its treatment, may predispose to conditions causing strokes such as inflammation, metabolic derangements, and obesity. The small study mentioned above found a higher incidence of silent cerebral infarcts in individuals with late-onset bipolar illness. This study also demonstrated that 47 % of patients in their 60s with early-onset bipolar illness had silent infarcts on brain imaging compared to 20 % of healthy people the same age [47], suggesting ischemia as both a trigger for and a consequence of bipolar illness.

The hypothesis that vascular injury to the brain may contribute to the onset of bipolar illness in a subset of individuals is particularly intriguing because it suggests that screening for and treating vascular risk factors could potentially delay or prevent onset of mania, and is an important question for future research. In addition, the increased risk for vascular disease in those with EOBD needs to be factored into treatment.

In addition to the possibility that symptomatic or silent cerebrovascular injury can cause new-onset mania in later life, the phenomenon of mania secondary to medication, somatic illness, delirium, or dementia is well established (Fig. 1.1) [11,

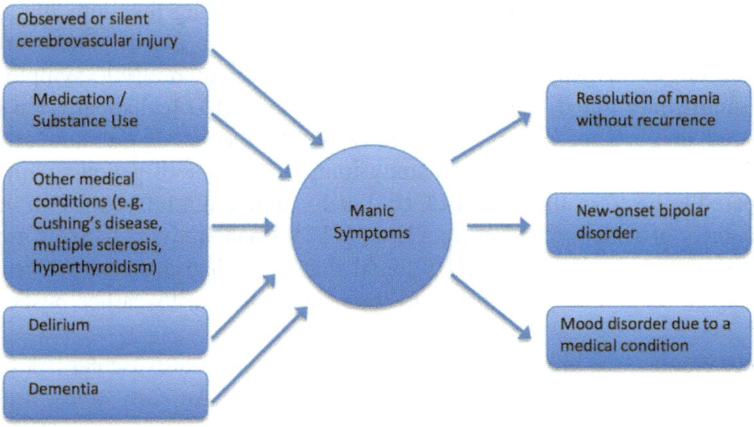

Fig. 1.1 Possible causes of late-life mania

50, 51]. In some cases, when the offending agent or illness is removed or successfully treated, mania resolves and does not recur. However, other patients may recover from the inciting factor but go on to develop repeating patterns of mania and depression best characterized as bipolar disorder, that we may think of as having been unmasked or triggered by the event. Others still may have chronic illnesses which cause a manic-like syndrome best thought of as a mood disorder secondary to a medical condition. Medications implicated are numerous and include corticosteroids, isoniazid, dopaminergic agents, and antidepressants [50]. Drugs of abuse including alcohol, cocaine, stimulants, and hallucinogens can also incite mania [52]. Illnesses-causing mania are likewise numerous and include Cushing's disease, influenza, HIV, neurosyphilis, multiple sclerosis, hyperthyroidism, brain tumors, and seizure disorders among others [52]. Delirium is an acute state of global confusion that can present with manic symptoms but should be resolved before diagnosis of ongoing mania is made. Dementias, especially frontal-temporal dementia, can present with manic-like syndromes and have cerebrovascular injury as an overlapping risk factor (Fig. 1.1).

Clinical Vignette 1.1

Ms. S is a 70-year-old married African American woman who was diagnosed with bipolar disorder in her 60s after experiencing a steroid-induced psychosis.

Her family history was notable for dementia in her mother. Her personal history was notable for an unremarkable birth and development; she successfully completed college and worked as a nurse until retirement in her 50s, and was married with one child. Her medical history was significant for giant cell arteritis requiring treatment with steroids.

Her psychiatric history was notable for the absence of mental illness until her 60s, when Ms. S was brought to the emergency department by her husband for talking fast and not making sense. A psychiatric consult attributed her abnormal behavior to high-dose prednisone she was taking at the time. This was tapered off and she returned to baseline. Six years later, she began having increased energy, with problems falling asleep, and increased cleaning at night while again on steroid medication. She was hospitalized on a medical service, diagnosed with steroid-induced psychosis, treated with low-dose neuroleptic medication, and discharged on a lower dose of steroids. Two months later, Ms. S presented with her first episode of depression marked by low mood, low appetite with weight loss, low energy, sadness, loss of confidence, isolation, and poor concentration. She was diagnosed with major depression and started on nortriptyline and after two months had resolution of depression but then began to experience decreased sleep and increased energy. Lithium was added to her regimen and her diagnosis was changed to bipolar disorder. Eventually, nortriptyline was tapered and discontinued and her mood remained stable on lithium alone for years with no further episodes of mania or depression.

Learning Points

- Steroids are an example of a medication that can trigger manic episodes which respond to antipsychotic treatment.
- Some patients will go on to develop recurrent mood episodes which may be managed with usual treatments for bipolar disorder such as mood stabilizers.

1.9 Bipolar 1 Disorder Versus Bipolar 2 Disorder

The majority of studies of OABD do not distinguish between bipolar 1 and bipolar 2 disorders, and the use of mania as a convenient defining feature of bipolar disorder naturally skews samples toward those with bipolar 1 disease. Bipolar spectrum disorders are a relatively recent area of interest post-dating many studies and will not be discussed here.

There have been relatively few studies looking specifically at older age or late-onset bipolar 2 disorder. One study of 525 outpatients in Italy noted a statistically significant reduced prevalence of late-life (defined as age 50) bipolar 2 disorder similar to the reduced prevalence of bipolar 1 disorder found elsewhere [6]. An additional observation was that features of atypical depression (defined in DSM-IV as hypersomnia, increased appetite or weight gain, leaden paralysis, and rejection sensitivity), which were seen more frequently in younger patients with bipolar 2 illness, seemed to diminish as patients aged.

1.10 Natural History and Course of Illness

1.10.1 Initial Presentation

As previously discussed, mania, the hallmark of bipolar illness, can occur for the first time at any age, with elders in their 90s experiencing new-onset mania [39, 53–55]. When the first manic episode arises in the context of a lifetime of unipolar depression, the clinical diagnosis is changed to bipolar illness. However, there is disagreement about whether to define bipolar disorder onset as occurring at the time of first depression, decades prior, or whether to consider the later onset of mania as initiating bipolar disorder, representing a change or evolution in illness course.

There may be important differences in the way older and younger patients first present with mania. An older study that defined late-onset bipolar illness as occurring after age 40 found the late-onset group to present less acutely, with less violence, irritability, and psychosis, but with more visual, olfactory, and somatic hallucinations [25]. A population-wide Danish study of 1719 inpatients and outpatients found that of those diagnosed with bipolar disorder by the end of their first hospital admission, those with late-onset bipolar illness (defined as beginning after age 50) presented with more psychosis related to depressions and less psychosis related to manias when compared to other inpatients with early onset disease [10]. However, these are relative differences between those with EOBD and LOBD and should not give the impression that those with LOBD do not frequently present with manias or that these manias do not feature psychotic symptoms. Notably, the same study, one of the few looking at a large group of older outpatients, found no differences in initial presentation for outpatients with late-onset compared with early-onset bipolar illness, suggesting that differences between the two groups may be less prominent among individuals with milder disease.

Clinical Vignette 1.2

Mr. J is a 74-year-old Caucasian widowed man who presented with his first episode of mania at the age of 73.

His family history was notable only for later life dementia in his mother. He had an unremarkable birth and development, did well in school, graduated from college, and had a career as a college professor with a successful marriage and two children. Mr. J had no history of substance abuse and his medical history was notable only for hypertension. When he was in his late 60s, his wife died suddenly of an aneurysm and he started seeing a counselor for difficulty coping with this loss. He was started on citalopram after a one-time visit with a psychiatrist and was then continued on this medication subsequently by his primary care physician. His intense feelings of sadness were not accompanied by changes in sleep, appetite, concentration, or self-attitude, and his depressed mood remitted after 1 year. He continued to take citalopram over the next five years.

Five years later, Mr. J experienced a number of difficult events over the course of several months: His brother died, his daughter-in-law was diagnosed with cancer, and he himself had a knee surgery with slow recovery. He began having trouble sleeping with increased energy, late-night reading, and began sending 3 a.m. emails to family members. His primary care doctor continued citalopram and started trazodone to help with sleep. The patient felt over-caffeinated and stimulated. He had an elevated self-attitude, became more talkative than normal, and began having conversations out loud when others were not present. Normally frugal, he started purchasing expensive items for himself and began considering investing in new business propositions.

Mr. J was diagnosed with bipolar 1 disorder. Citalopram and trazodone were stopped, and he was treated with lithium and olanzapine during an outpatient partial hospitalization. Over the course of a month, he became less pressured in speech, began sleeping 7–8 hours regularly, and was able to curb his spending. He experienced increased fatigue for which his olanzapine was decreased and he was discharged to outpatient care. He remains on medications and has had no further episodes of either depression or hypomania.

Learning Points

- Bipolar illness should be considered in elders of any age presenting with manic or hypomanic behavior even in the absence of prior mental illness.
- Antidepressants may contribute to flares of bipolar illness even years after their initiation.

1.10.2 Natural Course

It is clear that for many individuals with bipolar disorder, "the illness does not 'burn out' or attenuate over time" [2, 7]. Even among outpatient samples, which tend to have individuals with less severe illness, up to 5 % per year of older patients with diagnosed bipolar illness flare into mania or hypomania [11].

One recent large study of 2257 outpatients with bipolar I disorder that compared patients younger and older than 60 found no statistically significant difference in acute symptoms of depression or elevated mood, beyond younger people having more distractibility [8]. However, this study did not categorize patients by the age of bipolar disease onset and focused on outpatients with insurance, who may have been a healthier cohort. A recent midsize study of almost 600 outpatients found that those individuals over 65 years of age with bipolar 1 or 2 disorder had more depressive and catatonic episodes than hypomanic/manic episodes compared with their younger counterparts [56].

In general, in older age, bipolar disorder is likely to feature more frequent episodes of illness and decreasing time spent at baseline [12, 40]. One small prospective study found that older patients had a more "fragile recovery" with a significantly greater proportion who had been hospitalized for mania relapsing into depression prior to discharge [24].

The European Mania in Bipolar Longitudinal Evaluation of Medication (EMBLEM) study, one of the few large prospective studies comparing both older and younger adults being treated for mania, found that adults over 60 were less likely to present with psychosis, were more likely to have experienced rapid cycling of a least 4 episodes in the last year, and were more likely to have been treated with antidepressants [38]. The same study found that by 3 months after an acute mania, late-onset patients, while having equally severe mania scores at the outset (though less severe than younger patients), recovered faster and were discharged more frequently than early-onset older patients. After 2 years of psychiatric follow-up, significantly more older patients had recurrence of illness than younger patients and recurred in fewer days [37]. Older patients who had early onset of their illness fared the worst: Compared with younger patients, fewer recovered and of those that did, more relapsed into illness [37]. An earlier study found that, similar to younger populations, medication non-adherence remains a common trigger of relapse or rehospitalization for this older age group [7].

Frequent recurrence of illness with briefer remissions may partly explain the greater healthcare use among older adults with bipolar illness. One study comparing patients over the age of 60 with either unipolar or bipolar depression found that those with bipolar illness used almost 4 times the total amount of mental health services and were three times more likely to have been hospitalized in the 6 months prior to the study than those with unipolar depression [2]. Additionally, although the mechanisms remain unclear, some research suggests that bipolar disorder is a neuroprogressive disease, in which episodes of illness leave a lasting legacy on the brain, contributing to medical comorbidities, cognitive and functional decline, and poor response to treatment [1, 3].

Clinical Vignette 1.3

Ms. M is a 69-year-old divorced Caucasian woman who was diagnosed with bipolar 1 disorder in her mid-30s, who with advancing age has become increasingly challenging to effectively treat, with longer periods of illness duration and only brief periods of illness remission.

Her family history was notable for bipolar disorder and dementia in her father and bipolar disorder in a half-sister. Ms. M had an uneventful birth and development, graduated high school, worked in clerical jobs, later was on disability for her bipolar disorder, was married and divorced 2 times, and had 4 adult children, one with whom she lived. She had no history of alcohol or illicit substance abuse but was a lifelong cigarette smoker. Her medical history was notable for high blood pressure, diabetes type II, and osteoarthritis. After her diagnosis with bipolar 1 disorder in her late 30s, she had numerous hospitalizations for manic episodes marked by increased energy, paranoia, delusional thinking, and aggressive behavior toward family members alternating with hospitalizations for severe depressive episodes. Lithium was a mainstay of her psychiatric treatment along with antipsychotic or antidepressant medications during episodes of illness.

When younger, Ms. M returned to her baseline with independent functioning after each mood episode. In her 60s, she experienced more functional and cognitive decline with longer psychiatric hospitalizations when ill. In addition, she required more day-to-day supervision from family members when at home, and also started attending an adult day care.

Ms. M presented for acute psychiatric care after vigorous paranoid complaints about her day care facility and her family, accusing them of mistreating her and stealing her money. She was guarded, fearful, and felt guilty and was experiencing auditory hallucinations of dead relatives. She was thought initially to be in a mixed state and started on olanzapine, but later switched to risperidone due to drug-induced Parkinsonism. Her standing treatment with lithium was temporarily discontinued due to concerns that a high serum level had caused ataxia and confusion. Over the course of a 4-month hospitalization, she developed catatonia with minimal verbal responses, thought due to depression. Sertraline was added to her regimen. After several weeks, Ms. M became more active and engaged but then became agitated with reduced sleep and aggressive behavior toward staff with paranoid accusations and yelling and was diagnosed with mania. Sertraline was stopped and lithium was restarted along with multiple trials of different antipsychotic medications, including aripiprazole and ziprasidone. Valproic acid had previously resulted in neutropenia and, therefore, was not a therapeutic option during this hospitalization. Her family, already under significant stress unrelated to the patient, was not able to support the frequent blood draws and other measures necessary for a clozapine trial at the time.

After several months, her mood and sleep normalized and she was successfully discharged home, with scheduled outpatient follow-up, under the care of her family on a medication regimen of lithium, quetiapine, and low-dose haloperidol. Ms. M relapsed, however, within 12 months and returned to the emergency room due to severe paranoid delusions.

Learning Points

- With advancing age, bipolar illness can present with fewer periods of euthymia as well as functional decline.
- Older adults are more likely to experience adverse effects of medication and doses should be titrated cautiously.

1.10.3 Increased Morbidity and Mortality

Bipolar disorder in older age significantly increases the risk of functional decline. One study of community-dwelling adults over the age of 45 found that those with bipolar disorder had health care-related quality-of-life scores similar to or worse than individuals with schizophrenia, and greater medical comorbidity and prevalence of alcohol use disorder than control subjects with similar education and occupational achievements [57]. Although younger adults with bipolar disorder have a relatively better overall prognosis than those with schizophrenia, bipolar disorder in advancing age is associated with increasing functional impairment, attenuating these earlier distinctions.

A large study of more than 54,000 patients hospitalized for depression or bipolar disorder in Sweden compared mortality rates and causes of death with the general population and found that those with bipolar disorder had more deaths than expected or "excess mortality" even over those with unipolar depression, with standardized mortality ratios of 2.5 in men and 2.7 in women for all causes [58]. Notably, compared to individuals with unipolar depression, those with bipolar disorder had more deaths from natural causes and less from suicide, suggesting that either bipolar disorder, the behaviors associated with it, or its treatment shortens life span [58]. This premature mortality may partly account for the decreased prevalence of bipolar disorder in later life and samples of older adults with early-onset bipolar disorder may be considered a survivor cohort [1].

Other studies have shown similarly increased mortality likely due to bipolar illness [16, 59]. A 26-year follow-up analysis of the original five-center Epidemiologic Catchment Area (ECA) study found that those with any bipolar spectrum illness had 1.42 greater odds of having died in the follow-up period when compared to those with no bipolar illness after adjusting for age [60]. The association between bipolar illness and increased mortality remained statistically significant even after adjusting for increased depressive episodes and drug and alcohol abuse in the group with bipolar illness. However, when stratified by age and adjusted for drug and alcohol abuse, the association for those age 30–44 rose above the threshold for statistical significance, suggesting that if drug and alcohol use can be reduced or prevented in this younger population, some excess mortality may decline.

1.10.4 Medical Comorbidity

In later life, comorbid medical conditions are common in older adults with bipolar disorder, including an increased prevalence of hypertension, diabetes, cardiac disease, and dementia [3]. Despite a similar degree of medical comorbidity, including cardiovascular disease, those with bipolar illness, compared with unipolar major depression, have a greater prevalence of endocrine and metabolic disorders, specifically, hypothyroidism, diabetes, and obesity [61]. It remains unclear how much of this difference can be attributed to use of medications, such as lithium and antipsychotics, versus the contribution of factors related to bipolar illness itself.

1.10.5 Psychiatric Comorbidity

Results from the five-center ECA study found that individuals of any age with bipolar I disorder have a substantially higher risk of drug and alcohol use—with a substance abuse prevalence rate of 61 % and a lifetime prevalence of drug and alcohol dependence double that of those with major depression [62]. Another community sample demonstrated that those living with bipolar disorder in later life continue to report more alcohol use disorder, dysthymia, generalized anxiety disorder, and panic disorder than their age cohort without bipolar disorder. Although screening elders for psychiatric and substance use disorder comorbidity is recommended, the prevalence of lifetime and 12-month alcohol use disorder, dysthymia, and panic disorder in this group was less than in those under 65 with bipolar disorder [63]. One study that divided age of onset into three groups found that those who developed bipolar disorder before age 21 showed a greater prevalence of drug use disorders than those with later onset disease [33].

1.11 Summary

Although the prevalence of bipolar illness decreases with age, the need for mental health services among elderly patients with bipolar illness rises. Older patients may have more frequent recurrences of depressions and hypomanias or manias with briefer remissions when compared to younger patients. They also have disproportionately high rates of healthcare utilization when compared to older patients with unipolar depression. Clinical management of older age bipolar disorder will be discussed in Chap. 4, but is frequently complicated by medical comorbidity, psychiatric comorbidity, functional and cognitive decline, loss of social supports, and age-related physiologic changes in renal and liver function affecting drug pharmacokinetics and pharmacodynamics. Research has identified EOBD and LOBD as groups with likely different etiologies of bipolar disorder, but the significance for prognosis and treatment remains unclear. Perhaps to a degree greater than for any other mood disorder, the clinical complexity of OABD requires thoughtful and consistent psychiatric care.

Clinical Pearls

- The numbers of older adults with bipolar disorder are expected to increase in the future.
- While prevalence rates of older age bipolar disorder are low in community samples, older adults with bipolar disorder are frequently seen in clinical treatment settings and have high rates of psychiatric service utilization.
- OABD represents a heterogeneous group of individuals and includes adults with EOBD and LOBD, who may differ in terms of clinical course as well as illness pathogenesis.
- Individuals with late-onset bipolar illness are more likely to be women, less likely to have a family history of bipolar disorder, and more likely to have cerebrovascular risk factors or disease.

- Bipolar disorder does not "burn out" with advancing age. Rather, older adults with bipolar disorder may experience more frequent periods of illness with less time spent euthymic and at baseline levels of functioning.
- Individuals with OABD frequently have medical and psychiatric comorbidities which complicate treatment.

References

1. Sajatovic M, Strejilevich SA, Gildengers AG, Dols A, Al Jurdi RK, Forester BP, et al. A report on older-age bipolar disorder from the International Society for Bipolar Disorders Task Force. Bipolar Disord. 2015;17(7):689–704.
2. Bartels SJ, Forester B, Miles KM, Joyce T. Mental health service use by elderly patients with bipolar disorder and unipolar major depression. Am J Geriatr Psychiatry. 2000;8(2):160–6.
3. Sajatovic M, Forester BP, Gildengers A, Mulsant BH. Aging changes and medical complexity in late-life bipolar disorder: emerging research findings that may help advance care. Neuropsychiatry (London). 2013;3(6):621–33.
4. Forester BP, Ajilore O, Spino C, Lehmann SW. Clinical characteristics of patients with late life bipolar disorder in the community: data from the NNDC registry. Am J Geriatr Psychiatry. 2015;23(9):977–84.
5. Depp CA, Jeste DV. Bipolar disorder in older adults: a critical review. Bipolar Disord. 2004;6(5):343–67.
6. Benazzi F. Bipolar II depression in late life: prevalence and clinical features in 525 depressed outpatients. J Affect Disord. 2001;66(1):13–8.
7. Lehmann SW, Rabins PV. Factors related to hospitalization in elderly manic patients with early and late-onset bipolar disorder. Int J Geriatr Psychiatry. 2006;21(11):1060–4.
8. Al Jurdi RK, Nguyen QX, Petersen NJ, Pilgrim P, Gyulai L, Sajatovic M. Acute bipolar I affective episode presentation across life span. J Geriatr Psychiatry Neurol. 2012;25(1):6–14.
9. Kessing LV. Gender differences in subtypes of late-onset depression and mania. Int Psychogeriatr. 2006;18(4):727–38.
10. Kessing LV. Diagnostic subtypes of bipolar disorder in older versus younger adults. Bipolar Disord. 2006;8(1):56–64.
11. Dols A, Kupka RW, van Lammeren A, Beekman AT, Sajatovic M, Stek ML. The prevalence of late-life mania: a review. Bipolar Disord. 2014;16(2):113–8.
12. Chen ST, Altshuler LL, Spar JE. Bipolar disorder in late life: a review. J Geriatr Psychiatry Neurol. 1998;11(1):29–35.
13. Sajatovic M, Chen P. Geriatric bipolar disorder. Psychiatr Clin North Am. 2011;34(2):319–33.
14. Weissman MM, Leaf PJ, Tischler GL, Blazer DG, Karno M, Bruce ML, et al. Affective disorders in five United States communities. Psychol Med. 1988;18(1):141–53.
15. Kessler RC, Berglund P, Demler O, Jin R, Merikangas KR, Walters EE. Lifetime prevalence and age-of-onset distributions of DSM-IV disorders in the National Comorbidity Survey Replication. Arch Gen Psychiatry. 2005;62(6):593–602.
16. Miller C, Bauer MS. Excess mortality in bipolar disorders. Curr Psychiatry Rep. 2014;16(11):499-014-0499-z.

17. Koenig HG, Blazer DG. Epidemiology of geriatric affective disorders. Clin Geriatr Med. 1992;8(2):235–51.
18. Merikangas KR, Akiskal HS, Angst J, Greenberg PE, Hirschfeld RM, Petukhova M, et al. Lifetime and 12-month prevalence of bipolar spectrum disorder in the National Comorbidity Survey replication. Arch Gen Psychiatry. 2007;64(5):543–52.
19. Sheeran T, Greenberg RL, Davan LA, Dealy JA, Young RC, Bruce ML. A descriptive study of older bipolar disorder residents living in New York City's adult congregate facilities. Bipolar Disord. 2012;14(7):756–63.
20. Sajatovic M, Blow FC, Ignacio RV, Kales HC. New-onset bipolar disorder in later life. Am J Geriatr Psychiatry. 2005;13(4):282–9.
21. Yassa R, Nair V, Nastase C, Camille Y, Belzile L. Prevalence of bipolar disorder in a psychogeriatric population. J Affect Disord. 1988;14(3):197–201.
22. Wingerson D, Russo J, Ries R, Dagadakis C, Roy-Byrne P. Use of psychiatric emergency services and enrollment status in a public managed mental health care plan. Psychiatr Serv. 2001;52(11):1494–501.
23. Shulman RW, Marton P, Fisher A, Cohen C. Characteristics of psychogeriatric patient visits to a general hospital emergency room. Can J Psychiatry. 1996;41(3):175–80.
24. Broadhead J, Jacoby R. Mania in old age: a First Prospective Study. Int J Geriatr Psychiatry. 1990;5(4):215–22.
25. Kennedy N, Everitt B, Boydell J, Van Os J, Jones PB, Murray RM. Incidence and distribution of first-episode mania by age: results from a 35-year study. Psychol Med. 2005;35(6):855–63.
26. Hays JC, Krishnan KR, George LK, Blazer DG. Age of first onset of bipolar disorder: demographic, family history, and psychosocial correlates. Depress Anxiety. 1998;7(2):76–82.
27. Shulman K, Post F. Bipolar affective disorder in old age. Br J Psychiatry. 1980;136:26–32.
28. Almeida OP, Fenner S. Bipolar disorder: similarities and differences between patients with illness onset before and after 65 years of age. Int Psychogeriatr. 2002;14(3):311–22.
29. Cassidy F, Carroll BJ. Vascular risk factors in late onset mania. Psychol Med. 2002; 32(2):359–62.
30. Subramaniam H, Dennis MS, Byrne EJ. The role of vascular risk factors in late onset bipolar disorder. Int J Geriatr Psychiatry. 2007;22(8):733–7.
31. Schurhoff F, Bellivier F, Jouvent R, Mouren-Simeoni MC, Bouvard M, Allilaire JF, et al. Early and late onset bipolar disorders: two different forms of manic-depressive illness? J Affect Disord. 2000;58(3):215–21.
32. Wylie ME, Mulsant BH, Pollock BG, Sweet RA, Zubenko GS, Begley AE, et al. Age at onset in geriatric bipolar disorder. Effects on clinical presentation and treatment outcomes in an inpatient sample. Am J Geriatr Psychiatry. 1999;7(1):77–83.
33. Coryell W, Fiedorowicz J, Leon AC, Endicott J, Keller MB. Age of onset and the prospectively observed course of illness in bipolar disorder. J Affect Disord. 2013; 146(1):34–8.
34. Bellivier F, Golmard JL, Rietschel M, Schulze TG, Malafosse A, Preisig M, et al. Age at onset in bipolar I affective disorder: further evidence for three subgroups. Am J Psychiatry. 2003;160(5):999–1001.
35. Azorin JM, Bellivier F, Kaladjian A, Adida M, Belzeaux R, Fakra E, et al. Characteristics and profiles of bipolar I patients according to age-at-onset: findings from an admixture analysis. J Affect Disord. 2013;150(3):993–1000.
36. Leboyer M, Henry C, Paillere-Martinot ML, Bellivier F. Age at onset in bipolar affective disorders: a review. Bipolar Disord. 2005;7(2):111–8.
37. Oostervink F, Nolen WA, Kok RM. EMBLEM Advisory Board. Two years' outcome of acute mania in bipolar disorder: different effects of age and age of onset. Int J Geriatr Psychiatry. 2015;30(2):201–9.

38. Oostervink F, Boomsma MM, Nolen WA. Bipolar disorder in the elderly; different effects of age and of age of onset. J Affect Disord. 2009;116(3):176–83.
39. Sibisi CD. Sex differences in the age of onset of bipolar affective illness. Br J Psychiatry. 1990;156:842–5.
40. Goodwin FK, Jamison KR, Ghaemi SN. Manic-depressive illness: bipolar disorders and recurrent depression. 2nd ed. New York: Oxford University Press; 2007.
41. Celik Y, Erdogan E, Tuglu C, Utku U. Post-stroke mania in late life due to right temporoparietal infarction. Psychiatry Clin Neurosci. 2004;58(4):446–7.
42. Robinson RG. Mood disorders secondary to stroke. Semin Clin Neuropsychiatry. 1997; 2(4):244–51.
43. Robinson RG, Boston JD, Starkstein SE, Price TR. Comparison of mania and depression after brain injury: causal factors. Am J Psychiatry. 1988;145(2):172–8.
44. Santos CO, Caeiro L, Ferro JM, Figueira ML. Mania and stroke: a systematic review. Cerebrovasc Dis. 2011;32(1):11–21.
45. Starkstein SE, Boston JD, Robinson RG. Mechanisms of mania after brain injury. 12 case reports and review of the literature. J Nerv Ment Dis. 1988;176(2):87–100.
46. Fujikawa T, Yamawaki S, Touhouda Y. Silent cerebral infarctions in patients with late-onset mania. Stroke. 1995;26(6):946–9.
47. Huang SH, Chung KH, Hsu JL, Wu JY, Huang YL, Tsai SY. The risk factors for elderly patients with bipolar disorder having cerebral infarction. J Geriatr Psychiatry Neurol. 2012; 25(1):15–9.
48. Tohen M, Shulman KI, Satlin A. First-episode mania in late life. Am J Psychiatry. 1994; 151(1):130–2.
49. Nilsson FM, Kessing LV, Sorensen TM, Andersen PK, Bolwig TG. Enduring increased risk of developing depression and mania in patients with dementia. J Neurol Neurosurg Psychiatry. 2002;73(1):40–4.
50. Krauthammer C, Klerman GL. Secondary mania: manic syndromes associated with antecedent physical illness or drugs. Arch Gen Psychiatry. 1978;35(11):1333–9.
51. Evans DL, Byerly MJ, Greer RA. Secondary mania: diagnosis and treatment. J Clin Psychiatry. 1995;56(Suppl 3):31–7.
52. Van Gerpen MW, Johnson JE, Winstead DK. Mania in the geriatric patient population: a review of the literature. Am J Geriatr Psychiatry. 1999;7(3):188–202.
53. Kellner MB, Neher F. A first episode of mania after age 80. Can J Psychiatry. 1991;36 (8):607–8.
54. Summers WK. Mania with onset in the eighth decade: two cases and a review. J Clin Psychiatry. 1983;44(4):141–3.
55. Walter-Ryan WG. Mania with onset in the ninth decade. J Clin Psychiatry. 1983;44(11): 430–1.
56. Nivoli AM, Murru A, Pacchiarotti I, Valenti M, Rosa AR, Hidalgo D, et al. Bipolar disorder in the elderly: a cohort study comparing older and younger patients. Acta Psychiatr Scand. 2014;130(5):364–73.
57. Depp CA, Davis CE, Mittal D, Patterson TL, Jeste DV. Health-related quality of life and functioning of middle-aged and elderly adults with bipolar disorder. J Clin Psychiatry. 2006;67(2):215–21.
58. Osby U, Brandt L, Correia N, Ekbom A, Sparen P. Excess mortality in bipolar and unipolar disorder in Sweden. Arch Gen Psychiatry. 2001;58(9):844–50.
59. Shulman KI, Tohen M, Satlin A, Mallya G, Kalunian D. Mania compared with unipolar depression in old age. Am J Psychiatry. 1992;149(3):341–5.
60. Ramsey CM, Spira AP, Mojtabai R, Eaton WW, Roth K, Lee HB. Lifetime manic spectrum episodes and all-cause mortality: 26-year follow-up of the NIMH Epidemiologic Catchment Area Study. J Affect Disord. 2013;151(1):337–42.

61. Gildengers AG, Whyte EM, Drayer RA, Soreca I, Fagiolini A, Kilbourne AM, et al. Medical burden in late-life bipolar and major depressive disorders. Am J Geriatr Psychiatry. 2008; 16(3):194–200.
62. Regier DA, Farmer ME, Rae DS, Locke BZ, Keith SJ, Judd LL, et al. Comorbidity of mental disorders with alcohol and other drug abuse. Results from the epidemiologic catchment area (ECA) study. JAMA. 1990;264(19):2511–8.
63. Goldstein BI, Herrmann N, Shulman KI. Comorbidity in bipolar disorder among the elderly: results from an epidemiological community sample. Am J Psychiatry. 2006;163(2):319–21.

Clinical Assessment of Older Adults with Bipolar Disorder

2

Annemiek Dols, Peijun Chen, Rayan K. Al Jurdi and Martha Sajatovic

2.1 Introduction

Among older individuals with bipolar disorder, there may be substantial variability in clinical presentation and outcomes [1, 2]. Medical comorbidity is the norm rather than the exception, and cardiovascular disease, metabolic abnormalities, and cognitive impairment are particularly relevant across the life span [3–5]. Cognitive dysfunction may occur in at least 1/3 of older people with bipolar disorder [6]. Over time, bipolar disorder might act in concert with other neuropathological mechanisms such as vascular disease to accelerate aging and cognitive deterioration [1–6].

This chapter on clinical assessment of older adults with bipolar disorder will discuss the differential diagnosis of manic presentation in older individuals as well as the elements of a clinical evaluation appropriate for the older adult who may

A. Dols
Department of Old Age Psychiatry, GGZinGeest, VU Medical Center, Amstelveenseweg 589, 1081JC Amsterdam, The Netherlands
e-mail: a.dols@ggzingeest.nl

P. Chen
Department of Psychiatry, Louis Stokes Cleveland VA Medical Center, 10701 East Boulevard, Psychiatry 116 W, Cleveland, OH 44106, USA
e-mail: peijun.chen@va.gov

R.K. Al Jurdi
Department of Psychiatry and Behavioral Sciences, Baylon College of Medicine, 24 Greenway Plaza Suite 2020, Houston, TX 77046, USA
e-mail: drraj@brainhealthconsultants.com

M. Sajatovic (✉)
Department of Psychiatry, School of Medicine, Case Western Reserve University, 10524 Euclid Avenue, Cleveland, OH 44106, USA
e-mail: martha.sajatovic@UHhospitals.org

S.W. Lehmann and B.P. Forester (eds.), *Bipolar Disorder in Older Age Patients*, DOI 10.1007/978-3-319-48912-4_2 have bipolar disorder. This includes the psychiatric clinical interview, history-taking, risk assessment, application of standardized techniques in the assessment of mood symptoms, and that of cognition as well as the assessment of medical and psychiatric comorbidities.

Clinical Vignette 2.1

Introduction

Ms. K is a 62-year-old married woman with type I bipolar disorder, maintained on lithium 1200 mg/day for the past 25 years. She has had 2 psychiatric hospitalizations in her lifetime—the first related to a manic episode in her mid-twenties and then a post-partum depression after the birth of her second child at the age of 30. She successfully responded to electroconvulsive therapy (ECT) for the episode of post-partum depression.

Ms. K has maintained a relatively stable euthymic state over the past decade although she has had some difficulty in her performance as a clerk in an insurance company over the last year since the company implemented a new electronic record system which she has found hard to master. She feels frustrated that some of her younger coworkers have no problems with the new computer system, while she continues to struggle.

Relevant Medical History

Ms. K is 18 kg overweight with a history of type II diabetes mellitus, treated with an oral hypoglycemic agent. Her most recent laboratory testing demonstrated $HbA1_c = 7$. She has hypertension and is prescribed a beta-blocker. At times she forgets to take her antihypertensive medication, although her adherence has improved somewhat over the past 6 months after her daughter recommended that she use a weekly pill-minder. Ms. K has a history of migraines, which have been well controlled with as-needed use of a triptan drug. Her clinician recently checked a basic metabolic serum panel which was unremarkable except for a serum creatinine value of 1.1 mg/dL. Ms. K has been smoking ½ pack of cigarettes/day for the past 4 decades. Her mother had a history of recurrent depression and developed Alzheimer's disease in her 70s.

A New Problem

Approximately 6 months ago, Ms. K noticed a mild bilateral hand tremor that caused her embarrassment and slightly interfered with her ability to conduct her clerical duties. Her primary care clinician checked a basic serum chemistry panel and told her that labs looked "fine" except for "very mild impairment in kidney functioning," but did not recommend further medical work-up or evaluation. Worried about both the tremor and the abnormal laboratory testing, Ms. K reduced her lithium on her own to 900 mg/day. Her tremor resolved within the next week.

In the Last Several Weeks

Ms. K has become increasingly irritable at home. She is waking up approximately twice during the night to use the toilet, but unlike her previous usual pattern has found it difficult to get back to sleep readily when she returns back to bed. Last week, Ms. K made a few inappropriate comments to a coworker in the employee lounge which was out of character for her. Now, her concerned husband accompanies her to the clinician's office. He states that Ms. K seems "forgetful" at times in addition to being irritable and wonders if she is developing dementia like her mother.

2.2 Differential Diagnosis

Manic symptoms, such as disturbed sleep, irritability, and impaired attention, in later life have a broad differential diagnosis including (late-onset) bipolar disorder (LOBD) and schizoaffective disorder (primary mania), mania due to a specific medical cause (secondary mania) as well as delirium and dementia. Older age mania is not rare; the overall prevalence is estimated to be 6.0 % in older psychiatric inpatients with about one-third experiencing their first manic episode (i.e., late-onset mania) [7]. Although the management of both primary mania and secondary mania may be similar, the etiology of mania is of importance as the appropriate treatment of secondary mania includes addressing the cause [8].

2.2.1 Mania and Physical Health

Older age manic symptoms and physical health are highly linked. Somatic factors may be a true cause of mania (secondary mania) or may trigger mania as a first manifestation of bipolar disorder in a person with a latent vulnerability, either with or without a history of depressive episodes. Somatic comorbidity may also be present in an individual without any causal relationship to mania.

The concept of secondary mania was introduced by Krauthammer and Klerman in 1978 [8] as a condition with manic symptomatology resulting from an underlying medical illness that could develop in people with no history of mood disorder. For manic symptoms to be classified as secondary mania, the patient should have no history of primary mood disorder or evidence of delirium. As noted in Table 2.1, the list of various neurological conditions, systemic disturbances, and medications that have been described to cause secondary mania is extensive [9] Mania has been linked to cerebrovascular accidents, primary or metastatic brain tumors, and traumatic brain injury. Temporal lobe epilepsy, encephalitis, meningitis, HIV encephalopathy, and tertiary syphilis have all been associated with mania [10]. In

Table 2.1 Possible causes of secondary mania

Neurological	Dementia/neurocognitive disorders
	Traumatic brain injury
	Epilepsy
	Infectious encephalitis
	Cerebrovascular disease
	Brain tumors
	Movement disorders
Systemic	Infections
	Thyroid abnormalities
	Illicit Drugs: i.e., cocaine
Medication	Antidepressants
	Benzodiazepines
	Corticosteroids
	Thyroid replacements
	Dopamine agonists
	Antibiotics

addition, thyrotoxicosis, Cushing's disease, vitamin B12, and niacin deficiency can produce symptoms which mimic mania [11]. While secondary mania can occur at any age, it is more common in older patients given the higher prevalence of potentially causative medical conditions and medications.

Presently, data are lacking to label "due to a somatic condition or medication" as a diagnostic specifier in bipolar disorder. As we know from other psychiatric disorders (e.g., schizophrenia), certain substances (e.g., cannabis) can prime the development of psychiatric disease. As with delirium, many somatic conditions can cause mania; however, some patients seem more at risk. For example, vascular risk factors may prime older patients and patients with vascular (non-symptomatic) brain damage to develop manic-type symptoms.

2.2.2 Mania as a Symptom of Dementia

Particularly relevant to the clinical assessment of older adults, depending on the location of neurodegeneration, disinhibited behavior can be a symptom of Alzheimer's disease [12] or vascular dementia [13]. Disinhibition is also one of the core symptoms of the behavioral variant of frontotemporal dementia (bvFTD) [14]. According to the recent International Consensus criteria for bvFTD, at least 3 of the 6 core symptoms of behavioral disinhibition-apathy, stereotyped or compulsive behavior, loss of empathy, hyper-orality, and executive deficits are needed to make the diagnosis [14]. Neuroimaging and cerebrospinal fluid (CSF) biomarkers may help in possibly understanding potential cause of dementing illness [15, 16]; however, the differential diagnosis for FTD currently relies on clinical judgment. Frontal lobe syndrome, a positive history of psychiatric illness, male gender, a relative absence of stereotypy, and presence of depressive symptoms are predictive for psychiatric origin symptoms rather than bvFTD [17].

A possible link between bipolar disorder and bvFTD has also been suggested by case reports of patients presenting with manic symptoms as a first manifestation of bvFTD [18, 19] and patients with a lifetime diagnosis of bipolar disorder evolving into bvFTD [20, 21]. This large clinical overlap in social cognition, executive disturbances, and behavioral profiles might be explained by the involvement of common functional neuro-anatomical networks [22–24]. A proportion of bvFTD patients have a slow course with relatively normal neuroimaging, particularly those carrying a C9orf72 repeat expansion [25]. This repeat expansion has been found in patients with bipolar disorder preceding FTD [26, 27]; however, this mutation was not detected in a cohort of 206 patients with bipolar disorder [28].

The condition fulfilling criteria for *possible* bvFTD failing to convert to *probable* bvFTD over time is labeled the benign bvFTD phenocopy syndrome [29, 30]. These patients exhibit behavioral and functional impairments consistent with a frontal lobe syndrome but fail to progress over time and have no frontal or anterior temporal atrophy or hypo-perfusion at follow-up. Although an alternative explanation is generally lacking in these cases, it is possible that this could be an end-stage manifestation of bipolar disorder.

2.2.3 Secondary Mania with a Neurological Cause

Although far less common than depression, mania can occur in 1 % of stroke patients, in 2–12 % of patients with movement disorders such as Huntington's disease, in patients with epilepsy or infections of the brain [31]. Tumors, neurosurgery, and traumatic head injury can result in manic symptoms [10], occasionally with a delay of up to 12 months before the manic symptoms develop [32, 33]. Focal brain lesions in the right hemisphere have been associated with mania [34]. Steffens and Krishnan [35] proposed criteria for vascular mania and depression subtype specifiers, and their concept of vascular mania appears to have some overlap with the neurological disinhibition syndrome. Late-life mania may occur in patients with non-symptomatic vascular brain damage.

Differentiating between frontal disinhibition and bipolar mania can be challenging. While many symptoms are overlapping between the two conditions, bipolar mania may be more characterized by elevated mood and decreased need for sleep, rather than disturbed sleep. The presence of a positive family history of affective disorder may indicate that a somatic cause resulted in mania by triggering an existing bipolar predisposition [8].

2.2.4 Mania in the Context of Established Older Age Bipolar Disorder

In general, medical comorbidities are a substantial burden in older age bipolar disorder patients [36, 37]. A retrospective chart review of 73 patients over age 65 admitted for a manic episode revealed that 86.3 % had medical comorbidity [38].

Clinical emphasis on maintaining optimal physical health and avoiding polypharmacy may optimize the likelihood for better outcomes.

Clinical Vignette 2.1, Continued

Ms. K's new symptoms of irritability, disturbed sleep, and disinhibited behavior in the context of her history of bipolar 1 disorder, diabetes, hypertension, and medication use warrant closer evaluation. Her symptoms of irritability, decreased sleep, and disinhibition are consistent with a manic episode. Her husband mentioned concern about memory problems, and her difficulties in mastering the new computer system could indicate executive dysfunction. Her behavioral changes and cognitive impairment could also suggest possible early dementia and several etiologies could be considered. Hypertension, diabetes, and smoking are all risk factors for vascular dementia, and her family history is positive for Alzheimer's disease. With her disinhibited behavior, diminished social empathy, and problems in executive functioning, she could fulfill the criteria for bvFTD.

Ms. K's inadequate medication adherence, an untreated medical condition, or a new somatic comorbidity presenting as secondary mania should all be considered.

The clinical picture of older age bipolar mania can present as a mild confusional state, with disturbed attention as a key symptom. Additionally, the first priority should be to check her lithium serum levels, as toxicity can cause a variety of symptoms and subtherapeutic serum levels can induce a relapse.

Learning Points

- Medical comorbidity is common in older people with bipolar disorder.
- New onset physical symptoms, such as tremor, may represent emerging and aging-related, drug-related side effects or new medical or neurological comorbidity. This needs careful clinical evaluation that includes obtaining collateral history.
- Treatments for bipolar disorder need to be monitored and periodically reassessed as individuals age. Over time, some individuals may develop adverse effects or relative intolerability to specific therapeutic agents.

2.3 Assessment

2.3.1 The Clinical Interview and History-Taking

Recognizing and accurately diagnosing bipolar disorder in the geriatric population can be challenging. This is due to a number of factors, including the influence of culture and concomitant medical comorbidities, as well as the cyclical and chronic nature of bipolar disorder. From a diagnostic perspective, the presence of bipolar depression or psychotic symptoms may complicate the clinical presentation and distinguishing between mixed episodes, agitated depression, or mania with psychotic symptoms or a schizoaffective disorder adds to the complexity of diagnosis. Additionally, co-occurring psychiatric conditions (e.g., substance abuse) may distract clinical focus from symptoms of bipolar disorder, especially if the presenting symptoms for the other condition are more severe and prominent. Accurate diagnosis can be complicated in patients presenting with concurrent cognitive symptoms. For example, to return to our clinical vignette, it is very important for the clinician to determine whether Ms. K's new complaints of forgetfulness and frustration with the new electronic record system are the outcome of distractibility—as part of an acute manic episode exacerbation—or due to new neurological etiology such as Alzheimer's disease or FTD.

The literature is not clear as to whether there are symptom profile and severity differences between patients with OABD and younger individuals with bipolar disorder. Studies have suggested that some mood symptoms—namely anorexia, anxiety, somatic complaints, psychomotor agitation, suicidal behavior, hallucination, and delusions—are more severe in older age bipolar disorder [39]. However, Al Jurdi et al. [40] found that neither the severity nor the prevalence of bipolar manic or depressive symptoms differed when comparing young bipolar patients with older bipolar patients. Importantly, the *DSM-5* has no age-specific variations in diagnostic criteria for bipolar disorders.

The success of a clinical interview depends on collecting all relevant information through effective communication. This is especially important when interviewing older patients. Box 2.1 provides suggestions to guide the clinician's interaction with older patients. During the interview of a geriatric patient, atypical, subsyndromal, and vague symptoms can be expected. Clinicians should make thorough inquiries about symptoms that patients may perceive to be expected aspects of aging. These include sleep disturbances, lethargy or decreased energy, and changes in appetite. Using a structured format and in consideration of the patient's symptoms, a psychiatric review of systems should be part of the initial interview.

Box 2.1 Tips for interviewing geriatric patients

- Address the patient by last name (family name), using the title patient prefers.
- Speak slowly in a clear, low-pitched voice.
- Face the patient directly at eye level to allow for lip reading in those who may be hard of hearing or hearing-impaired.
- Pay attention to verbal and nonverbal clues (tempo of speech, tone of voice, eye contact).
- Remember that the exam starts in the waiting area, Observe movements walking into room, gait, ability to sit and rise from the waiting room chair.

- Allow adequate time for the patient to respond (information processing and memory retrieval may be slow, but unimpaired).
- Include family and support-system members as appropriate for the patients cognitive, functional and sociocultural status.
- Don't rush and try not to interrupt.
- Use active listening skills.
- Eliminate visual and auditory distractions (background office noises).
- Use adequate lighting (including sufficient light on your face).

Clinicians should explore the patient's current and past hypomanic, syndromal manic, mixed, or major depressive episodes as well as observed euthymic and subsyndromal symptoms. The interviewer should address onset, frequency, prodromes, precipitants of symptoms, and the impact of patients' symptoms on their daily social and occupational activities.

In the case of the clinical vignette, Ms. K's struggles with the new computerized system could reflect cognitive symptoms, while her relationship with her colleagues could reflect mood symptoms. Additionally, the existence of other psychiatric conditions during prior mood episodes should be characterized as well as both adverse and therapeutic responses to past treatment approaches. A depressed patient's ability to describe and recall past elevated mood events may be impaired. Similarly, during a manic episode, patients tend to have a suboptimal insight on the nature of manic symptoms. Patients with chronic illness characterized by numerous episodes of mood illness may find remembering the details about a specific episode to be problematic. In these instances, collaborative sources, such as family or close informants, can fill in the gaps to ensure diagnostic accuracy.

As noted in Box 2.2, medical history and current medical status are crucial components of the clinical interview of the older patient. Because some psychiatric conditions arise due to comorbid physical conditions, and because medical disorders can worsen symptom severity of a primary psychiatric condition, prior and existing medical conditions and treatments must be evaluated in detail. Co-occurring psychiatric conditions, past and current treatments, and treatment response as well as adherence to treatment regimens and lifestyle factors such as physical activity levels and use of tobacco or other substances must all be incorporated into the assessment and plan of care.

Box 2.2 Elements of the clinical interview for an older patient

- Chief complaint (s).
- Current symptoms and history of present illness.
- Psychiatric review of systems.
- Past psychiatric history.

- Family psychiatric history.
- Family medical history.
- Social history.
- Developmental history.
- Current and past medical history including medications prescribed, medication adherence and list of current healthcare providers as well as previous diagnostic procedures such as neuroimaging and neurocognitive evaluations.
- Assessment of lifestyle factors (drugs and alcohol, smoking, exercise and other healthy or unhealthy behaviors).
- Assessment of past and recent functional status including driving history, independent living skills, and guardianship status.

Addressing biopsychosocial stressors is a priority in the evaluation of the older patient with known or suspected bipolar disorder. The interview should assess current employment if applicable, sources of social support (including guardianship status), religious beliefs and participation, cultural experience, marital status, living situation, and an assessment of functioning including any changes in social and occupational functioning or activities of daily living, such as ability to prepare meals or drive. Because of the chronicity and the involvement of multiple organ systems in bipolar disorder, the context in which a patient is experiencing and attempting to cope with cognitive dysfunction, comorbid medical conditions, and difficulty with activities of daily life is highly relevant.

When taking the family history, priority should be given to obtaining information about first-degree relatives and/or others who have received diagnoses of and undergone treatment for psychiatric disorders or symptoms (e.g., suicidal ideation and attempts, and psychotic disorders and symptoms, etc.).

As warranted by the history and presentation, reviewing recent or implementing new imaging and laboratory workup is recommended. As discussed previously, many neurological and systemic diseases can present as mania. Accordingly, frequently ordered tests in the evaluation of the geriatric patient with what appears to be bipolar symptoms include complete blood count blood electrolytes, kidney and liver function tests, thyroid function tests, urinalysis and urine drug screen, EKG, and $B_{12,}$ folate, fasting lipid profile, and fasting blood glucose [41–44] (Table 2.2). More specialized testing may warranted depending on the clinical presentation and differential diagnosis. For example, brain imaging [brain-computed tomography (CT) or magnetic resonance imaging (MRI)], an electroencephalogram (EEG), or lumbar puncture with cerebrospinal fluid analysis may be ordered to rule out cerebrovascular accidents seizures or meningoencephalitis presenting with manic symptoms [42–44].

Table 2.2 Assessment of physical health in older bipolar patients

Recommendations	
History	Medical history
	Medications including over the counter medications
	Cigarette smoking
	Alcohol and illicit drug use
	Family history for somatic illnesses History of medication/other allergies
Physical examination	Blood pressure and pulse
	Waist circumference if there is concern for possible metabolic syndrome
	Weight and height ECG
laboratory studies	Full blood count
	Electrolytes, urea, creatinine
	Liver function tests
	Fasting blood glucose
	Fasting lipid profile Thyroid screening B12, folate (if there is concern about cognitive impairment) Serum blood levels of current medications such as lithium and anticonvulsant medications

Used with permission from Ng et al. [41]

2.3.2 Risk Assessment

Care should be taken when evaluating older patients for risk of self-harm. In 2014, the suicide rate of elderly men older than 65 years was reported to be 16.6 per 100,000. Among white men over 85 years, the suicide rate is 50.67 per 100,000 the highest of any age-gender-race group [45]. Suicidal ideas or fantasies as well as recent actions, religious and cultural beliefs, and any previous history of disinhibition impulsivity should all be assessed. Access to weapons and other methods of self-harm must be evaluated, especially if the patient reports having considered such methods. Information on prior incidents of self-harm, including aborted or actual suicide attempts, is crucial. Intervention is warranted when patients present with anhedonia, feelings of hopelessness, a history of suicide attempts [46], impulsivity [47], anxiety [48], psychosis [48, 49], or substance use [50, 51]. Patients who can find no reason to continue living or have stopped planning for the future such as the individual with severe chronic and/or terminal illnesses are at high risk for suicide [52]. Hospitalization or other high-intensity interventions should be pursued as determined by careful risk assessment.

2.3.3 Cognitive Assessment

Cognitive dysfunction is well recognized as a core component of bipolar disorder [53, 54–56]. Cognitive deficits occur in approximately 40–50 % of euthymic, geriatric bipolar patients [6, 57, 58] and have been noted to occur across mood states, and to persist through the euthymic phase [59–63]. Dysfunction is found in attention, cognitive flexibility, information process speed, memory, semantic fluency, and verbal fluency [54, 64, 65]. Numerous individual neuropsychological tasks have been evaluated in studies addressing cognitive function in bipolar disorder. More vascular burden and more psychiatric hospital admissions in addition to age are associated with cognitive dysfunction in older age bipolar disorder [66]. Cognitive dysfunction in older people is associated with worse clinical outcomes [67].

The area of cognitive assessment in bipolar disorder generally has expanded in recent years. While most general psychiatrists will not administer neuropsychological testing, it may be helpful to understand some of the key domains where cognitive impairment may occur. Recently, studies of bipolar disorder in the general population have included core measures from the Measurement and Treatment Research to Improve Cognition in Schizophrenia (MATRICS) for Consensus Cognitive Battery (MCCB) [54], with some modifications specific to bipolar disorder [68]. The MATRICS Consensus Cognitive Battery (MCCB) was initially designed to be uniformly applied to clinical trials targeting cognitive function in patients with schizophrenia [69, 70]. MCCB assesses the domains of attention/vigilance, processing speed, working memory, verbal learning, visual learning, reasoning and problem solving, and social cognition. MCCB has been tested in mixed-age patients with bipolar disorder [71, 72]. The Brief Assessment of Cognition in Affective Disorders (BAC-A) is composed of 6 subtests of the Brief Assessment of Cognition (BAC) and Brief Assessment of Cognition in Schizophrenia (BAC-S) and 2 additional tests: affective interference and emotion inhibition. A composite score is derived from the 6 subtests of the BAC-A, as well as the BAC and BAC-S [73].

The International Society for Bipolar Disorders–Battery for Assessment of Neurocognition (ISBD-BANC) is a cognitive battery developed to address specific cognitive issues in bipolar disorder in order to be more applicable for international use in broad bipolar disorders research. ISBD-BANC includes subtests from the MCCB and the Stroop Test and TMT-B, while flexible components include the use of either the HVLT-R or CVLT, as well as the optional inclusion of the WCST [68].

Specific to the older age bipolar population, a general neuropsychological battery by Gildengers et al. [74] encompassed 21 well-established and validated individual tests measuring multiple cognitive domains, and grouped into four distinct cognitive domains based on factor analysis: Delayed Memory, Information Processing Speed/Executive Function (Trails A, Stroop, Executive Interview, Animal Fluency, Digit Symbol Substitution Test), Language (Spot the Word, Letter Fluency, Silly Sentences), and the Visuomotor (Rey-Osterrieth Complex Figure Copy, Simple Drawings, Finger Tapping, Block Design, Trails B). While most office-based clinical evaluations do not include an extensive neurocognitive battery, a comprehensive evaluation of the older adult with bipolar disorder that seeks to answer important questions such as current and future support needs should include at least a subset of cognitive evaluations for task-specific domains.

2.4 Symptom Rating Scales

Standardized rating scales have been critical for studying bipolar disorder and a number of these scales are useful in an office setting for both evaluating and monitoring patients. In research, assessment of bipolar disorder and psychiatric comorbidities can be done through a semistructured diagnostic interview, as the Mini-International Neuropsychiatric Interview Plus (MINI) [75] or Structured Clinical Interview for DSM Disorders (SCID) [76]. Several scales are available to rate comorbid symptoms, such as the Beck Anxiety Inventory (BAI) [77] and Hamilton Anxiety Rating Scale (HAM-A) [78] for anxiety symptoms, or Alcohol Use Disorders Identification Test (AUDIT) [79] for alcohol use. A major function of rating scales, particularly in clinical trials, is to assess bipolar symptom severity. Some of the briefer rating scales, especially those that are self-rated tools such as the Quick Inventory of Depressive Symptomatology (QIDS) and the Beck Depression Inventory (BDI), can be used in clinical settings. Commonly used bipolar symptom rating scales, including those that can be self-rated by patients, are summarized in Table 2.3. In the era of growingly sophisticated information technology, electronic self-monitoring instruments using computers, personal digital assistants, Web interfaces, and smartphones have recently been explored. A recent review by Fauholt-Jepsen et al. [80] suggested that electronic self-monitoring of depression is more robust than that of mania and that more rigorous studies on its benefits and harm are needed.

2.4.1 Assessment of Comorbidities

2.4.1.1 Psychiatric Comorbidities

The definition of comorbidity is the occurrence of 2 syndromes in the same patient, and presupposes that they are distinct categorical entities. Psychiatric symptoms, fitting the criteria for an anxiety disorder, substance abuse, or personality disorder may be part of bipolar disorder or occur alongside of it as a comorbid condition. This explains why rates vary among studies, with up to 65 % of bipolar patients meting DSM-IV criteria for at least 1 comorbid Axis I disorder [82]. Common psychiatric comorbidities in studies among younger adults with bipolar disorder include substance abuse, anxiety disorders, attention-deficit/hyperactivity disorder, eating disorders, and personality disorders [83]. In contrast, the rates of psychiatric comorbid conditions in older adults with bipolar disorder appear lower (anxiety disorders up to 9.8 %) [84, 85], except for lifetime alcohol dependence and abuse and lifetime substance dependence (latter ranging from 9 to 29 %). Psychiatric comorbidities in bipolar disorder are associated with more severe symptoms,

Table 2.3 Common symptom rating scales in bipolar disorder

Scale	Key Features
BDRS	20 items for bipolar depression; includes items that are more common in bipolar versus unipolar depression; rater-administered; 15 min
HAM-D	17 items version, and 21 items version for depression; heavily influenced by physical symptoms; rater-administered; 20–30 min
IDS-C30	30 items for depression; has both self-rated version; and rater-administered version; 30 min
MADRS	10 items for depression; minimal focus on physical symptoms rater-administered; 15–20 min
QIDS	16 items for depression; has QIDS-SR (self-rated version); and QIDS-C (rater-administered version); 5–10 min
BDI	21 items for depression; self-rated; 5–10 min
BRMS	11 items for mania; rater-administered; 15–30 min
CARS-M	15 items for mania; rater-administered; 15–30 min
CGI-BP	3 domains: mania, depression, overall; each with 3 items; rater-administered; less than 5 min
MADS	23 items for mania; rater-administered; 60 min
MMRS	28 items for mania; rater-administered; 30–45 min
MRS	11 items for mania; rater-administered; 15 min
MSRS	26 items for mania; rater-administered; 15–30 min
PS	7 items for mania; rater-administered; 15–30 min
YMRS	11 items for mania; rater-administered; 15 min

Used with permission from Sajatovic et al. [81]

BDRS Bipolar Depression Rating Scale; *HAM-D* Hamilton Depression Rating Scale; *IDS-C30* Inventory of Depressive Symptomatology-30-Item Clinician Version; *MADRS* Montgomery Äsberg Depression Rating Scale; *MDD* major depressive disorder; *QIDS* Quick Inventory of Depressive Symptomatology; *BDI* Beck Depression Inventory; *BRMS* Bech-Rafaelsen Scale; *CARS-M* Clinician Administered Rating Scale for Mania; *CGI-BP* Clinical Global Impression-Bipolar Disorder; *MADS* Mania Diagnostic and Severity Scale; *MMRS* Modified Manic Rating Scale; *MRS* Mania Rating Scale; *MSRS* Manic State Rating Scale; *PS* Peterson Scale; *SADS* Schedule for Affective Disorders and Schizophrenia; *YMRS* Young Mania Rating Scale; *MDS* Manic Depressiveness Scale; and *MDQ* Mood Disorder Questionnaire

increased suicidality, poor adherence, and an overall more complicated course of illness. The need for appropriate treatment of substance use is underlined by the findings that bipolar patients who achieved sustained remission of their comorbid substance abuse had better outcomes in the area of role functioning [86]. In turn, effectively treating bipolar patients with mood stabilizers has been shown to reduce their engagement in substance abuse [87, 88].

2.4.1.2 Recognizing and Assessing Somatic Comorbidities

Medical conditions coexisting with bipolar disorder may be truly comorbid, related to the treatment of bipolar disorder, or a combination of both. Since few studies have studied medical comorbidities in bipolar older patients [84], knowledge on somatic comorbidities in bipolar disorder is mainly derived from studies in younger or mixed aged samples. A review of comorbidity in older patients with bipolar disorder found an average of 3–4 medical comorbidities [84], including: metabolic syndrome (up to 50 %); hypertension (45–69 %); diabetes mellitus (18–31 %); cardiovascular disease (9–49 %); respiratory illness (4–15 %); arthritis (16–21 %); and endocrine abnormalities (17–22 %) [83], as well as atopic diseases such as allergic rhinitis and asthma (6–20 %), which can greatly impact quality of life [84, 89, 90]. The number of somatic comorbidities is reported to increase with each decade of life, to 11 comorbid somatic conditions in those older than 70 years [56].

Although older bipolar patients have a greater burden of physical illnesses than similarly aged unipolar depressed peers [91], the overall prevalence of somatic comorbidity in patients with bipolar disorder appears comparable to rates reported in community-based geriatric samples [84]. Nevertheless, bipolar patients have much higher mortality rates: death due to cardiovascular and other physical illnesses on average of 10 years earlier than the general population [92]. In light of this early mortality, patients with bipolar disorder who survive into old age likely represent a disproportionately healthier subpopulation. This was illustrated by a report on metabolic syndrome in older bipolar and schizophrenia patients with rates comparable with healthy elderly [93].

Comorbid medical conditions will limit treatment options for bipolar disorder by drug-interactions and altered drug metabolisms. Polypharmacy is frequent, with 31.7 % of patients reported to be on six or more medications [85]. As some psychiatric patients have a limited access to physical health care, screening, and prevention [94], their somatic care should have the attention of mental health professionals. The recommendations for somatic workup have been defined by the International Society for Bipolar Disorders [41] and are summarized in Table 2.2. They include history-taking, physical examination, and laboratory studies. For older patients with bipolar disorder, screening for side effects and/or complications of medication and evaluating their general physical health are recommended more frequently (2–4 times a year) [41]. In patients using antipsychotics screening for metabolic syndrome is advised (fasting lipid profile, fasting blood glucose, blood pressure, and waist circumference).

Close collaboration between mental health, primary care, and medical speciality clinicians is strongly recommended.

2.5 Summary and Directions for Future Research

As illustrated in the preceding text, the clinical assessment of the older adult with bipolar disorder requires careful consideration of aging-related factors such as increased risk of dementia, medical and psychiatric comorbidities and the psychological sequelae of cumulative medical burden, cognitive decline, and functional impairment. Mania, particularly when it is of new onset in an older individual, should be evaluated for the presence of medical and neurological conditions as well as medications that may cause secondary mania. The clinical interview and history-taking is essential to the evaluation of the older adult with bipolar disorder as is supplemental laboratory, radiologic, and neuropsychological evaluation. Standardized tools for evaluating symptom severity, comorbidity, and neurocognitive status can be helpful in informing treatment planning and prognosis.

There is still insufficient research on assessment methods of the older individual who presents with bipolar symptoms. A recent report on older age bipolar disorder by the International Society for Bipolar Disorder (ISBD) notes that there is a critical need for studying a variety of aspects of bipolar disorder in elderly individuals, particularly as this will be helpful in health policy planning given the general global demographic trends [2]. A challenge in interpreting existing research studies is substantial sample heterogeneity and disparate measures used to evaluate symptoms, comorbidity, functional status, cognition, and other outcomes. Developing minimum data set recommendations such as use of specific symptom measures and medical burden evaluation as well as a cognitive assessment battery relevant to older individuals could help to address some of these methodological limitations and pave the way for more standardized evaluations. This is turn has potential to inform a prognosis on the individual and population level and advance understanding bipolar disorder trajectory in the second half of life.

Clinical Pearls

Differential Diagnosis

- Somatic conditions can cause late-life mania; a full somatic work-up is warranted, especially in patients who first present with mania in later life.
- Secondary mania can be caused by an extensive list of medications, metabolic disturbances and neurological conditions.
- Tumors, neurosurgery and traumatic head injury can result in manic symptoms described as vascular/neurological mania or neurological disinhibition syndrome.
- Dementia with involvement of the frontal circuit can present with manic symptoms, most specific in bvFTD.

Clinical Interview, History Taking, Risk Assessment

- The clinical interview and history-taking is essential to appropriately assess older individuals who appear to present with possible bipolar disorder.
- Collateral information from care givers and family members is an essential component of the clinical evaluation of the older individual with bipolar disorder.

- As many systemic illnesses presentation can mimic bipolar disorder, clinicians should be diligent in evaluating whether the presenting symptoms are exacerbation of a primary bipolar disorder or due to a systemic disease.
- Compared to the general population, elderly patients are at higher risk for suicide. Risk assessment is an essential element of every clinical encounter.

Cognitive Assessment

- Cognitive dysfunction is a common and core feature of bipolar disorder that is associated with disability and poor outcome. Older bipolar patients may be particularly at risk for cognitive impairment and focused cognitive assessment should be part of a comprehensive evaluation.
- Neurocognitive assessments used in later-life bipolar disorder should be sensitive enough to detect impairment and track meaningful change, and at the same time, should be practical for implementation.
- There have been a variety of neuropsychological instruments in studies of adults with bipolar disorder. The MATRICS Consensus Cognitive Battery (MCCB) appears to include reasonable core components with additional measures that have been included in the International Society for Bipolar Disorders–Battery for Assessment of Neurocognition (ISBD-BANC). Recent studies have identified neuropsychological batteries that may identify impairments most common in older adults.

Assessment of Comorbidities

- Clinicians providing care for bipolar elderly patients should carefully assess for comorbid conditions, choose treatment options that take into account these comorbid states, minimize side effects and treatment burden.
- Given the high prevalence of medical comorbidity in older bipolar patients, general medical conditions should be regularly screened for to enable timely diagnosis and treatment.
- Close collaboration between mental health, primary care, and medical speciality clinicians is strongly recommended to optimize care in these patients with high psychiatric and medical complexity.

References

1. Depp CA, Jeste DV. Bipolar disorder in older adults: a critical review. Bipolar Disord. 2004;6:343–67.
2. Sajatovic M, Strejilevich S, Gildengers A, Dols A, Al Jurdi RK, Forester B, et al. A report on older-age bipolar disorder from the international society for bipolar disorders task force. Bipolar Disord. 2015;17(7):689–704.
3. Lala SV, Sajatovic M. Medical and psychiatric comorbidities among elderly individuals with bipolar disorder: a literature review. J Geriatr Psychiatry Neurol. 2012;25:20–5.
4. Goldstein BI, Schaffer A, Wang S, Blanco C. Excessive and premature new-onset cardiovascular disease among adults with bipolar disorder in the US NESARC cohort. J Clin Psychiatry. 2015;76:163–9.
5. Kessing LV, Nilsson FM. Increased risk of developing dementia in patients with major affective disorders compared to patients with other medical illnesses. J Affect Disord. 2003;73:261–9.
6. Tsai SY, Lee HC, Chen CC, Huang YL. Cognitive impairment in later life in patients with early-onset bipolar disorder. Bipolar Disord. 2007;9:868–75.
7. Dols A, Kupka RW, van Lammeren A, Beekman AT, Sajatovic M, Stek ML. The prevalence of late-life mania: a review. Bipolar Disord. 2014;16(2):113–8.
8. Krauthammer C, Klerman GL. Secondary mania: manic syndromes associated with antecedent physical illness or drugs. Arch Gen Psychiatry. 1978;35(11):1333–9.
9. Van Gerpen MW, Johnson JE, Winstead DK. Mania in the geriatric patient population: a review of the literature. Am J Geriatr Psychiatry. 1999;7(3):188–202.
10. Brooks JO 3rd, Hoblyn JC. Secondary mania in older adults. Am J Psychiatry. 2005;162 (11):2033–8.
11. Wise MG, Rundell JR. Consultation psychiatry: concise guide. Washington: American Psychiatric; 1998.
12. Woodward M, Jacova C, Black SE, Kertesz A, Mackenzie IR, Feldman H. Differentiating the frontal variant of Alzheimer's disease. Int J Geriatr Psychiatry. 2010;25(7):732–8.
13. Staekenborg SS, Su T, van Straaten EC, Lane R, Scheltens P, Barkhof F, et al. Behavioural and psychological symptoms in vascular dementia; differences between small- and large-vessel disease. J Neurol Neurosurg Psychiatry. 2010;81(5):547–51.
14. Rascovsky K, Hodges JR, Knopman D, Mendez MF, Kramer JH, Neuhaus J, et al. Sensitivity of revised diagnostic criteria for the behavioral variant of frontotemporal dementia. Brain. 2011;134(9):2456–77.
15. Roman GC, Tatemichi TK, Erkinjuntti T, Cummings JL, Masdeu JC, Garcia JH, et al. Vascular dementia: diagnostic criteria for research studies. Report of the NINDS-AIREN international workshop. Neurology. 1993;43(2):250–60.
16. McKhann GM, Knopman DS, Chertkow H, Hyman BT, Jack CR Jr, Kawas CH, et al. The diagnosis of dementia due to Alzheimer's disease: recommendations from the National Institute on Aging-Alzheimer's Association workgroups on diagnostic guidelines for Alzheimer's disease. Alzheimers Dement. 2011;7(3):263–9.
17. Dols A, van Liempt S, Gossink F, Krudop WA, Sikkes S, Pijnenburg YAL et al. Identifying specific clinical symptoms of bvFTD versus differential psychiatric disorders in patients presenting with a late onset frontal lobe syndrome. J Clin Psychiatry. 2016. [Epub ahead of print].
18. Vorspan F, Bertoux M, Brichant-Petitjean C, Dubois B, Lepine JP. Relapsing-remitting behavioral variant of frontotemporal dementia in a bipolar patient. Funct Neurol. 2012;27 (3):193–6.
19. Kerstein AH, Schroeder RW, Baade LE, Lincoln J, Khan AY. Frontotemporal dementia mimicking bipolar disorder. J Psychiatr Pract. 2013;19(6):498–500.

20. Cerami C, Marcone A, Galimberti D, Villa C, Scarpini E, Cappa SF. From genotype to phenotype: two cases of genetic frontotemporal lobar degeneration with premorbid bipolar disorder. J Alzheimers Dis. 2011;27(4):791–7.
21. Pavlovic A, Marley J, Sivakumar V. Development of frontotemporal dementia in a case of bipolar affective disorder: is there a link? BMJ Case Rep. 2011;2011.
22. Zhou J, Seeley WW. Network dysfunction in Alzheimer's disease and frontotemporal dementia: implications for psychiatry. Biol Psychiatry. 2014;75(7):565–73.
23. Rashid B, Damaraju E, Pearlson GD, Calhoun VD. Dynamic connectivity states estimated from resting fMRI identify differences among Schizophrenia, bipolar disorder, and healthy control subjects. Front Hum Neurosci. 2014;8:897.
24. Lois G, Linke J, Wessa M. Altered functional connectivity between emotional and cognitive resting state networks in euthymic bipolar I disorder patients. PLoS ONE. 2014;9(10): e107829.
25. Khan BK, Yokoyama JS, Takada LT, Sha SJ, Rutherford NJ, Fong JC, et al. Atypical, slowly progressive behavioral variant frontotemporal dementia associated with C9ORF72 hexanucleotide expansion. J Neurol Neurosurg Psychiatry. 2012;83(4):358–64.
26. Meisler MH, Grant AE, Jones JM, Lenk GM, He F, Todd PK, et al. C9ORF72 expansion in a family with bipolar disorder. Bipolar Disord. 2013;15(3):326–32.
27. Floris G, Di Stefano F, Pisanu C, Chillotti C, Murru MR, Congiu D, et al. C9ORF72 repeat expansion and bipolar disorder—is there a link? No mutation detected in a Sardinian cohort of patients with bipolar disorder. Bipolar Disord. 2014;16(6):667–8.
28. Floris G, Borghero G, Cannas A, Stefano FD, Murru MR, Corongiu D, et al. Bipolar affective disorder preceding frontotemporal dementia in a patient with C9ORF72 mutation: is there a genetic link between these two disorders? J Neurol. 2013;260(4):1155–7.
29. Kipps CM, Hodges JR, Hornberger M. Nonprogressive behavioral frontotemporal dementia: recent developments and clinical implications of the bvFTD phenocopy syndrome. Curr Opin Neurol. 2010;23(6):628–32.
30. Davies RR, Kipps CM, Mitchell J, Kril JJ, Halliday GM, Hodges JR. Progression in frontotemporal dementia: identifying a benign behavioral variant by magnetic resonance imaging. Arch Neurol. 2006;63(11):1627–31.
31. Mendez MF. Mania in neurologic disorders. Curr Psychiatry Rep. 2000;2(5):440–5.
32. Jorge RE, Robinson RG, Starkstein SE, Arndt SV, Forrester AW, Geisler FH. Secondary mania following traumatic brain injury. Am J Psychiatry. 1993;150(6):916–21.
33. Robinson RG, Boston JD, Starkstein SE, Price TR. Comparison of mania and depression after brain injury: causal factors. Am J Psychiatry. 1988;145(2):172–8.
34. Braun CM, Larocque C, Daigneault S, Montour-Proulx I. Mania, pseudomania, depression, and pseudodepression resulting from focal unilateral cortical lesions. Neuropsychiatry Neuropsychol Behav Neurol. 1999;12(1):35–51.
35. Steffens DC, Krishnan KR. Structural neuroimaging and mood disorders: recent findings, implications for classification, and future directions. Biol Psychiatry. 1998;43(10):705–12.
36. Kilbourne AM, Cornelius JR, Han X, Pincus HA, Shad M, Salloum I, et al. Burden of general medical conditions among individuals with bipolar disorder. Bipolar Disord. 2004;6(5):368–73.
37. Perron BE, Howard MO, Nienhuis JK, Bauer MS, Woodward AT, Kilbourne AM. Prevalence and burden of general medical conditions among adults with bipolar I disorder: results from the National Epidemiologic Survey on Alcohol and Related Conditions. J Clin Psychiatry. 2009;70(10):1407–15.
38. Lehmann SW, Rabins PV. Factors related to hospitalization in elderly manic patients with early and late-onset bipolar disorder. Int J Geriatr Psychiatry. 2006;21(11):1060–4.
39. Brodaty H, Luscombe G, Parker G, Wilhelm K, Hickie I, Austin MP, et al. Increased rate of psychosis and psychomotor change in depression with age. Psychol Med. 1997;27(5):1205–13.
40. Al Jurdi RK, Nguyen QX, Petersen NJ, Pilgrim P, Gyulai L, Sajatovic M. Acute bipolar I affective episode presentation across life span. J Geriatr Psychiatry Neurol. 2012;25(1):6–14.

41. Ng F, Mammen OK, Wilting I, Sachs GS, Ferrier IN, Cassidy F, et al. The International Society for Bipolar Disorders (ISBD) consensus guidelines for the safety monitoring of bipolar disorder treatments. Bipolar Disord. 2009;11(6):559–95.
42. Sajatovic M, Blow FC. Bipolar disorder in later life. Baltimore: John Hopkins UP; 2007.
43. Ketter TA. Handbook of diagnosis and treatment of bipolar disorders. Washington, DC: American Psychiatric Pub; 2010.
44. Hales RE, Yudofsky SC, Weiss L. The American psychiatric publishing textbook of psychiatry. Washington, DC: American Psychiatric Pub; 2008.
45. American Association of Suicidology [cited 2016 January]. http://www.suicidology.org/.
46. Wiktorsson S, Runeson B, Skoog I, Ostling S, Waern M. Attempted suicide in the elderly: characteristics of suicide attempters 70 years and older and a general population comparison group. Am J Geriatr Psychiatry. 2010;18(1):57–67.
47. Vanyukov PM, Szanto K, Siegle GJ, Hallquist MN, Reynolds CF 3rd, Aizenstein HJ, et al. Impulsive traits and unplanned suicide attempts predict exaggerated prefrontal response to angry faces in the elderly. Am J Geriatr Psychiatry. 2015;23(8):829–39.
48. Waern M, Runeson BS, Allebeck P, Beskow J, Rubenowitz E, Skoog I, et al. Mental disorder in elderly suicides: a case-control study. Am J Psychiatry. 2002;159(3):450–5.
49. Chiu HF, Yip PS, Chi I, Chan S, Tsoh J, Kwan CW, et al. Elderly suicide in Hong Kong—a case-controlled psychological autopsy study. Acta Psychiatr Scand. 2004;109(4):299–305.
50. Quinlivan L, Cooper J, Steeg S, Davies L, Hawton K, Gunnell D, et al. Scales for predicting risk following self-harm: an observational study in 32 hospitals in England. BMJ Open. 2014;4(5):e004732.
51. Warden S, Spiwak R, Sareen J, Bolton JM. The SAD PERSONS scale for suicide risk assessment: a systematic review. Arch Suicide Res. 2014;18(4):313–26.
52. Conwell Y, Van Orden K, Caine ED. Suicide in older adults. Psychiatr Clin N Am. 2011;34 (2):451–68.
53. Schouws SN, Comijs HC, Stek ML, Beekman AT. Self-reported cognitive complaints in elderly bipolar patients. Am J Geriatr. 2012;20(8):700–6.
54. Bora E, Yucel M, Pantelis C. Cognitive impairment in affective psychoses: a meta-analysis. Schizophr Bull. 2010;36:112–25.
55. Sajatovic M, Chen PJ. Geriatric bipolar disorder: epidemiology, clinical features, assessment, and diagnosis. UpToDate: Feb 2012; updated on August 2016 www.uptodate.com. Philadelphia: Wolters Kluwer Health.
56. Tsitsipa E, Fountoulakis KN. The neurocognitive functioning in bipolar disorder: a systematic review of data. Ann Gen Psychiatry. 2015;14:42.
57. Schouws SN, Comijs HC, Stek ML, Dekker J, Oostervink F, Naarding P, et al. Cognitive impairment in early and late bipolar disorder. Am J Geriatr Psychiatry. 2009;17(6):508–15.
58. Gildengers AG, Butters MA, Seligman K, McShea M, Miller MD, Mulsant BH, et al. Cognitive functioning in late-life bipolar disorder. Am J Psychiatry. 2004;161:736.
59. Malhi GS, Ivanovski B, Hadzi-Pavlovic D, Mitchell PB, Vieta E, Sachdev P. Neuropsychological deficits and functional impairment in bipolar depression, hypomania and euthymia. Bipolar Disord. 2007;9:114–25.
60. Bora E, Yucel M, Pantelis C. Cognitive endophenotypes of bipolar disorder: a meta-analysis of neuropsychological deficits in euthymic patients and their first-degree relatives. J Affect Disord. 2009;113:1–20.
61. Adida M, Jollant F, Clark L, Besnier N, Guillaume S, Kaladjian A, et al. Trait-related decision-making impairment in the three phases of bipolar disorder. Biol Psychiatry. 2011;70:357–65.
62. Mann-Wrobel MC, Carreno JT, Dickinson D. Meta-analysis of neuropsychological functioning in euthymic bipolar disorder: an update and investigation of moderator variables. Bipolar Disord. 2011;13:334–42.

63. Santos JL, Aparicio A, Bagney A, Sánchez-Morla EM, Rodríguez-Jiménez R, Mateo J, et al. A five-year follow-up study of neurocognitive functioning in bipolar disorder. Bipolar Disord. 2014;16:722–31.
64. Samamé C, Martino DJ, Strejilevich SA. A quantitative review of neurocognition in euthymic late-life bipolar disorder. Bipolar Disord. 2013;15:633.
65. Bourne C, Aydemir O, Balanza-Martinez V, Bora E, Brissos S, Cavanagh JT, et al. Neuro-psychological testing of cognitive impairment in euthymic bipolar disorder: an individual patient data meta-analysis. Acta Psychiatr Scand. 2013;128:149–62.
66. Schouws SN, Stek ML, Comijs HC, Beekman AT. Risk factors for cognitive impairment in elderly bipolar patients. J Affect Disord. 2010;125(1–3):330–5.
67. Burdick KE, Goldberg JF, Harrow M. Neurocognitive dysfunction and psychosocial outcome in patients with bipolar I disorder at 15-year follow-up. Acta Psychiatr Scand. 2010;122 (6):499–506.
68. Yatham LN, Torres IJ, Malhi GS, Frangou S, Glahn DC, Bearden CE, et al. The international society for bipolar disorders-battery for assessment of neurocognition (ISBD-BANC). Bipolar Disord. 2010;12(4):351–63.
69. Nuechterlein KH, Green MF, Kern RS, Baade LE, Barch DM, Cohen JD, et al. The MATRICS consensus cognitive battery, part 1: test selection, reliability, and validity. Am J Psychiatry. 2008;165(2):203–13.
70. Kern RS, Nuechterlein KH, Green MF, Baade LE, Fenton WS, Gold JM, et al. The MATRICS consensus cognitive battery: part 2: co-norming and standardization. Am J Psychiatry. 2008;165:214–20.
71. Burdick KE, Goldberg TE, Cornblatt BA, Keefe RS, Gopin CB, Derosse P, et al. The MATRICS consensus cognitive battery in patients with bipolar I disorder. Neuropsychopharmacology. 2011;36(8):1587–92.
72. Kessler U, Schoeyen HK, Andreassen OA, Eide GE, Hammar A, Malt UF, et al. Neurocognitive profiles in treatment-resistant bipolar I and bipolar II disorder depression. BMC Psychiatry. 2013;13:105.
73. Fox KH, Burdick KE, Lombardo L, Keefef RSE. Cognitive impairment in patients with bipolar disorder: an overview of some assessment tools. Psychiatry Times. 2009;26(12).
74. Gildengers AG, Butters MA, Chisholm D, Rogers JC, Holm MB, Bhalla RK, et al. Cognitive functioning and instrumental activities of daily living in late-life bipolar disorder. Am J Geriatr Psychiatry. 2007;15:174–9.
75. Sheehan DV, Lecrubier Y, Sheehan KH, Amorim P, Janavs J, Weiller E et al. The Mini-International Neuropsychiatric Interview (M.I.N.I.): the development and validation of a structured diagnostic psychiatric interview for DSM-IV and ICD-10. J Clin Psychiatry. 1998;59 (Suppl 20):22–33; quiz 4–57.
76. Spitzer RL, Williams JB, Gibbon M, First MB. The Structured Clinical Interview for DSM-III-R (SCID). I: history, rationale, and description. Arch Gen Psychiatry. 1992;49 (8):624–9.
77. Beck AT, Epstein N, Brown G, Steer RA. An inventory for measuring clinical anxiety: psychometric properties. J Consult Clin Psychol. 1988;56(6):893–7.
78. Hamilton M. The assessment of anxiety states by rating. Br J Med Psychol. 1959;32(1):50–5.
79. Babor TF, Kranzler HR, Lauerman RJ. Early detection of harmful alcohol consumption: comparison of clinical, laboratory, and self-report screening procedures. Addict Behav. 1989;14(2):139–57.
80. Fauholt-Jepsen M, Munkholm K, Frost M, Bardram JE, Kessing LV. Electronic self-monitoring of mood using IT platforms in adult patients with bipolar disorder: A systematic review of the validity and evidence. BMC Psychiatry. 2016;16:7.
81. Sajatovic M, Chen PJ, Young RC. Rating scales in bipolar disorder. In: Tohen M, Bowden C, Neirenberg A, Geddes J, editors. The international society for bipolar disorders clinical trial designs in mood disorders. San Diego: Academic Press; 2015. p. 105–136.

82. McElroy SL, Altshuler LL, Suppes T, Keck PE Jr, Frye MA, Denicoff KD, et al. Axis I psychiatric comorbidity and its relationship to historical illness variables in 288 patients with bipolar disorder. Am J Psychiatry. 2001;158(3):420–6.
83. Krishnan KR. Psychiatric and medical comorbidities of bipolar disorder. Psychosom Med. 2005;67(1):1–8.
84. Lala SV, Sajatovic M. Medical and psychiatric comorbidities among elderly individuals with bipolar disorder: a literature review. J Geriatr Psychiatry Neurol. 2012;25(1):20–5.
85. Dols A, Rhebergen D, Beekman A, Kupka R, Sajatovic M, Stek ML. Psychiatric and medical comorbidities: results from a bipolar elderly cohort study. Am J Geriatr Psychiatry. 2014;22 (11):1066–74.
86. Weiss RD, Ostacher MJ, Otto MW, Calabrese JR, Fossey M, Wisniewski SR 7 et al. Does recovery from substance use disorder matter in patients with bipolar disorder? J Clin Psychiatry. 2005;66(6):730–5; quiz 808–9.
87. Geller B, Cooper TB, Sun K, Zimerman B, Frazier J, Williams M, et al. Double-blind and placebo-controlled study of lithium for adolescent bipolar disorders with secondary substance dependency. J Am Acad Child Adolesc Psychiatry. 1998;37(2):171–8.
88. Salloum IM, Cornelius JR, Daley DC, Kirisci L, Himmelhoch JM, Thase ME. Efficacy of valproate maintenance in patients with bipolar disorder and alcoholism: a double-blind placebo-controlled study. Arch Gen Psychiatry. 2005;62(1):37–45.
89. Tsai SY, Kuo CJ, Chung KH, Huang YL, Lee HC, Chen CC. Cognitive dysfunction and medical morbidity in elderly outpatients with bipolar disorder. Am J Geriatr Psychiatry. 2009;17(12):1004–11.
90. Fenn HH, Bauer MS, Altshuler L, Evans DR, Williford WO, Kilbourne AM, et al. Medical comorbidity and health-related quality of life in bipolar disorder across the adult age span. J Affect Disord. 2005;86(1):47–60.
91. Gildengers AG, Whyte EM, Drayer RA, Soreca I, Fagiolini A, Kilbourne AM, et al. Medical burden in late-life bipolar and major depressive disorders. Am J Geriatr Psychiatry. 2008;16 (3):194–200.
92. Westman J, Hallgren J, Wahlbeck K, Erlinge D, Alfredsson L, Osby U. Cardiovascular mortality in bipolar disorder: a population-based cohort study in Sweden. BMJ Open. 2013;3(4).
93. Konz HW, Meesters PD, Paans NP, van Grootheest DS, Comijs HC, Stek ML, et al. Screening for metabolic syndrome in older patients with severe mental illness. Am J Geriatr Psychiatry. 2014;22(11):1116–20.
94. De Hert M, Dekker JM, Wood D, Kahl KG, Holt RI, Moller HJ. Cardiovascular disease and diabetes in people with severe mental illness position statement from the European Psychiatric Association (EPA), supported by the European Association for the Study of Diabetes (EASD) and the European Society of Cardiology (ESC). Eur Psychiatry. 2009;24(6):412–24.

Neurobiology of Older Age Bipolar Disorder

3

Eulogio Eclarinal and Olusola Ajilore

Clinical Vignette 3.1

Mr. F is a 60-year-old Caucasian male with a history of hypertension, chronic back pain, diverticulitis, abdominal hernia, and bipolar disorder, type I for 20 years. At the time, he presented to the clinic, he had worsening worsening symptoms over the past 5 years, characterized by emotional lability, irritability, and physical aggression. His daughter indicated that his reactions had been "obsessive and overboard" which the patient acknowledged as "bad mood swings." These symptoms occurred while the patient was on lithium 600 mg twice daily with a recent serum lithium level of 0.4 mmol/L. Lithium was increased to 600 mg in the morning and 900 mg in the evening. After 1 month at the increased dose, the serum level was 0.7 mmol/L and the patient reported significant symptomatic improvement in mood. Over the next 2 years, the patient remained stable but his lithium levels increased to 0.9 mmol/L without a change in dose. The patient was reluctant to consider a dose reduction given his current stable mood. One month later, Mr. F was hospitalized for an episode of intention tremors in his hands and syncope. Per his admission note, he had "shaking in his hands" which started 5 months prior, progressively worsened, and spread to his legs leading to a shuffling gait. On examination, he was bradycardic (heart rate 26) and his lithium level on admission was 2.4 mmol/L. The patient was unintentionally taking more

E. Eclarinal
Ambulatory Clinic, Neuropsychiatric Institute, University of Illinois at Chicago, 912 S. Wood Street, Chicago, IL 60612, USA
e-mail: eeclarinal@psych.uic.edu

O. Ajilore (✉)
Psychiatric Institute, University of Illinois at Chicago, 1601 W. Taylor Street, Chicago, IL 60612, USA
e-mail: oajilore@psych.uic.edu

S.W. Lehmann and B.P. Forester (eds.), *Bipolar Disorder in Older Age Patients*,
DOI 10.1007/978-3-319-48912-4_3

than the prescribed dose and had severe lithium toxicity. He reported that he was "confused about lithium dosing" which led to the accidental overdose. On admission, he had a creatinine of 2.7 and the fractional excretion of sodium of 0.16 %, indicative of a pre-renal etiology. It was believed that his lithium toxicity was due to a combination of pre-renal acute renal insufficiency and an unintentional overdose. After intravenous hydration and the normalization of his lithium levels, Mr. F was discharged in stable condition.

Learning Points

- Lithium levels require frequent monitoring in older patients.
- Severe cardiac complications can arise from toxic lithium levels.

3.1 Introduction

Bipolar disorder is a leading cause of disability (globally 6th), affecting approximately 3 % of the world's population [1] and depending on criteria used, this value can be as high as 6.4 % within the inclusion of bipolar spectrum disorder [2]. Its incidence is similar between genders and even across different cultural and ethnic groups though there may be a larger disparity in terms of severity [3]. It is widely accepted that the peak of onset frequency is late adolescence or early adulthood.

Bipolar disorder itself is a psychiatric disorder that consists of alternating episodes of depression and elevated mood and is associated with higher incidences of morbidity and mortality [4], especially with regard to suicide in patients in mixed episode states [5]. Etiological factors for bipolar disorder (BD) are not clearly explicated, indeed some researchers have noted that its treatment advanced as a result of serendipitous discovery as opposed to understood pathophysiology [6], though it appears environmental and hereditary factors are important players in its development [4]. Despite the prevalence of the disorder, BD in midlife remains widely misdiagnosed, with a gap of 5–10 years between onset and accurate diagnosis with consequence of delayed appropriate treatment [7].

The identification and diagnosis of bipolar disorder is often a difficult challenge as the disorder itself can present on a spectrum of severity. The diagnosis of BD can also prove elusive due to its dependence on the variability of clinical rating measurements. Improvements in diagnostic challenges could be realized with the identification of objective biomarkers that serve as signals for the disorder. Researchers argue that these objective biomarkers could be discovered through use of neuroimaging studies [8].

Recent emergence of neuroimaging technology and its relative advancement over the years has led to a deeper understanding of the structural, functional, and chemical markers of bipolar disorder. Most studies reveal correlations between abnormal brain structure and bipolar disorder diagnosis, but cautiously limit their conclusions regarding neuroimaging and its potential role in identifying or differentiating psychiatric disease [9]. However, in a more recent review of neuroimaging studies of bipolar disorder by Phillips and Kupfer [8], investigators examining studies involving fMRI, volumetric analysis, and diffusion neuroimaging discovered abnormalities in neural circuits involved in affective regulation for individuals with bipolar disorder. Other groups hypothesize that neuroimaging could reveal distinguishing patterns to be used for diagnosis in comparison with healthy controls [7].

While the role of neuroimaging in bipolar disorder continues to be studied in the general population, there have been relatively fewer neuroimaging studies in the geriatric population, in particular for Older Age Bipolar Disorder (OABD). This particular subset has become increasingly prominent due to the aging of the population and the rising proportion of patients contributing to this age group. Sajatovic and coworkers highlighted the increasing importance of this in a recent report featuring OABD as an important step in tracking BD across a life span. This group also reflected that limited studies in the older adult cohort reduce the potential impact of neuroimaging in the geriatric patient population.

In spite of limited studies, geriatric individuals with BD provide an apt and unique population to study the long-term, neuroprogressive effects of the disorder [10]. Although BD accounts for approximately 25 % of all geriatric patients with mood disorders [11], the presentation of such individuals in clinical studies has been reported to be a meager 2–17 % [12]. With a dearth of published studies regarding OABD, many aspects of the disorder remain to be further elucidated. This section will summarize current and pertinent findings regarding neuroimaging studies of late-onset and early-onset BD, as well as discusses implications for future studies.

3.2 White Matter Hyperintensities, Vascular Risk, and Cognitive Function

Magnetic resonance imaging (MRI) studies have suggested a relationship between late-onset BD and a higher prevalence of white matter hyper intensities [13]. On T2 or intermediate-weighted MR images, WMHs exhibit high-intensity signals and appear as bright areas [14]. Increased prevalence of WMHs, however, are often also associated with aging [15]; several studies have found higher rates of WMH in non-BD elderly with vascular, cognitive, and neuropsychological problems. While aging, vascular insults, and BD are associated with WMHs, the relationship between these insults and development of BD needs further study.

Some studies focusing on WMH and BD have suggested that the cognitive defects experienced by some late-onset BD individuals are also caused by cerebral vascular disorders and risks. Tamashiro et al. [16] for instance, reported that unlike elderly controls or early-onset BD, individuals with late-onset BD exhibited hyperintense lesions around the deep white matter of the parietal, frontal, and subcortical basal ganglia regions. The study proposed that the presence of WMHs in these regions supports a link between vascular risk factors and late-onset bipolar disorder. This group also reported that although there was no significant difference in Periventricular White Matter WMHs, late-onset individuals had more Deep White Matter WMHs than controls and those with early-onset BD [16].

Other studies, however, have found conflicting findings regarding late-onset BD and the incidence of WMHs. In a recent study by Rej et al. [10], for example, a cohort of BD subjects greater than or equal to 50 years of age had reduced WMH burden compared with controls, despite poor performance on cognitive tests. These findings seem to suggest that cognitive dysfunction in OABD individuals does not necessarily arise as a result of processes (including those that are vascular) related to increased prevalence of WMHs. Similarly, Delaloye et al. [17] found that despite significantly diminished cognitive function in older individuals with BD, there were no significant changes in white matter volume for the group in comparison with controls over a 2-year follow-up. In summary, results of studies to date vary and suggest that white matter hyperintensities in elderly individuals with BD still require further investigation through longitudinal neuroimaging studies.

3.3 Volumetric Differences in Particular Regions of the Brain

In addition to increased white matter hyperintensities, neuroimaging studies of OABD (early- and late-onset BD) or late-onset only BD individuals have observed structural and volumetric abnormalities in specific brain regions (Fig. 3.1). One study by Beyer et al. [18] for example, reported reduced right caudate and total caudate volume in older bipolar subjects compared to controls. In a different study, Beyer et al. [19] also observed no difference in hippocampal volume between late-onset and early-onset BD subjects. Interestingly, however, Huang et al. [20] observed opposite effects in a more recent study. In particular, individuals with late-onset BD were reported to have a larger left caudate in addition to a larger volume in the left middle frontal gyrus in comparison with subjects with early-onset BD.

The temporal lobe is another brain region of interest for researchers because of its cortical and subcortical connections to areas of the brain that regulate emotion, mood, and memory [21]. Jones et al. [22] reported increased temporal lobe volumes in adult patients with BD. In another study, amygdala volumes were found to be significantly larger in the bipolar group (average age 50.2 ± 12.7) compared to normal and schizophrenic groups [23].

A relatively recent review of MRI imaging studies from 2009 also showed whole brain and prefrontal lobe volume reductions and increased volume of the globus pallidus and lateral ventricles [24]. Wijeratne et al. [25] recently demonstrated that older patients with BD had smaller amygdala and hippocampal volumes, and that

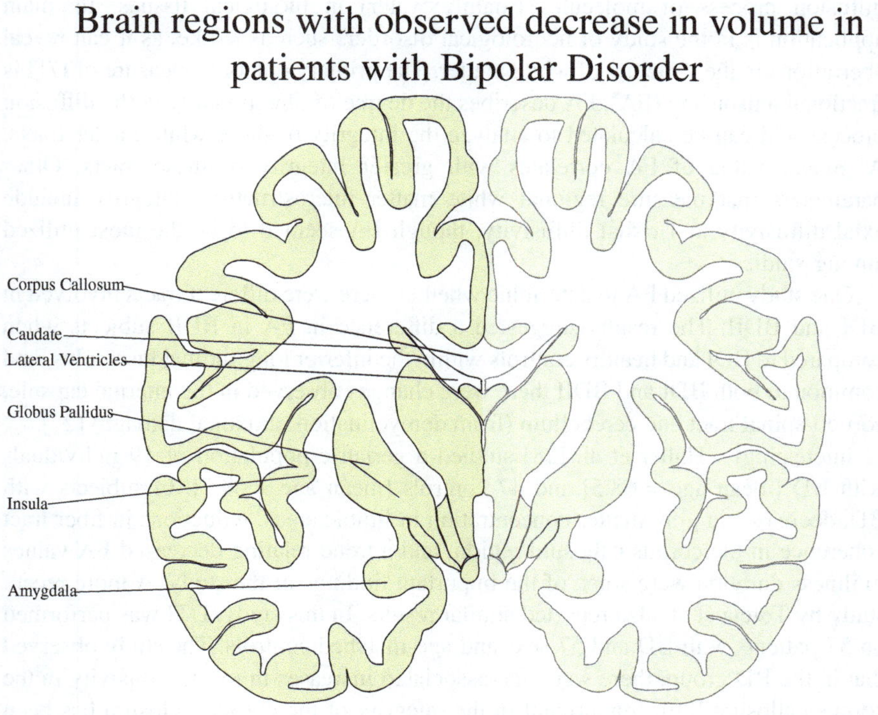

Fig. 3.1 Imaging from research has shown decrease in the volume of *gray* matter in patients with bipolar disorder in the right cudate, globus palidus, lateral ventricles, insula, and amygdale. *White* matter hyperintensities have been observed in the corpus callosum, parietal, frontal, and subcortical basal ganglia

the latter was negatively associated with the duration of manic and depressive episodes in these individuals. Other studies have discovered decreased gray matter concentration in the right anterior insula, nucleus accumbens, ventral putamen, and frontal orbital cortex. In contrast, in a study comparing 71 older BD individuals to 82 controls, the OABD group showed no significant age-associated volumetric changes in gray matter [26]. Nevertheless, despite some conflicting studies, the current evidence suggests that bipolar disorder does involve a reduction in brain volume, though the pathophysiology of this change requires further elucidation.

3.4 Diffusion Tensor Imaging

Diffusion tensor imaging (DTI)/diffusion MRI, and the subsequent calculation of fractional anisotropy (FA), demonstrates microstructural alterations of white matter in Older Age Bipolar Disorder. Diffusion MRI permits the in vivo mapping of the diffusion process of molecules (mainly water) in biological tissues. Its main application is in the study of neurological disorders such as stroke, as it can reveal aberrations in the structure of white matter. The primary outcome measure of DTI is fractional anisotropy (FA). FA describes the degree of directionality in the diffusion process and can be calculated to analyze the integrity of these white matter tracts. A greater value of FA correlates with greater integrity of these tracts. Other parameters that measure regional white matter microstructural integrity include axial diffusivity and radial diffusivity, though FA seemed to be the most utilized among studies.

One study utilized FA to determine whether there were different tracts involved in BDI and BDII. The results suggested a difference in FA in BDII subjects when compared to BDI and healthy controls within the inferior longitudinal fasciculus, and common to both BDI and BDII there were changes observed in the internal capsule, cortico-spinal tract and cerebellum (from demyelination or axonal damage) [27].

Interestingly, Haller et al. [28] studied a geriatric population of 19 individuals with BD [mean age = 68.5] and 47 controls [mean age = 69.7]. In subjects with BD, decreases in gray matter concentration in limbic areas, reductions in fiber tract coherence in the corpus callosum region, and a trend relating decreased FA values to illness duration were some of the important findings of the study. A more recent study by Toteja et al. also reported similar results. In this study, DTI was performed on 57 patients with BD and 57 sex- and age-matched controls. The study observed that in the BD group, there were age-associated increases in mean diffusivity in the corpus callosum [29]. Impairment in the integrity of the corpus callosum has been specifically implicated in late-life bipolar disorder [30].

3.5 Magnetic Resonance Spectroscopy

Of note, in a lithium-7 magnetic resonance spectroscopy (MRS) study focused on the corpus callosum, Forester et al. [31] found that the relationship between brain and serum lithium levels was moderated by age such that serum lithium levels were not associated with brain levels in patients 50 years of age or older. Furthermore, higher brain lithium levels were associated with frontal lobe dysfunction. Thus, neurochemical abnormalities and the disruption in these white matter tracts and the regions of the brain they connect are thought to be a contributor to the mood dysregulation that occurs in bipolar disorder [27].

3.6 Functional Neuroimaging: PET, SPECT, and fMRI

In addition to structural neuroimaging analyses, some studies in BD research have utilized functional neuroimaging techniques such as positron emission topography (PET), single photon emission topography (SPECT), and functional MRI (fMRI).

However, compared to the literature examining gray and white matter changes, functional studies in BD, especially in OABD, are quite sparse. In a comprehensive review of neuroimaging findings in bipolar disorder, Phillips and Swartz [32] suggest that BD is characterized by state-specific alterations in circuits underlying emotion processing and emotion regulation (amygdala, insula, orbitofrontal cortex, dorsolateral prefrontal cortex). Additionally, they report that in resting-state fMRI studies, there is a pattern of altered intrinsic connectivity in fronto-temporal-striatal circuits. Their review also highlights a critical gap in the literature by the fact that to date, there are no published functional imaging studies in OABD.

3.7 Bipolar Disorder as a Neuroprogressive Disorder

Stemming from these abnormal imaging findings is the concept of neuroprogression that has been proposed for bipolar disorder and OABD. Neuroprogression is a relatively new term that describes the detrimental changes (defined as increase in proinflammatory cytokines, oxidative stress products, decrease in anti-inflammatory cytokines, decrease in treatment response, and decrease in cognitive and functioning performance) that occur along the natural history of bipolar disorder as it progresses [33]. Though more studies are needed, imaging has increased our understanding of the structural and connective changes in the brain that have been observed in OABD [34]. One study by Gildengers and coworkers, for example, studied fifty-four adults with BD [mean age = 64.4 years] for the purpose of investigating whether BD is a neuroprogressive disorder. Using MR imaging, the study found that lower total gray matter volume was related to longer duration of bipolar illness, even when controlling for age [35]. The findings of this study provide evidence for the theory of neuroprogression in older adults with BD.

The neuroprogression hypothesis postulates that neurochemical dysregulation, neuroinflammation, oxidative stress, and mitochondrial dysfunction contribute to changes in brain structure and function (Fig. 3.2). For example, excessive dopamine and glutamate neurotransmission may lead to a decrease in brain derived neurotrophic factor (BDNF) and secondary structural changes in gray and white matter [13]. Neuroprogression may also explain the clinical observation of decreased treatment response and increased risk of future recurring episodes for individuals with severe bipolar disorder. Researchers also posit that with neuroprogression, the different processes that cause these structural and functional changes may represent stages with the progression of BD.

Some neuroimaging studies have demonstrated neuroprotective effects of various treatments for bipolar disorder including lithium, omega 3 fatty acids, statins, and anti-inflammatory medications. Giakoumatos et al. studied patient populations with BD that were lithium-free versus lithium-treated. Findings suggest that patients without lithium treatment had substantially smaller hippocampal subfield volumes than patients treated with Lithium. Based on this evidence, the authors postulated

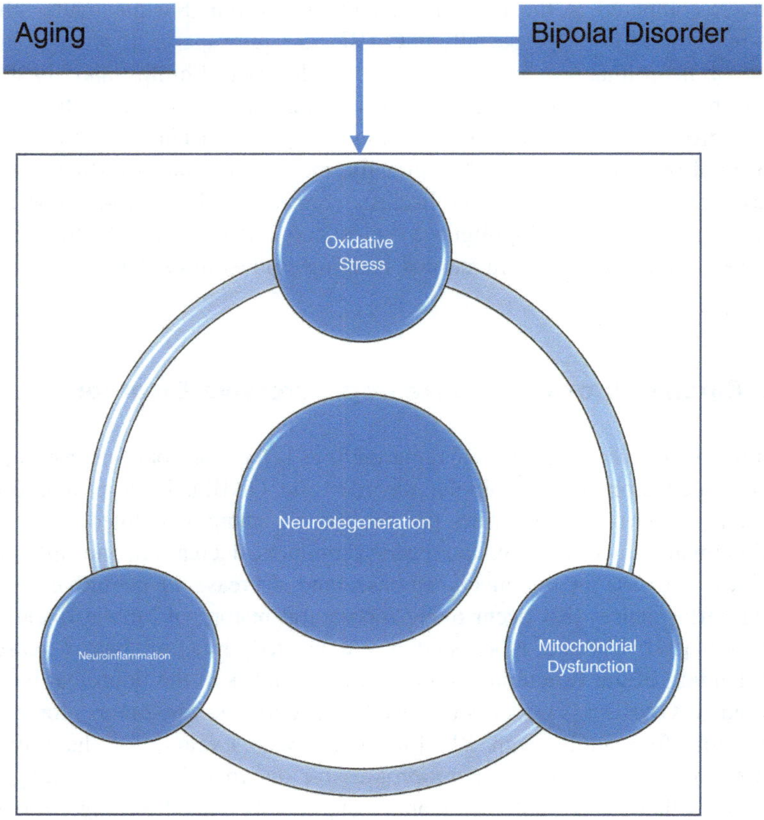

Fig. 3.2 Schematic demonstrating how aging and bipolar disorder contribute to linked processes underlying neurodegeneration: oxidative stress, mitochondrial dysfunction, and neuroinflammation

that lithium may counteract the gray matter changes and cortical thickness changes found in bipolar disorder [36, 37].

3.7.1 Biomarkers of Oxidative Stress and Mitochondrial Dysfunction

Oxidative stress and mitochondrial dysfunction have been identified as key components in the mechanisms underlying neuroprogression in BD [38]. Oxidative stress arises from the imbalance in generating reactive oxygen species (ROS) and the body's ability to remove or repair ROS. It is believed that oxidative stress is associated with systemic changes involved in the aging process [39]. Oxidative stress has been implicated in the pathophysiology of BD and has been suggested as a possible biomarker involved in different stages of the illness. In one of the first meta-analyses of oxidative stress and bipolar disorder, Andreazza et al. [40] found that specific biomarkers of oxidative stress, thiobarbituric acid reactive substance (TBARS, a marker of lipid peroxidation), and nitric oxide (NO) were significantly elevated in patients with bipolar disorder. More specifically, elevations in TBARS appear to be related to the manic state. Tsai and Huang [41] showed that elevated TBARS levels in manic patients were reduced after treatment. Additionally, NO has been shown to correlate with the number of manic episodes in euthymic BD patients [42]. Furthermore, late-stage bipolar disorder (at least 10 years of illness) has been associated with an increased activity of the antioxidant enzymes glutathione reductase and glutathione S-transferase [43]. The evidence of oxidative stress in BD appears to persist into later life. These findings have been replicated in a number of studies, and recent meta-analysis identified lipid peroxidation, DNA/RNA damage, and NO as significantly increased in BD patients compared to controls [44].

Another pathophysiological process that could contribute to neuroprogression in bipolar disorder and the neuroimaging findings previously described is mitochondrial dysfunction. Mitochondrial dysfunction is a major source of oxidative stress and has been implicated in the pathophysiology of bipolar disorder. Specifically, higher levels of mitochondrial DNA oxidative damage have been demonstrated in BD [45]. Furthermore, BD patients exhibit abnormalities in peripheral mitochondrial morphology and distribution. Specifically, BD patients were found to have smaller mitochondria that were more likely located in the perinuclear region as opposed to distal processes [46]. Researchers have used innovative neuroimaging techniques to probe in vivo neuronal mitochondrial function in BD. Using magnetic resonance spectroscopy (MRS), studies have shown alterations in metabolites associated with neuronal energetics such as pH changes, reductions in high-energy phosphates, and n-acetyl aspartate (a marker of mitochondrial function) [47–50].

The notion that oxidative damage is a key component in the pathophysiology of BD has led to a number of interesting treatment trials targeting oxidative damage and mitochondrial dysfunction. Since cysteine is an important precursor to glutathione, an antioxidant, it was thought that n-acetylcysteine (NAC) could be beneficial in the treatment of bipolar depression. In a series of studies, Berk et al. [51, 52] demonstrated that NAC was associated with a decrease in depressive symptoms in bipolar patients. Of relevance to older patients with BD, it was shown that medical comorbidity moderates the benefits of NAC in bipolar depression [53]. In OABD, 4 weeks of treatment with CoEnzyme Q10, an effective antioxidant known to enhance mitochondrial function, improved depression severity scores [48, 54].

In addition to novel treatments for BD, the notion of oxidative stress has implications for the effects of existing treatments for BD. For example, in tissue culture, lithium has been shown to increase mitochondrial oxidative phosphorylation activity, suggesting a neuroprotective effect [55]. Lithium also increases mitochondrial complex I activity in the context of bipolar depression [56]. The role of oxidative stress has not been limited to lithium. In a study of the treatment response in OABD, Gildengers et al. [57] found that lamotrigine was most effective in patients with high cardiometabolic risk, a risk factor associated with damage from oxidative stress.

3.8 Clinical Implications Present and Future

The clinical implications from recent studies of the neurobiology of bipolar disorder in late-life suggest novel targets for intervention, as well as alternative mechanisms of actions for existing treatments as described above. Future implications of these studies indicate an opportunity to personalize BD treatments according to specific clinical profiles. For example, BD patients with significant medical comorbidities may benefit from adjunctive treatments that target oxidative stress, such as NAC. Additionally, neuroimaging techniques like MRS could be used to track treatment response to antioxidants measuring metabolites that reflect mitochondrial function. As highlighted by the work of Forester et al. [31], MRS could also be used to determine brain levels of lithium, which may be more sensitive in detecting lithium toxicity than current practice focusing on serum lithium levels. This notion is of particular relevance for the clinical vignette at the beginning of the chapter since serum lithium levels may not reliably reflect brain levels in older patients.

Furthermore, an expanded knowledge base of neural networks that are characterized by neuroimaging methods and involved in BD could guide non-invasive neuromodulatory treatments, such as transcranial magnetic stimulation or transcranial current stimulation, that are designed to engage or enhance specific brain circuits.

3.9 Summary and Conclusion

The advent of neuroimaging and its increasing sophistication has helped to bring about a better understanding of the structural and functional changes that occur in bipolar disorder. Many of the studies reviewed highlighted the potential importance of neuroimaging for bipolar disorder particularly as a conduit for discovering clinically relevant biomarkers of disease state and predictors of treatment response. However, the current clinical role for neuroimaging remains yet to be clearly defined. Neuroimaging research to date in OABD is limited in that there are not enough bipolar studies involving imaging, and among those that are available, there are very few longitudinal studies. While bipolar disorder is, in general, challenging to diagnose, the reality of high medical comorbidity and cognitive impairment in OABD may explain the dearth of longitudinal studies. In addition, longitudinal structural MRI studies, an examination of longitudinal functional MRI, and DTI studies would help to further elucidate our understanding of the neuroprogression hypothesis of BD. Although bipolar disorder is associated with significant morbidity and mortality, further research utilizing neuroimaging modalities may shed light on neurobiological mechanisms to target for therapeutic interventions designed to reduce the adverse impact of this psychiatric illness that persists into later life with often devastating consequences.

Clinical Pearls

- Neuroimaging studies in OABD show gray matter volume reductions, increases in white matter hyperintensities, and neurochemical alterations.
- Neuroprogression may serve as model to understand longitudinal changes in brain function associated with pathophysiology of OABD.
- Better characterization of pathophysiological processes such as oxidative stress and mitochondrial dysfunction could lead to more biologically informed interventions for late-life bipolar disorder.

References

1. Schmitt A, Malchow B, Hasan A, Falkai P. The impact of environmental factors in severe psychiatric disorders. Front Neurosci. 2014;8:19.
2. Judd LL, Akiskal HS. The prevalence and disability of bipolar spectrum disorders in the US population: re-analysis of the ECA database taking into account subthreshold cases. J Affect Disord. 2003;73(1):123–31.
3. Ayuso-Mateos JL. Global burden of bipolar disorder in the year 2000. Geneva: World Health Organization; 2002.
4. Anderson IM, Haddad PM, Scott J. Bipolar disorder. BMJ. 2012;345:e8508.
5. Holma KM, Haukka J, Suominen K, Valtonen HM, Mantere O, Melartin TK, Sokero TP, Oquendo MA, Isometsä ET. Differences in incidence of suicide attempts between bipolar I and II disorders and major depressive disorder. Bipolar Disord. 2014;16(6):652–61.
6. Brady RO, Keshavan M. Emergent treatments based on the pathophysiology of bipolar disorder: a selective review. Asian J Psychiatry. 2015;18:15–21.
7. Rocha-Rego V, Jogia J, Marquand A, Mourao-Miranda J, Simmons A, Frangou S. Examination of the predictive value of structural magnetic resonance scans in bipolar disorder: a pattern classification approach. Psychol Med. 2014;44(03):519–32.
8. Phillips ML, Kupfer DJ. Bipolar disorder diagnosis: challenges and future directions. The Lancet. 2013;381(9878):1663–71.
9. Keener MT, Phillips ML. Neuroimaging in bipolar disorder: a critical review of current findings. Curr Psychiatry Rep. 2007;9(6):512–20.
10. Rej S, Butters MA, Aizenstein HJ, Begley A, Tsay J, Reynolds CF 3rd, Mulsant BH, Gildengers A. Neuroimaging and neurocognitive abnormalities associated with bipolar disorder in old age. Int J Geriatr Psychiatry. 2014;29(4):421–7.
11. Aziz R, Lorberg B, Tampi RR. Treatments for late-life bipolar disorder. Am J Geriatr Pharmacother. 2006;4(4):347–64.
12. Sajatovic M, Forester BP, Gildengers A, Mulsant BH. Aging changes and medical complexity in late-life bipolar disorder: emerging research findings that may help advance care. Neuropsychiatry. 2013;3(6):621–33.
13. Sajatovic M, Strejilevich SA, Gildengers AG, Dols A, Al Jurdi RK, Forester BP, Kessing LV, Beyer J, Manes F, Rej S, Rosa AR, Schouws SN, Tsai SY, Young RC, Shulman KI. A report on older-age bipolar disorder from the International Society for Bipolar Disorders Task Force. Bipolar Disord. 2015;17(7):689–704.

14. Murray AD, Staff RT, Shenkin SD, Deary IJ, Starr JM, Whalley LJ. Brain white matter hyperintensities: relative importance of vascular risk factors in nondemented elderly people. Radiology. 2005;237(1):251–7.
15. Maniega SM, Valdes Hernandez MC, Clayden JD, Royle NA, Murray C, Morris Z, Aribisala BS, Gow AJ, Starr JM, Bastin ME, Deary IJ, Wardlaw JM. White matter hyperintensities and normal-appearing white matter integrity in the aging brain. Neurobiol Aging. 2015;36(2):909–18.
16. Tamashiro JH, Zung S, Zanetti MV, deCastro CC, Vallada H, Busatto GF, deToledoFerrazAlves TC. Increased rates of white matter hyperintensities in late-onset bipolar disorder. Bipolar Disord. 2008;10(7):765–75.
17. Delaloye C, Moy G, de Bilbao F, Weber K, Baudois S, Haller S, Xekardaki A, Canuto A, Giardini U, Lovblad KO, Gold G, Giannakopoulos P. Longitudinal analysis of cognitive performances and structural brain changes in late-life bipolar disorder. Int J Geriatr Psychiatry. 2011;26(12):1309–18.
18. Beyer JL, Kuchibhatla M, Payne M, Moo-Young M, Cassidy F, MacFall J, Krishnan KR. Caudate volume measurement in older adults with bipolar disorder. Int J Geriatr Psychiatry. 2004;19(2):109–14.
19. Beyer JL, Kuchibhatla M, Payne ME, Moo-Young M, Cassidy F, Macfall J, Krishnan KR. Hippocampal volume measurement in older adults with bipolar disorder. Am J Geriatr Psychiatry. 2004;12(6):613–20.
20. Huang SH, Tsai SY, Hsu JL, Huang YL. Volumetric reduction in various cortical regions of elderly patients with early-onset and late-onset mania. Int Psychogeriatr. 2011;23(1):149–54.
21. Dening T, Thomas A. Oxford textbook of old age psychiatry. Oxford: Oxford University Press; 2013.
22. Jones LD, Payne ME, Messer DF, Beyer JL, MacFall JR, Krishnan KRR, Taylor WD. Temporal lobe volume in bipolar disorder: relationship with diagnosis and antipsychotic medication use. J Affect Disord. 2009;114(1):50–7.
23. Altshuler LL, Bartzokis G, Grieder T, Curran J, Jimenez T, Leight K, Wilkins J, Gerner R, Mintz J. An MRI study of temporal lobe structures in men with bipolar disorder or schizophrenia. Biol Psychiatry. 2000;48(2):147–62.
24. Arnone D, Cavanagh J, Gerber D, Lawrie S, Ebmeier K, McIntosh A. Magnetic resonance imaging studies in bipolar disorder and schizophrenia: meta-analysis. Br J Psychiatry. 2009;195(3):194–201.
25. Wijeratne C, Sachdev S, Wen W, Piguet O, Lipnicki DM, Malhi GS, Mitchell PB, Sachdev PS. Hippocampal and amygdala volumes in an older bipolar disorder sample. Int Psychogeriatr. 2013;25(01):54–60.
26. Sarnicola A, Kempton M, Germana C, Haldane M, Hadjulis M, Christodoulou T, Koukopoulos A, Girardi P, Tatarelli R, Frangou S. No differential effect of age on brain matter volume and cognition in bipolar patients and healthy individuals. Bipolar Disord. 2009;11(3):316–22.
27. Karababa IF, Bayazıt H, Kılıçaslan N, Celik M, Cece H, Karakas E, Selek S. Microstructural changes of anterior corona radiata in bipolar depression. Psychiatry Investig. 2015;12(3):367–71.
28. Haller S, Xekardaki A, Delaloye C, Canuto A, Lovblad KO, Gold G, Giannakopoulos P. Combined analysis of grey matter voxel-based morphometry and white matter tract-based spatial statistics in late-life bipolar disorder. J Psychiatry Neurosci. 2011;36(1):100140.
29. Toteja N, Guvenek-Cokol P, Ikuta T, Kafantaris V, Peters BD, Burdick KE, John M, Malhotra AK, Szeszko PR. Age-associated alterations in corpus callosum white matter integrity in bipolar disorder assessed using probabilistic tractography. Bipolar Disord. 2015;17(4):381–91.
30. Sexton CE, Allan CL, Mackay CE, Ebmeier KP. White matter integrity within the corpus callosum differentiates late-life bipolar and unipolar depression. Bipolar Disord. 2012;14(7):790-1.

31. Forester BP, Streeter CC, Berlow YA, Tian H, Wardrop M, Finn CT, Harper D, Renshaw PF, Moore CM. Brain lithium levels and effects on cognition and mood in geriatric bipolar disorder: a lithium-7 magnetic resonance spectroscopy study. Am J Geriatr Psychiatry. 2009;17(1):13–23.
32. Phillips ML, Swartz HA. A critical appraisal of neuroimaging studies of bipolar disorder: toward a new conceptualization of underlying neural circuitry and a road map for future research. Am J Psychiatry. 2014;171(8):829–43.
33. Gama CS, Kunz M, Magalhaes PV, Kapczinski F. Staging and neuroprogression in bipolar disorder: a systematic review of the literature. Rev Brasil Psiquiatr. 2013;35(1):70–4.
34. Schneider MR, DelBello MP, McNamara RK, Strakowski SM, Adler CM. Neuroprogression in bipolar disorder. Bipolar Disord. 2012;14(4):356–74.
35. Gildengers AG, Chung KH, Huang SH, Begley A, Aizenstein HJ, Tsai SY. Neuroprogressive effects of lifetime illness duration in older adults with bipolar disorder. Bipolar Disord. 2014;16(6):617–23.
36. Giakoumatos C, Nanda P, Mathew I, Tandon N, Shah J, Bishop J, Clementz B, Pearlson G, Sweeney J, Tamminga C. Effects of lithium on cortical thickness and hippocampal subfield volumes in psychotic bipolar disorder. J Psychiatr Res. 2015;61:180–7.
37. Lan MJ, Chhetry BT, Oquendo MA, Sublette ME, Sullivan G, Mann JJ, Parsey RV. Cortical thickness differences between bipolar depression and major depressive disorder. Bipolar Disord. 2014;16(4):378–88.
38. Berk M, Kapczinski F, Andreazza AC, Dean OM, Giorlando F, Maes M, Yücel M, Gama CS, Dodd S, Dean B, Magalhães PVS, Amminger P, McGorry P, Malhi GS. Pathways underlying neuroprogression in bipolar disorder: focus on inflammation, oxidative stress and neurotrophic factors. Neurosci Biobehav Rev. 2011;35(3):804–17.
39. Sohal RS, Weindruch R. Oxidative stress, caloric restriction, and aging. Science. 1996;273(5271):59–63.
40. Andreazza AC, Kauer-Sant'anna M, Frey BN, Bond DJ, Kapczinski F, Young LT, Yatham LN. Oxidative stress markers in bipolar disorder: a meta-analysis. J Affect Disord. 2008;111(2–3):135–44.
41. Tsai M-C, Huang T-L. Thiobarbituric acid reactive substances (TBARS) is a state biomarker of oxidative stress in bipolar patients in a manic phase. J Affect Disord. 2015;173:22–6.
42. Savas HA, Gergerlioglu HS, Armutcu F, Herken H, Yilmaz HR, Kocoglu E, Selek S, Tutkun H, Zoroglu SS, Akyol O. Elevated serum nitric oxide and superoxide dismutase in euthymic bipolar patients: impact of past episodes. World J Biol Psychiatry. 2006;7(1):51–5.
43. Andreazza AC, Kapczinski F, Kauer-Sant'Anna M, Walz JC, Bond DJ, Goncalves CA, Young LT, Yatham LN. 3-Nitrotyrosine and glutathione antioxidant system in patients in the early and late stages of bipolar disorder. J Psychiatry Neurosci. 2009;34(4):263–71.
44. Brown NC, Andreazza AC, Young LT. An updated meta-analysis of oxidative stress markers in bipolar disorder. Psychiatry Res. 2014;218(1–2):61–8.
45. Chang CC, Jou SH, Lin TT, Liu CS. Mitochondrial DNA variation and increased oxidative damage in euthymic patients with bipolar disorder. Psychiatry Clin Neurosci. 2014;68(7):551–7.
46. Cataldo AM, McPhie DL, Lange NT, Punzell S, Elmiligy S, Ye NZ, Froimowitz MP, Hassinger LC, Menesale EB, Sargent LW, Logan DJ, Carpenter AE, Cohen BM. Abnormalities in mitochondrial structure in cells from patients with bipolar disorder. Am J Pathol. 2010;177(2):575–85.
47. Kato T, Takahashi S, Shioiri T, Murashita J, Hamakawa H, Inubushi T. Reduction of brain phosphocreatine in bipolar II disorder detected by phosphorus-31 magnetic resonance spectroscopy. J Affect Disord. 1994;31(2):125–33.
48. Forester BP, Zuo CS, Ravichandran C, Harper DG, Du F, Kim S, Cohen BM, Renshaw PF. Coenzyme Q10 effects on creatine kinase activity and mood in geriatric bipolar depression. J Geriatr Psychiatry Neurol. 2012;25(1):43–50.

49. Kato T, Murashita J, Kamiya A, Shioiri T, Kato N, Inubushi T. Decreased brain intracellular pH measured by 31P-MRS in bipolar disorder: a confirmation in drug-free patients and correlation with white matter hyperintensity. Eur Arch Psychiatry Clin Neurosci. 1998;248(6):301–6.
50. Frye MA, Thomas MA, Yue K, Binesh N, Davanzo P, Ventura J, O'Neill J, Guze B, Curran JG, Mintz J. Reduced concentrations of N-acetylaspartate (NAA) and the NAA-creatine ratio in the basal ganglia in bipolar disorder: a study using 3-Tesla proton magnetic resonance spectroscopy. Psychiatry Res. 2007;154(3):259–65.
51. Berk M, Copolov DL, Dean O, Lu K, Jeavons S, Schapkaitz I, Anderson-Hunt M, Bush AI. N-acetyl cysteine for depressive symptoms in bipolar disorder—a double-blind randomized placebo-controlled trial. Biol Psychiatry. 2008;64(6):468–75.
52. Berk M, Dean O, Cotton SM, Gama CS, Kapczinski F, Fernandes BS, Kohlmann K, Jeavons S, Hewitt K, Allwang C, Cobb H, Bush AI, Schapkaitz I, Dodd S, Malhi GS. The efficacy of N-acetylcysteine as an adjunctive treatment in bipolar depression: an open label trial. J Affect Disord. 2011;135(1–3):389–94.
53. Magalhaes PV, Dean OM, Bush AI, Copolov DL, Weisinger D, Malhi GS, Kohlmann K, Jeavons S, Schapkaitz I, Anderson-Hunt M, Berk M. Systemic illness moderates the impact of N-acetyl cysteine in bipolar disorder. Prog Neuropsychopharmacol Biol Psychiatry. 2012;37 (1):132–5.
54. Forester BP, Harper DG, Georgakas J, Ravichandran C, Madurai N, Cohen BM. Antidepressant effects of open label treatment with coenzyme Q10 in geriatric bipolar depression. J Clin Psychopharmacol. 2015;35(3):338–40.
55. Maurer IC, Schippel P, Volz HP. Lithium-induced enhancement of mitochondrial oxidative phosphorylation in human brain tissue. Bipolar Disord. 2009;11(5):515–22.
56. de Sousa RT, Streck EL, Zanetti MV, Ferreira GK, Diniz BS, Brunoni AR, Busatto GF, Gattaz WF, Machado-Vieira R. Lithium increases leukocyte mitochondrial complex I activity in bipolar disorder during depressive episodes. Psychopharmacology. 2015;232(1):245–50.
57. Gildengers A, Tatsuoka C, Bialko C, Cassidy KA, Al Jurdi RK, Gyulai L, Mulsant BH, Young RC, Sajatovic M. Correlates of treatment response in depressed older adults with bipolar disorder. J Geriatr Psychiatry Neurol. 2012;25(1):37–42.

Clinical Management of Older Age Bipolar Disorder

4

Annemiek Dols, Megan Y.S. Chan and Kenneth Shulman

4.1 Introduction

The management of older adults with bipolar disorder (OABD) has several unique aspects. During this phase of life, there may be loss of physical health and cognitive performance. The usual routines of work, education and caring for children may also undergo change. Lastly, such older people may also experience the loss of their loved ones. Life events triggering mood episodes may be just as frequent as younger adults [1], while the increase in somatic illnesses and use of multiple medications are known to disrupt mood. In addition, impaired cognitive performance may limit the ability to stabilize mood swings and function effectively with respect to independent activities of daily living (IADL).

A. Dols (✉)
Department of Old Age Psychiatry, VU Medical Center, GGZinGeest,
Amstelveenseweg 589, 1081JC Amsterdam, The Netherlands
e-mail: a.dols@ggzingeest.nl

M.Y.S. Chan
Department of Psychological Medicine, Tan Tock Seng Hospital,
11 Jalan Tan Tock Seng, Singapore 308433, Singapore
e-mail: yuen_sze_chan@ttsh.com.sg

K. Shulman
Department of Psychiatry, Sunnybrook Health Sciences Centre,
2075 Bayview Avenue, Toronto, ON M4N3M5, Canada
e-mail: ken.shulman@sunnybrook.ca

S.W. Lehmann and B.P. Forester (eds.), *Bipolar Disorder in Older Age Patients*,
DOI 10.1007/978-3-319-48912-4_4

4.2 Organizing Care

Bipolar disorder is characterized by a heterogeneous course with distinct mood phases (euthymic, (hypo) mania, and depression) and wide interindividual variation of frequency, severity, and duration of episodes. Level of functioning is influenced by comorbid psychiatric and somatic illnesses, personality traits, and psychosocial factors. Treatment may vary in intensity and focus depending on the phase of illness (acute, symptomatic remission, and relapse prevention). In the acute phase of a mood episode, the main goal will be to achieve symptomatic remission and to prevent or limit the psychiatric, medical, psychological, relational, financial, and social complications. Once symptomatic remission is achieved, the focus should shift to preventing relapses, stimulation of self-management, aiding functional recovery, as well as reintegration of social roles. During the maintenance phase, pharmacological treatment can be optimized with a reduction of subclinical symptoms, treatment of comorbid illness and restoration of psychosocial function.

Limited evidence suggests that a multidisciplinary approach is advantageous, resulting in reduction of symptoms, fewer relapses, better overall functioning, and higher quality of life [2–5].

Caring for OABD requires attention to somatic comorbidities, cognitive decline, polypharmacy, and specific phase of dealing with multiple losses including loved ones, occupational, and social status. The worldwide shortage of geriatric psychiatrists will grow, while the number of older patients with mental disorders increases; many (if not most) older adults with bipolar disorder will be treated by general psychiatrists and family physicians. The number of clinics specialized in caring for the older patients with bipolar disorder are very limited.

A study of 78 older adults with bipolar disorder employing the Camberwell Assessment of Need in the Elderly (CANE) [6] assessed met and unmet needs, both from a patient and a staff perspective. They reported a mean of 4.3 needs from a patient perspective compared to 4.4 reported by staff, of which 0.8 were unmet according to patients and 0.5 according to staff [7]. Patients frequently rated social interactions and daytime activities as unmet needs. More current mood symptoms were associated with a higher total number of needs. Less social participation was associated with a higher total number of needs and greater unmet needs. The CANE can provide valuable information about the needs of the patients, and can include a caregiver and staff perspective.

Furthermore, organizing care for these vulnerable OABD requires close collaboration with their family physician, pharmacist, and other medical specialists in order to provide comprehensive and integrated care.

4.3 Self-management, Psychoeducation, and Psychotherapy

Self-management is the cornerstone of treating bipolar disorder. In OABD, self-management should be emphasized by encouraging patients to manage their illness and care. Self-management is the individual strength to cope with symptoms, treatment, physical, psychosocial consequences, and lifestyle changes that are inherent to living with a chronic illness [8]. Empowerment and successful aging are popular terms that are meant to encourage patients to deal with their illness and feel independent of their caregivers and health professionals, and not to highlight their lack of competence while ill.

Professionals need to aid patients in their self-management by providing them with knowledge about their illness (psychoeducation), insight into their illness (self-reflection), and self-interventions.

Psychoeducation can and should be provided with every consultation of individuals with bipolar disorder, even patients who were diagnosed with bipolar disorder since early adulthood. Keeping a life chart can provide patients with valuable knowledge about their own disease. A crisis management plan, including prodromal symptoms and actions to be taken, is a mandatory part of the treatment of bipolar disorder. Self-management can be supported, as in younger adults with bipolar disorder, by stimulating contra-behavior (behavior opposite of the mood episode), organizing social support, encouraging active coping, and lifestyle advice on dealing with psychosocial stressors.

Few psychosocial interventions including specific psychotherapies for OABD have been studied systematically. Current practice is informed primarily by extrapolation from mixed-age studies or based on "clinical experience." The Helping Older People Experience Success (HOPES) was compared in a two-year randomized trial with treatment as usual (TAU) and found to improve social skills, community functioning, self-efficacy, leisure, and recreation [9]. Another focus of psychosocial intervention is medication adherence. A small study aimed at improving medication adherence skills, showed feasibility, acceptability, and improvement in depression and some indices of health-related quality of life [10]. Other psychosocial interventions hold promise for improving health and functioning in older adults with serious mental illnesses [11]. A specific psychoeducation course of approximately 12 sessions for OABD and their caregivers are valued [12–14], even more when sessions are shortened and planned during daytime.

4.4 Drug Interactions and Tolerance

As a result of aging, decreases in drug absorption, body distribution, metabolism, and excretion complicated by polypharmacy will impact the pharmacokinetics and pharmacodynamics of drugs affecting the central nervous system. Medical comorbidity may also increase risk of drug-drug interactions due to polypharmacy. These changes associated with aging may affect the rate of absorption, metabolism, or excretion of a drug and hence also affect drug serum levels and influence rates of toxicity or drops to subtherapeutic levels. Clinicians must be hypervigilant to possible drug interactions as well as pharmacokinetic and dynamic alterations when prescribing new drugs or when adjusting dosage in OABD.

Side effects increase in direct proportion to the number of prescribed medications [15]. Side effects are among the most important reasons that patients stop taking their medications. Discussing possible side effects will encourage patients to report them. Most side effects are temporary, or diminish after dose reductions. Divided dosing throughout the day instead of prescribing medications once a day has not been shown to reduce side effects [16]. The prevalence and treatment options for the most common side effects of lithium, valproate, carbamazepine, and lamotrigine are described below [17].

4.5 Interactions of Drugs Frequently Used in Bipolar Disorder

4.5.1 Lithium

Lithium serum levels will be influenced by simultaneous use of other agents that interfere with renal clearance (Table 4.1). In clinical practice, it is advisable to anticipate the increasing or decreasing effects of interacting medications by adjusting the lithium dose by 30–50 % based on pharmacokinetic studies of lithium in older adults [18]. The risk for serotonin syndrome is increased when prescribing a SSRI or MAO inhibitor with lithium.

4.5.2 Valproate

Valproate inhibits liver enzymes, e.g., CYP2C9, and increases the availability of several antipsychotics, benzodiazepines, moclobemide, and antidepressants. It reduces the metabolism of lamotrigine. The most probable explanation for this effect is hepatic competition between valproate and lamotrigine for glucuronidation [19].

4.5.3 Carbamazepine

Interactions are caused by induction of the liver enzymes CYP2C9 and CYP3A4. Carbamazepine increases the metabolism of haloperidol and valproate, and the neurotoxicity of lithium [20].

Table 4.1 Effect of concomitant medication on serum levels of mood stabilizers

Increase	No effect	Decrease
Lithium		
Loop diuretics	Aspirin	Mannitol
Thiazide diuretics	Paracetamol	Aminophylline
Calcium blockers	Nefazodone	Theophylline
ACE inhibitors	Mirtazepine	
AT II receptor blockers	Valproate	
COX2 inhibitors	Lamotrigine	
Trimethoprim	Amisulpride	
Metronidazole	Ziprasidone	
Spectinomycin	Risperidone	
Levofloxacin	Quetiapine	
Alprazolam	Carbamazepine	
NSAIDs	Acetazolamide	
Topiramate		
Valproate		
Stiripentol	Orlistat	Carbamazepine
Bupropion	Cholestyramine	Phenytoin
	Colesevelam	Rifampicin
		Carbapenems
		Ritonavir
		Chemotherapeutics (temporary)
Carbamazepine		
Cimetidine (temporary)	Valproate (variable effect)	Efavirenz
Ciprofloxacin	Tramadol	Nevirapine
Claritromycin	Hypericum	Rifampicin
Danazol		Chemotherapeutics (temporary)
Diltiazem		Valproate (variable effect)
Erythromycin		
Fluconazole		
Fluoxetine		
Fluvoxamine		
Isoniazid		
HIV protease inhibitor		
Terbinafine		
Verapamil		
Stiripentol		
Ketoconazole		
Valproate (variable effect)		
Trazodone		

(continued)

Table 4.1 (continued)

Increase	No effect	Decrease
Lamotrigine		
Valproate	Retigabine	Carbamazepine
	Orlistat	Phenobarbital
	Bupropion	Phenytoin
	Olanzapine	Oxcarbazepine
	Aripiprazole	Rifampicin
	Risperidone	Lopinavir
	Lithium	Primidone

Acknowledgments to J.L.W. Pot, MS, pharmacologist, and P. Bet, PhD, pharmacologist, for their help in formulating this table

4.5.4 Lamotrigine

Valproate reduces the metabolism of lamotrigine and requires a 50 % dose reduction even in the start-up phase. Carbamazepine increases the metabolism of lamotrigine. Therefore, doubling the dose of lamotrigine is required when coprescribed with carbamazepine.

4.5.5 Antipsychotics

All antipsychotics can prolong the QTc interval.

4.6 Specific Pharmacotherapies and Electroconvulsive Therapy

4.6.1 General Recommendations

Research on pharmacotherapy in OABD is limited as older adults are often excluded from randomized controlled registration trials (RCTs) due to the increasing risk of medical complications with advancing age. In fact, the mean age of most RCTs investigating the efficacy and safety of atypical antipsychotic medications for the treatment of acute mania, for example, is approximately 40 years of age. Nevertheless, post hoc analyses of older adult cohorts from such trials support the use of similar first line treatments recommended for younger adults with bipolar disorder. However, due to changes in pharmacokinetic and pharmacodynamic properties, older adults are more vulnerable to side effects and drug interactions which increase with the number of medications prescribed [15]. Although a specific medication may have been tolerated for many years, new side effects may develop with aging or the onset of medical comorbidities. Clinical factors that may influence dose adjustment include age, medical comorbidity, and drug interactions. Polypharmacy is common in older adults with bipolar disorder. For example, 31.7 % of OABD are prescribed six or more medications [21]. Over the Counter (OTC) drugs and medications prescribed by other physicians may adversely interact with those medications used to treat symptoms of bipolar disorder (e.g., interaction between nonsteroidal anti-inflammatory medications (NSAIDs) and lithium) Interestingly, a prescription data study done with the Systematic Treatment Enhancement Program for Bipolar Disorder (STEP-BD) data revealed that recovery can be achieved in the elderly, though more than one medication is often required regardless of age [22]. Here, we describe the limited evidence on pharmacotherapy for acute mania, bipolar depression, and maintenance therapy in OABD.

We will describe and discuss the available research on pharmacotherapy in older patients with bipolar disorder and conclude with specific evidence-based recommendations for each mood phase.

4.6.2 Lithium

Lithium is described in more detail in Chap. 7, and we will provide only an overview of lithium therapy in older adults in this section. Clinicians have been widely prescribing lithium in OABD for the management of acute mania but with much less frequency in recent years [23]. Lithium has been demonstrated to be effective in placebo-controlled studies of mixed-age patients [24]. There are eight studies of lithium in manic patients [25–32]. No randomized placebo-controlled studies have been published to date. Nonetheless, available evidence supports the use and efficacy of lithium in the treatment of mania in OABD. In terms of efficacy of lithium compared to other classes of medications, lithium has been shown to be equally efficacious. Although there are several case studies suggesting that elderly patients respond to lower lithium levels, most studies have required treatment at conventional lithium levels to achieve optimal results [28].

In twelve small retrospective case series and open-label studies of the effectiveness of lithium in OABD (Table 4.2), methodological differences between the studies preclude comparisons. The study samples were relatively small (2–80 patients). Four studies included patients only treated with lithium as maintenance therapy [33–36]. Two prospective, open-label studies concluded that lithium is more effective than placebo [35] and valproate [36]. There are eight studies of lithium in manic patients [25–32]. No randomized placebo-controlled studies have been published to date. All studies concluded that lithium is effective in reducing manic symptoms. Five studies concluded that lithium is also effective in treating bipolar depression [25, 27, 29, 30, 32]. From the limited available evidence, we conclude that the effectiveness of lithium in OABD is not different than in younger adults.

4.6.2.1 Clinical Recommendations for Lithium Therapy

Therapeutic serum levels can be achieved with a 25–50 % lower dose compared to younger adults [35]. Lithium serum levels of 0.4–0.6 mmol/l can be effective, although levels of 0.8 mmol/l or higher may be needed for therapeutic efficacy. Lithium may also be effective at lower serum levels for certain individuals. Balancing toxicity and clinical efficacy is a great challenge when using lithium for the treatment of older adults with bipolar disorder.

Table 4.2 Studies of lithium in OABD

	N	Age (range)	Design	Dose-concentration	Duration (weeks)	Results (outcome measure)
Van der Velde [26]	12	67 (60–74)	R	Unknown	2–156	33 % recovery of mania (global rating scale)
Himmelhoch et al. [27]	81	63.3 (55–88)	R	Unknown	3–8	69 % response of depressive or manic symptoms (scale for clinical efficacy)
Abou-Saleh and Coppen [25]	7	57.1	P	Unknown	52	43 % remission of mania and depression (affective morbidity index)
Murray et al. [33]	25	(60–78)	P	Unknown	104	Compared to younger patients clinical effect on maintenance treatment was independent of age
Schaffer et al. [28]	14	69 (65–77)	P	900 mg–0.58 mEq/ml	>2	10 patients (71 %) had clinical improvement of manic symptoms
Stone [34]	48	70.3 (65–82)	R	Unknown	26	40 % had no relapse after 6 months, no difference in recovery of mania between lithium users ($n = 48$) and non-lithium users ($n = 44$)
Sharma et al. [29]	4	68.5 (66–71)	P	300–600 mg/day	40–78	Response in all rapid-cycling patients, 2/4 had a substantial recovery of depressive or manic symptoms
Sanderson [30]	41 (72)	67.2	R	Unknown	5	Duration of admission (mania and depression) was equal for lithium users ($n = 41$), valproate users ($n = 20$) and carbamazepine users ($n = 11$)

(continued)

Table 4.2 (continued)

	N	Age (range)	Design	Dose-concentration	Duration (weeks)	Results (outcome measure)
Chen et al. [31]	30	69.4 (>55)	R	Unknown	2.3	Mania improved in 67 % of lithium users (*n* = 30) versus 35 % of valproate users (*n* = 29). At therapeutic serum levels 83 % of lithium users improved (>0.8 mmol/l) versus 75 % of valproate users (65–90 micro g/l)
Goldberg et al. [32]	2	76; 71	P	600 mg/day–0.63 mmol/l; 900 mg/day–0.43 mmol/l	3	Remission of depressive and manic episodes after re-introduction of lithium following toxicity
Sajatovic et al. [35]	34	60.1 (55–82)	RCT	750 mg/day 0.8—1.1 mmol/l	76	Lithium (*n* = 34) is more effective than placebo (*n* = 31) in prevention of relapse into (hypo)mania, 29 % dropped out
Geddes et al. [36]	27	(>53)	P	0.4–1.0 mmol/l	104	Lithium is as effective (*n* = 27) as the combination lithium–valproate (*n* = 22) and more effective than valproate alone (*n* = 31) in preventing relapse

R Retrospective, *P* prospective, *RCT* randomized controlled trial

Due to the reduced renal function with normal aging, the elimination half-life of lithium can be prolonged to 36–48 h compared to 24 h in younger adults. Therefore, steady state of lithium serum levels may not be reached for up to 10 days [37]. Dosing should reflect the altered pharmacodynamics and pharmacokinetics of older adults resulting in the need for significantly lower doses. As always, treatment depends on effectiveness and tolerance, and lithium should be titrated accordingly. Unfortunately, we still do not have consensus or clear guidelines for the appropriate therapeutic range of lithium in older adults. As a rough guideline, half the dose used in younger adults should be adequate and much safer. Very careful monitoring of clinical status and serum levels are indicated, even more so in older adults as maintenance treatment with lithium as practiced in modern care with regular measurements of renal function and lithium serum levels is associated with less decline of renal function [38, 39].

In older patients, lithium serum levels can rapidly elevate due to dehydration (perspiration, diarrhea, or insufficient fluid intake) and drug interactions with commonly used medications in older adults (e.g., diuretics, ACE- inhibiters, and NSAIDs).

As in younger adults, lithium toxicity in older adults is diagnosed by careful assessment of patients' clinical symptoms and not solely quantified by serum lithium levels. Neurological and cardiovascular comorbidity and polypharmacy increase the risk of side effects, drug interactions, and therefore toxicity [40–42].

4.6.3 Anticonvulsants

The available research on anticonvulsants in older adults with bipolar disorder is summarized in Table 4.3. Older patients are more susceptible to side effects of anticonvulsants than younger adults with an increased risk for delirium and falls [43].

4.6.3.1 Carbamazepine

In two studies, the effectiveness of carbamazepine was evaluated in OABD. In one study, carbamazepine was effective in 2 of 3 treatment-resistant patients [44]. The other study showed that duration of admission was not different in patients on lithium ($n = 41$), valproate ($n = 20$), or carbamazepine ($n = 11$) [30]. In a subgroup analysis of a double-blind study in younger adults with bipolar disorder assessing both carbamazepine and lithium individually as an anti-manic drug, both drugs were shown to be equally effective [45].

4.6.3.2 Valproate

Clinicians have increasingly prescribed valproate over the years for the treatment of bipolar disorder. Retrospective studies have suggested its anti-manic effects in OABD [29–31, 46–53]. There are 12 small studies (4–31 patients) on the effectiveness of valproate in treating OABD, none are randomized placebo-controlled.

In eleven studies, valproate was effective in treating mania [29–31, 46–53], and in five studies, it was effective as add-on in treatment resistance [29, 36, 46, 50, 53]. Valproate monotherapy has been reported in several studies to improve manic symptoms in almost all OABD, with the duration of treatment ranging from 1 to 7 weeks [47, 48, 52]. The National Institute of Mental Health has also funded a multisite, randomized controlled trial of lithium and valproate for the management of acute mania, with the aim of assessing the tolerability and efficacy of lithium and valproate in acute mania, hypomania, or mixed episodes in elderly bipolar patients [54].

4.6.3.3 Lamotrigine

Three studies were found on lamotrigine in treating OABD [35, 55, 56]. In a randomized placebo-controlled study, lamotrigine was more effective in preventing relapse compared to placebo [35]. The other two studies showed a reduction of depressive symptoms of approximately 50 % [55, 56].

Table 4.3 Studies of anticonvulsants in OABD

	N	Age (range)	Design	Dose-concentration	Duration (weeks)	Results (outcome measure)
Valproate						
McFarland et al. [46]	6	66 (56–74)	R	500 mg/day 50–150 microg/ml	4	Significant improvement of manic symptoms after valproate addition in therapy-resistant patients
Sharma et al. [29]	4	68.5 (66–71)	P	1000–1250 mg/day	40–78	Combination of lithium and valproate results in response in all rapid-cycling patients, 2/4 had significant recovery
Risinger et al. [47]	4	70 (65–73)	R	1000–1500 mg/day 50–75 microg/ml	2–4	Recovery of manic symptoms in all patients
Puryear et al. [48]	7	70 (63–81)	R	1000 mg/day (100–1750) 57 nanog/ml (34–82)	>1	Significant improvement of mainly manic symptoms
Kando et al. [49]	24	71.3	R	743 mg/day (250–2000) 53 mg/l (11–102)	>2	Effective in 62 % of manic patients with adequate treatment
Schneider and Wilcox [50]	4	74.8 (65–81)	R	52–115 mg/l	72–156	Remission after addition of valproate to lithium therapy in manic rapid cyclers
Sanderson [30]	20	67.2	R	Unknown	4	Duration of admission was equal for lithium users (*n* = 41), valproate users (*n* = 20) and carbamazepine users (*n* = 11)
Niedermier and Nasrallah [51]	23	67 (60–86)	R	1.029 mg/day (500–2250) 72 mg/l (36–111)	>1	87 % response (CGI) in manic, depressive, and mixed episodes
Noaghiul et al. [52]	21	71 (60–82)	R	1.405 mg/day 72 mg/l	1–7	19 patients (90 %) had significant clinical recovery of mania (CGI)
Chen et al. [31]	29	71.2 (>55)	R	Unknown	2.3	Mania improved in 67 % of lithium users (*n* = 30) versus 35 % of valproate users (*n* = 29). At therapeutic serum levels, 83 % of lithium users improved (>0.8 mmol/l) versus 75 % of valproate users (65–90 microg/l)
Mordecai et al. [53]	6	70.8 (64–75)	R	250–1000 mg/day 23–51.7 meq/ml	2–43	3 patients stabilized with valproate monotherapy 2 lithium users improved after valproate addition Both manic and depressive symptoms

(continued)

Table 4.3 (continued)

	N	Age (range)	Design	Dose-concentration	Duration (weeks)	Results (outcome measure)
Geddes et al. [36]	31	(>53)	P	750–1250 mg/day	104	Lithium is as effective (n = 27) as the combination lithium–valproate (n = 22) and more effective than valproate alone (n = 31) in preventing relapse
Carbamazepine						
Cullen et al. [44]	3	57 (48–72)	R	200–1200 mg/day 2236 Umol/l	>1	2/3 patients recovered from therapy-resistant melancholic depression
Sanderson [30]	11	67.2	R	Unknown	4	Duration of admission was equal for lithium users (n = 41), valproate users (n = 20) and carbamazepine users (n = 11)
Lamotrigine						
Robillard and Conn [55]	5	71.5 (65–85)	P	25–100 mg/day	12	50 % reduction of depressive symptoms (HDRS) in 3 rapid cyclers
Sajatovic et al. [58]	33	60.1 (55–82)	RCT	100–400 mg/day	76	Lamotrigine (n = 34) is more effective than placebo (n = 31) in preventing relapse (mania/depression) 18 % dropped out
Sajatovic et al. [56]	57	66.5 (60–90)	P	150.9 mg/day		57.4 % remission (MADRS) 64.8 % response 33 % dropout
Gabapentin						
Sethi et al. [57]	7	72.7 (59–90)	R	1028.5 mg/day (600–1200 mg/day)		All patients experienced improvement in manic symptoms. On gabapentin in combination with antipsychotic medications, and in 1 case in combination with valproate

R Retrospective, *P* prospective, *RCT* randomized controlled trial, *CGI* Clinical Global Impression scale, *HDRS* Hamilton Depression Rating Scale, and *MADRS* Montgomery Asberg Depression Rating scale

4.6.3.4 Gabapentin

One study described 7 cases that were treated successfully for mania with gabapentin in addition to antipsychotics or valproate [57].

4.6.3.5 Recommendations for Anticonvulsants

The indication for anticonvulsants in OABD is similar to younger adults. As always, caution in older adults is necessary, starting with a low dose and slowly titrating to a higher dose depending on effectiveness and tolerance of side effects such as sedation, cognitive symptoms, ataxia, and tremor [43, 58].

4.6.4 Antipsychotics

The atypical antipsychotics aripiprazole, quetiapine, risperidone, olanzapine, and clozapine were studied in OABD (Table 4.4).

Aripiprazole was studied as add-on to mood stabilizers and found to be effective in reducing manic and depressive symptoms [59, 60].

In a randomized placebo-controlled study, quetiapine was more effective than placebo by day 4 and after 12 weeks in manic patients [61]. In an open-label study of 4 weeks, the majority of the 11 manic patients were successfully treated with asenapine [62].

The effectiveness of risperidone, olanzapine, clozapine, and most recently lurasidone in older patients with bipolar disorder are only described in case reports or very small case studies [63–67].

4.6.4.1 Recommendations for Antipsychotics

The indication for antipsychotics in older patients is similar to younger adults with bipolar disorder. However, caution is warranted when prescribing antipsychotics in older adults. For the atypical antipsychotics olanzapine and risperidone, an increased risk for stroke and mortality has been demonstrated. The risk for stroke increases from 0.8 to 3.1 %. Possibly, this risk is a class effect and caution should be taken for all antipsychotics [66, 68]. In typical antipsychotics, the risk of mortality is 30 % higher in the first 6 months compared to atypical antipsychotics. Studies of metabolic syndrome in older patients, as a complication of using atypical antipsychotics, are very limited. In 100 older patients with schizophrenia and bipolar disorder, the prevalence of metabolic syndrome was not higher than in healthy controls and not related to the use of a specific class of antipsychotics [69].

Antipsychotics can be used as a monotherapy or as an adjunctive therapy for acute mania. Quetiapine and olanzapine are the common atypical antipsychotics used for acute mania in the elderly. In a post hoc analysis of pooled data from two quetiapine monotherapy clinical trials, quetiapine was shown to be an effective treatment, with a reduction in the Young Mania Rating Scale (YMRS) score as early as day 4 of treatment [60, 61].

Table 4.4 Studies of antipsychotics in OABD

	N	Age (range)	Design	Dose-concentration	Duration (weeks)	Results
Aripiprazole						
Gupta et al. [59]	1	64	R	40 mg/day	56	Clinical improvement and improvement of Parkinson symptoms
Sajatovic et al. [60]	22	59.6 (50–83)	P	10.3 mg/day	12	Significant improvement of manic and depressive symptoms (YMRS and HAM-D)
Quetiapine						
Sajatovic et al. [60]	59	62.9 (55–79)	RCT	400–800 mg/day	3–12	Response on day 4 (YMRS) in quetiapine (n = 28) versus placebo (n = 31), sustained after 12 weeks
Risperidone						
Madhusoodanan et al. [63]	2	71–79	P	1–2 mg/day	2–3	1 patient recovered from mixed episode
Olanzapine						
Nicolato et al. [65]	1	85	R	2.5 mg/day	24	Remission of catatonic symptoms in 4 days, stable after 6 months
Clozapine						
Shulman et al. [64]	3	72 (70–74)	P	25–112.5 mg/day	44	Clinical response (CGI) of psychotic mania in therapy-resistant patients
Asenapine						
Baruch et al. [62]	11	67.7 (61–79)	P	20 mg/day	28	82 % response, 64 % remission on mania (YMRS)
Lurasidone						
Sajatovic et al. [67]	142	60.0	P	34.6 mg or 96.0 mg 76.2 mg as adjunctive	6	Both low dose and high dose were more effective than placebo (MADRS, effect size 0.83)
						As adjunctive, there was no significant difference from placebo

R Retrospective, *P* prospective, *RCT* randomized controlled trial, *CGI* Clinical Global Impression scale, *YMRS* Young Mania Rating Scale, and *HAM-D* Hamilton Depression scale

Asenapine has also been shown to be effective and well tolerated in a small open-label study of elderly patients with mania, with 63.6 % achieving remission [62]. Shulman et al. [64] also reported improvement of symptoms with clozapine in an open-label study of three treatment-resistant manic elderly patients.

4.6.5 Electroconvulsive Therapy

The effectiveness of electroconvulsive therapy (ECT) has been shown in bipolar disorder [70–72] for both manic and depressive symptoms. For treatment-resistant bipolar depression, ECT is the treatment option with the most evidence [73]. Nevertheless, in most guidelines, ECT is offered only as second or third line treatment for refractory depression [74, 75], possibly due to stigma and concern for cognitive side effects. There are no systematic studies on the effectiveness of ECT in older patients with bipolar disorder. However, extrapolating results of ECT in younger adults with bipolar disorder [70–72] and older adults with unipolar disorder [76, 77], a superior effect of ECT in older patients with bipolar disorder can be expected in the acute phases (mania, depression, and mixed episode). ECT is a treatment option in manic or depressive older patients with bipolar disorder who are pharmacotherapy resistant, have previously shown to be ECT responders, or in situations where urgent safety concerns exist (severe suicidality, physical exhaustion, or refusal of all foods and fluids).

Cognitive side effects of ECT have been studied in older patients with unipolar depression [78, 79]; postictal confusion has been described, but most studies report improvements of cognitive functions after ECT, most likely due to recovery of depressed mood, concentration, and attention. Therefore, special attention to baseline cognitive function is important with particular concern for bilateral ECT. As concluded in an expert consensus paper, ECT remains an important treatment option in OABD [80].

4.6.6 Pharmacotherapy of Bipolar Depression

Similar to the treatment of bipolar mania in the geriatric population, the availability of literature on the management of bipolar depression in this population is limited. The role of antidepressants in causing the switch from depression to mania has also always been a clinical concern [81]. There are studies that support the combination of antidepressants and a mood stabilizer in such treatment. One such study reported that the usage of both paroxetine and lithium was more efficacious than lithium alone for the treatment of depression in bipolar disorder. This study included patients aged 21–71 years old, but there was no age-dependent response noted [82]. In contrast, Schaffer et al. [28] reported that, in comparing a second mood stabilizer versus an antidepressant, to the existing mood stabilizer, there was no significant difference in the response to lamotrigine and citalopram.

4.6.7 Maintenance Pharmacotherapy

The available literature on maintenance therapy for maintenance/prophylactic treatment in OABD is even more scarce compared to acute therapy. The best evidence comes from two prospective studies. Sajatovic et al. [35] analyzed data of 98 older patients who were treated with lamotrigine, lithium, or placebo from a larger scale double-blind study. With the mean total daily dose of lamotrigine being

240 mg and lithium 750 mg, the two drugs were shown to be effective in delaying a depressive and manic relapse. In a randomized open-label study, both combination therapy with lithium plus valproate and lithium monotherapy were more effective in preventing relapse compared to valproate monotherapy [36].

Clinical Vignette 4.1
Balancing Familial Tremor with the Effectiveness of Mood Stabilizers

Reason for Referral
Mr. B, a 75-year-old married male, retired dentist with a lifelong history of bipolar disorder, Type II, was referred by his general practitioner because of worsening bilateral hand tremor. He had been maintained on lithium carbonate since the age of 40 for management of bipolar disorder and had gradually been experiencing worsening tremor that interfered with his ability to write, drink from a cup, or use a computer. It was his general practitioner (GP), not a psychiatrist, who had been following him during all of these years. The GP reduced the maintenance dose of lithium from 900 to 600 mg per day in divided doses with some improvement in tremor but the GP was concerned that the lithium level was subtherapeutic at 0.26 mmol/l. However, the serum lithium level was actually drawn 24 h after the last dose not the customary 12 h.

Family and Personal History
Mr. B was the only child of parents who both suffered from bipolar disorder. His mother committed suicide when he was less than a year old, presumably from a postpartum psychosis. His maternal grandfather was cyclothymic and two maternal cousins had also suicided. His father suffered from bipolar 1 disorder and was treated with electroconvulsive therapy. Ultimately, he died by suicide at the age of 50.

Mr. B was raised by his paternal aunt who provided a loving, nurturing, and supportive environment. His father eventually re-married but separated because of the impact of his persistent mood disorder until his eventual suicide.

Familial tremor was evident on his father's side of the family including his paternal grandfather and paternal uncles.

Mr. B never married but has lived for many years with a female partner who provided valuable observations of his mood and behavior.

Past Medical and Psychiatric History
Mr. B was healthy except for hypothyroidism since his early 40s secondary to lithium therapy.

There were no past psychiatric admissions. His first depression occurred at the age of 18 that affected his academic productivity at various times and limited educational achievement as a result. The pattern of mood disorder included intermittent depressions lasting six months in duration followed by a period of euthymia for three months and then a period of hypomania for three months. Mr. B had been followed primarily by his general practitioner as access to psychiatric follow-up was limited. He was maintained on lithium carbonate 900 mg on a t.i.d. regimen.

Initial Mental Status and Cognitive Examination
Mr. B presented as euthymic with no evidence of major psychiatric symptoms. His bilateral tremor was very obvious with mild cogwheel rigidity but no other features suggestive of Parkinson's disease.

Cognitive screening was done using the Montreal Cognitive Assessment (MoCA), and he scored 26/29. He was unable to copy the cube because of his tremor. Despite his tremor, he was able to complete the clock drawing test but only when a larger circle was provided compared to the one used on the standard MoCA form.

Laboratory investigations revealed normal renal function and a normal thyroid-stimulating hormone level.

Management
Initially, lithium dose was gradually reduced from 900 to 300 mg per day achieving 12 h serum levels of about 0.5 mmol/l. While the tremor was still quite evident, Mr. B remained euthymic.

Six months later, Mr. B presented with reports from his partner of hypomanic symptomatology lasting several weeks. This included singing to himself, loquaciousness, pressured speech, and a decreased need for sleep. Yet objectively, he appeared euthymic and without gross behavioral disturbance. Consequently, divalproex was added to the regimen initially at 250 mg b.i.d.

Almost a year later, the tremor was very much improved, although still evident. Lithium had been reduced further to 150 mg 2 days a week and 300 mg on all other days. This led to a mild recurrence of depressive symptoms. Eventually, Mr. B stabilized on a regimen of lithium 300 mg q.h.s. (0.5 mmol/l) and divalproex 125 mg q.h.s. Divalproex was used as an augmenting agent because hypomania was the primary target, and it did not pose the same metabolic concerns as atypical agents. On this much reduced regimen, a balance of tolerance of the familial tremor with stabilization of mood was achieved. Mr. B declared: "Life is good and I can live with the tremor."

Learning Points

- The importance of access to psychiatric services in bipolar disorder, especially with respect to lithium management and monitoring.
- Changing lithium needs in later life and appreciation of the risk of side effects and toxicity. Knowledge of appropriate lithium dosing and serum levels with aging.
- Patients with bipolar disorder typically have a positive family history in first-degree relatives with the secondary psychological impact of having parents with bipolar disorder, including the traumatic effects of premature death by suicide, divorce, and separation. Unfortunately, the psychologically poor do get poorer. Lack of family history and late age of onset increases the likelihood of an underlying neurological or systemic medical disorder.

- The challenge of distinguishing familial tremor from lithium-induced or lithium-exacerbated tremor.
- The challenge of distinguishing Parkinson's disease from familial tremor and from lithium-induced tremor and extrapyramidal side effects (EPS).
- The advantage of low-dose polypharmacy in bipolar disorder in older adults, versus high-dose monotherapy in controlling side effects and managing effectiveness.
- The need for careful and long-term monitoring of bipolar patients where there are subtle changes in behavior and mood reflecting cyclical changes in bipolar disorder.
- The fundamental importance of family involvement and input to provide independent observations in order to inform management. Clinicians also need to acknowledge the impact of bipolar disorder on family members and provide psychoeducation and support accordingly.

Clinical Vignette 4.2
To Continue or Not to Continue Lithium in Older Adults: Mood Stabilization and Renal Function

Reason for Referral
Mr. D was referred initially as a 65-year-old male who had been a successful businessman and was recently retired. His wife was unhappy with the lack of response to ongoing psychotherapy for his lifelong bipolar disorder and current prolonged depression and asked for a second opinion.

Family and Personal History
There was a very strong family history of mood disorder on the maternal side of Mr. D's family. Four out of seven maternal aunts and uncles suffered from significant mood disorder that required treatment. His one sibling was well.

Fluctuations in motivation and mood led to academic difficulties when Mr. D was a youth. This was episodic and associated with his recurrent mood changes. When he was euthymic or hypomanic, he was energetic, motivated, and showed initiative. This was reflected in academic success. When depressed, his functioning and performance declined.

Past Medical and Psychiatric History
Medical history included treatment for hypertension with an ACE Inhibitor and diuretics. Mr. D had evidence of peripheral vascular disease with intermittent claudication and elevated cholesterol treated with atorvastatin. Interstitial nephritis was diagnosed by a nephrologist.

Mr. D suffered from recurrent depressions for most of his adult life interspersed with prolonged periods of subtle hypomania. Depression was characterized by social avoidance, decreased motivation, and a tendency toward procrastination. Appetite was slightly reduced with associated weight loss, and he would develop periods of somatization and fleeting suicidal ideation. Hypomanic episodes were characterized by a change in mood and personality. He would become jocular, expansive, charming, and generous. His mood was variously euphoric and irritable. As a businessman, he would develop entrepreneurial ideas and creative projects during these cycles of hypomania that lasted between 18 and 24 months.

Mr. D was treated primarily with psychodynamic psychotherapy with no significant impact on his mood symptoms. He had refused lithium in the past and was also reluctant to take antidepressants which had not had a consistent positive impact on his mood or function.

Clinical Management

At the time of initial referral, Mr. D was stabilized on lithium carbonate alone and remained well for over 10 years with regular psychiatric follow-up. During that period of time, even with careful lithium monitoring and levels maintained below 0.8 mmol/l, renal function began to decline. There were no episodes of acute lithium toxicity. He was referred to a nephrologist who concluded that the trend toward chronic renal failure was secondary to interstitial nephritis due to lithium nephrotoxicity and suggested a decrease and eventual discontinuation of lithium. As a result, Mr. D became very concerned about the possibility of renal failure and discontinued lithium on his own. This led to a gradual and prolonged depression characterized by excessive financial concerns and a complete cessation of entrepreneurial ideas and projects. This was unresponsive to several trials of antidepressants and showed only a limited response to a trial of lamotrigine up to 300 mg daily. Mr. D continued to refuse re-challenge with lithium.

After a period of over two years, his depression gradually remitted. It is unclear whether this was simply a function of the natural history of his illness or whether lamotrigine had contributed to his mood stability. He remains off lithium at this time and on lamotrigine 200 mg per day. Renal function is relatively stable. Even though Mr. D remains off lithium, there is ongoing communication between psychiatrist and nephrologist in order to balance the risks and benefits of managing renal disease and mood disorder simultaneously.

Learning Points

- In this vignette, as in our first vignette, there is a strong family history of mood disorder as is expected in patients especially with early onset bipolar disorder.

- Input from family remains essential to describe subtle behavioral and mood changes that may not be evident on clinical examination. Family members are also profoundly affected by these changes and deserve to be supported and part of the management plan.
- The effectiveness of lithium as a mood stabilizer is clearly demonstrated in this vignette. When lithium was discontinued due to renal concerns, the destabilization that resulted was very significant and impacted on the quality of life of both patient and his spouse.
- A very common challenge is dealing with declining renal function with aging. The nephrologist concluded that the interstitial nephritis and declining renal function was due to lithium nephrotoxicity, even though there had been no prior episodes of acute lithium toxicity. The data on this issue remain limited and controversial.
- The issue of balancing declining renal function and unstable mood disorder simultaneously highlights the need for collaboration among medical specialties, especially between nephrologist and psychiatrist. Good communication and continuing assessment of the benefits and risks of maintenance of lithium or alternate forms of mood stabilization is essential. This is especially important in light of the ongoing controversy and uncertainty about the impact of chronic lithium therapy on renal function [83].
- The natural history of this disorder makes it difficult to tease out the possibility that lamotrigine had provided mood stability after considerable time versus the natural history of mood swings that were evident of this man's lifetime. Careful follow-up and monitoring with input from family will help to tease out these clinical challenges.
- Older adults with bipolar disorder require careful follow-up and monitoring of psychiatric and medical status within an interdisciplinary approach to health care.

4.7 Summary and Recommendations for Acute Bipolar Mania, Bipolar Depression, and Maintenance Therapy

We are very limited in our ability to make firm recommendations for any of these phases of OABD because of the lack of RCTs and even systematic data. We depend now on extrapolation from mixed-age populations, individual case reports, small case series, or expert consensus [80]. These recommendations must suffice for OABD with the caveats listed above regarding the unique aspects of pharmacotherapy in OABD.

For acute bipolar mania in OABD, lithium remains a first line treatment in all consensus guidelines for adults and hence for OABD until we have more direct evidence. We are awaiting publication of the results of the National Institute of Mental Health-funded multisite RCT of valproate compared to lithium for acute mania in type 1 OABD (age over 60 years). These data will help to shed light on the tolerability and efficacy of lithium compared to valproate in the treatment of OABD in acute mania, hypomania, and mixed episodes. Limited data are available for olanzapine, quetiapine, asenapine, carbamazepine, gabapentin, and clozapine [80].

Clinical Pearls

- Involvement of family in the management of older adults with bipolar disorder is essential for two reasons: firstly, they can provide important and sometime subtle clinical information, and secondly, they are profoundly affected by the disorder.
- Lithium carbonate remains a first line mood stabilizer in older adults but calls for special precautions including significantly lower serum levels (0.4–0.6 mmol/l are often effective) and concomitant lowering of dosing. The decline in its use is not backed by clinical evidence.
- Renal function declines normally with aging and care must be taken not to discontinue lithium prematurely in stable bipolar patients simply because of rising serum creatinine. This remains a controversial clinical issue inviting further research and a collaborative approach with nephrologists.
- Older adults may respond to the same therapeutic armamentarium as younger individuals including ECT which is generally well tolerated. ECT is sometimes safer than using high-dose drug monotherapy. Combining mood stabilizers at low dose is a therapeutic approach that may limit toxicity in those who do not respond to monotherapy. Polypharmacy is not always a bad thing if carefully monitored.

References

1. Thesing CS, Stek ML, van Grootheest DS, van de Ven PM, Beekman AT, Kupka RW, et al. Childhood abuse, family history and stressors in older patients with bipolar disorder in relation to age at onset. J Affect Disord. 2015;184:249–55.
2. Bauer MS, McBride L, Williford WO, Glick H, Kinosian B, Altshuler L, et al. Collaborative care for bipolar disorder: part I. Intervention and implementation in a randomized effectiveness trial. Psychiatr Serv. 2006;57(7):927–36.
3. Kessing LV, Hansen HV, Hvenegaard A, Christensen EM, Dam H, Gluud C, et al. Treatment in a specialised out-patient mood disorder clinic v. standard out-patient treatment in the early course of bipolar disorder: randomised clinical trial. Br J Psychiatry. 2013;202(3):212–9.

4. Kilbourne AM, Goodrich DE, Lai Z, Clogston J, Waxmonsky J, Bauer MS. Life goals collaborative care for patients with bipolar disorder and cardiovascular disease risk. Psychiatr Serv. 2012;63(12):1234–8.
5. Kilbourne AM, Post EP, Nossek A, Drill L, Cooley S, Bauer MS. Improving medical and psychiatric outcomes among individuals with bipolar disorder: a randomized controlled trial. Psychiatr Serv. 2008;59(7):760–8.
6. Reynolds T, Thornicroft G, Abas M, Woods B, Hoe J, Leese M, et al. Camberwell Assessment of Need for the Elderly (CANE). Development, validity and reliability. Br J Psychiatry. 2000;176:444–52.
7. Dautzenberg G, Lans L, Meesters PD, Kupka R, Beekman A, Stek ML, et al. The care needs of older patients with bipolar disorder. Aging Mental Health. 2015:1–9.
8. Barlow J, Wright C, Sheasby J, Turner A, Hainsworth J. Self-management approaches for people with chronic conditions: a review. Patient Educ Couns. 2002;48(2):177–87.
9. Mueser KT, Pratt SI, Bartels SJ, Swain K, Forester B, Cather C, et al. Randomized trial of social rehabilitation and integrated health care for older people with severe mental illness. J Consult Clin Psychol. 2010;78(4):561–73.
10. Depp CA, Lebowitz BD, Patterson TL, Lacro JP, Jeste DV. Medication adherence skills training for middle-aged and elderly adults with bipolar disorder: development and pilot study. Bipolar Disord. 2007;9(6):636–45.
11. Bartels SJ, Pratt SI. Psychosocial rehabilitation and quality of life for older adults with serious mental illness: recent findings and future research directions. Curr Opin Psychiatry. 2009; 22(4):381–5.
12. Colom F, Vieta E, Reinares M, Martinez-Aran A, Torrent C, Goikolea JM, et al. Psychoeducation efficacy in bipolar disorders: beyond compliance enhancement. J Clin Psychiatry. 2003;64(9):1101–5.
13. Colom F, Vieta E, Martinez-Aran A, Reinares M, Goikolea JM, Benabarre A, et al. A randomized trial on the efficacy of group psychoeducation in the prophylaxis of recurrences in bipolar patients whose disease is in remission. Arch Gen Psychiatry. 2003;60(4):402–7.
14. Castle D, White C, Chamberlain J, Berk M, Berk L, Lauder S, et al. Group-based psychosocial intervention for bipolar disorder: randomised controlled trial. Br J Psychiatry. 2010;196(5):383–8.
15. Ghose K. The need for a review journal of drug use and the elderly. Drugs Aging. 1991; 1(1):2–5.
16. Malhi GS, Tanious M. Optimal frequency of lithium administration in the treatment of bipolar disorder: clinical and dosing considerations. CNS Drugs. 2011;25(4):289–98.
17. Dols A, Sienaert P, van Gerven H, Schouws S, Stevens A, Kupka R, et al. The prevalence and management of side effects of lithium and anticonvulsants as mood stabilizers in bipolar disorder from a clinical perspective: a review. Int Clin Psychopharmacol. 2013;28(6):287–96.
18. Hardy B, Shulman K, Mackenzie S, Kutcher S, Silverberg J. Pharmacokinetics of lithium in the elderly. Psychopharmacology. 1987;7:153–8.
19. Yuen AW, et al. Sodium valproate acutely inhibits lamotrigine metabolism. Br J Clin Pharmacol. 1992;33:511–3.
20. Marcoux AW. Carbamazepine-lithium drug interaction. Ann Pharmacother. 1996;30(5):547.
21. Dols A, Rhebergen D, Beekman A, Kupka R, Sajatovic M, Stek ML. Psychiatric and medical comorbidities: results from a bipolar elderly cohort study. Am J Geriatr Psychiatry Off J Am Assoc Geriatr Psychiatry. 2014;22(11):1066–74.
22. Al Jurdi RK, Marangell LB, Petersen NJ, Martinez M, Gyulai L, Sajatovic M. Prescription patterns of psychotropic medications in elderly compared with younger participants who achieved a “recovered” status in the systematic treatment enhancement program for bipolar disorder. Am J Geriatr Psychiatry Off J Am Assoc Geriatr Psychiatry. 2008;16(11):922–33.
23. Shulman KI, Rochon P, Sykora K, Anderson G, Mamdani M, Bronskill S, et al. Changing prescription patterns for lithium and valproic acid in old age: shifting practice without evidence. BMJ. 2003;326(7396):960–1.

24. Goodwin FK, Jamison KR. Manic depressive illness. New York: Oxford Univ Press; 1990. pp. 603–29.
25. Abou-Saleh MT, Coppen A. The prognosis of depression in old age: the case for lithium therapy. Br J Psychiatry. 1983;143:527–8.
26. Van der Velde CD. Effectiveness of lithium carbonate in the treatment of manic-depressive illness. Am J Psychiatry. 1970;127(3):345–51.
27. Himmelhoch JM, Neil JF, May SJ, Fuchs CZ, Licata SM. Age, dementia, dyskinesias, and lithium response. Am J Psychiatry. 1980;137(8):941–5.
28. Schaffer CB, Batra K, Garvey MJ, Mungas DM, Schaffer LC. The effect of haloperidol on serum levels of lithium in adult manic patients. Biol Psychiatry. 1984;19(10):1495–9.
29. Sharma V, Persad E, Mazmanian D, Karunaratne K. Treatment of rapid cycling bipolar disorder with combination therapy of valproate and lithium. Can J Psychiatry. 1993; 38(2):137–9.
30. Sanderson DR. Use of mood stabilizers by hospitalized geriatric patients with bipolar disorder. Psychiatr Serv. 1998;49(9):1145–7.
31. Chen ST, Altshuler LL, Melnyk KA, Erhart SM, Miller E, Mintz J. Efficacy of lithium vs. valproate in the treatment of mania in the elderly: a retrospective study. J Clin Psychiatry. 1999;60(3):181–6.
32. Goldberg JF, Sacks MH, Kocsis JH. Low-dose lithium augmentation of divalproex in geriatric mania. J Clin Psychiatry. 2000;61(4):304.
33. Murray N, Hopwood S, Balfour DJ, Ogston S, Hewick DS. The influence of age on lithium efficacy and side-effects in out-patients. Psychol Med. 1983;13(1):53–60.
34. Stone K. Mania in the elderly. Br J Psychiatry. 1989;155:220–4.
35. Sajatovic M, Gyulai L, Calabrese JR, Thompson TR, Wilson BG, White R, et al. Maintenance treatment outcomes in older patients with bipolar I disorder. Am J Geriatr Psychiatry. 2005; 13(4):305–11.
36. Geddes JR, Goodwin GM, Rendell J, Azorin JM, Cipriani A, Ostacher MJ, et al. Lithium plus valproate combination therapy versus monotherapy for relapse prevention in bipolar I disorder (BALANCE): a randomised open-label trial. Lancet. 2010;375(9712):385–95.
37. Licht RW, Vestergaard P, Kessing LV, Larsen JK, Thomsen PH. Psychopharmacological treatment with lithium and antiepileptic drugs: suggested guidelines from the Danish Psychiatric Association and the Child and Adolescent Psychiatric Association in Denmark. Acta Psychiatr Scand. 2003; 108(Suppl 419):1–22.
38. Clos S, Rauchhaus P, Severn A, Cochrane L, Donnan PT. Long-term effect of lithium maintenance therapy on estimated glomerular filtration rate in patients with affective disorders: a population-based cohort study. Lancet Psychiatry. 2015;2(12):1075–83.
39. Kessing LV, Gerds TA, Feldt-Rasmussen B, Andersen PK, Licht RW. Use of lithium and anticonvulsants and the rate of chronic kidney disease: a nationwide population-based study. JAMA Psychiatry. 2015;72(12):1182–91.
40. Young RC, Murphy CF, Heo M, Schulberg HC, Alexopoulos GS. Cognitive impairment in bipolar disorder in old age: literature review and findings in manic patients. J Affect Disord. 2006;92(1):125–31.
41. Adityanjee, Munshi KR, Thampy A. The syndrome of irreversible lithium-effectuated neurotoxicity. Clin Neuropharmacol. 2005;28(1):38–49.
42. Freeman MP, Freeman SA. Lithium: clinical considerations in internal medicine. Am J Med. 2006;119(6):478–81.
43. Perucca E, Berlowitz D, Birnbaum A, Cloyd JC, Garrard J, Hanlon JT, et al. Pharmacological and clinical aspects of antiepileptic drug use in the elderly. Epilepsy Res. 2006;68(Suppl 1): S49–63.
44. Cullen M, Mitchell P, Brodaty H, Boyce P, Parker G, Hickie I, et al. Carbamazepine for treatment-resistant melancholia. J Clin Psychiatry. 1991;52(11):472–6.

45. Okuma T, Yamashita I, Takahashi R, Itoh H, Otsuki S, Watanabe S, et al. Comparison of the antimanic efficacy of carbamazepine and lithium carbonate by double-blind controlled study. Pharmacopsychiatry. 1990;23(3):143–50.
46. McFarland BH, Miller MR, Straumfjord AA. Valproate use in the older manic patient. J Clin Psychiatry. 1990;51(11):479–81.
47. Risinger RC, Risby ED, Risch SC. Safety and efficacy of divalproex sodium in elderly bipolar patients. J Clin Psychiatry. 1994;55(5):215.
48. Puryear LJ, Kunik ME, Workman R Jr. Tolerability of divalproex sodium in elderly psychiatric patients with mixed diagnoses. J Geriatr Psychiatry Neurol. 1995;8(4):234–7.
49. Kando JC, Tohen M, Castillo J, Zarate CA Jr. The use of valproate in an elderly population with affective symptoms. J Clin Psychiatry. 1996;57(6):238–40.
50. Schneider AL, Wilcox CS. Divalproate augmentation in lithium-resistant rapid cycling mania in four geriatric patients. J Affect Disord. 1998;47(1–3):201–5.
51. Niedermier JA, Nasrallah HA. Clinical correlates of response to valproate in geriatric inpatients. Ann Clin Psychiatry. 1998;10(4):165–8.
52. Noaghiul S, Narayan M, Nelson JC. Divalproex treatment of mania in elderly patients. Am J Geriatr Psychiatry. 1998;6(3):257–62.
53. Mordecai DJ, Sheikh JI, Glick ID. Divalproex for the treatment of geriatric bipolar disorder. Int J Geriatr Psychiatry. 1999;14(6):494–6.
54. Young AH, McElroy SL, Bauer M, Philips N, Chang W, Olausson B, et al. A double-blind, placebo-controlled study of quetiapine and lithium monotherapy in adults in the acute phase of bipolar depression (EMBOLDEN I). J Clin Psychiatry. 2010;71(2):150–62.
55. Robillard M, Conn DK. Lamotrigine use in geriatric patients with bipolar depression. Can J Psychiatry. 2002;47(8):767–70.
56. Sajatovic M, Gildengers A, Al Jurdi RK, Gyulai L, Cassidy KA, Greenberg RL, et al. Multisite, open-label, prospective trial of lamotrigine for geriatric bipolar depression: a preliminary report. Bipolar Disord. 2011;13(3):294–302.
57. Sethi MA, Mehta R, Devanand DP. Gabapentin in geriatric mania. J Geriatr Psychiatry Neurol. 2003;16(2):117–20.
58. Sajatovic M, Bingham CR, Campbell EA, Fletcher DF. Bipolar disorder in older adult inpatients. J Nerv Mental Dis. 2005;193(6):417–9.
59. Gupta S, Chohan M, Madhusoodanan S. Treatment of acute mania with aripiprazole in an older adult with noted improvement in coexisting Parkinson's disease. Prim Care Companion J Clin Psychiatry. 2004;6(1):50–1.
60. Sajatovic M, Coconcea N, Ignacio RV, Blow FC, Hays RW, Cassidy KA, et al. Aripiprazole therapy in 20 older adults with bipolar disorder: a 12-week, open-label trial. J Clin Psychiatry. 2008;69(1):41–6.
61. Sajatovic M, Calabrese JR, Mullen J. Quetiapine for the treatment of bipolar mania in older adults. Bipolar Disord. 2008;10(6):662–71.
62. Baruch Y, Tadger S, Plopski I, Barak Y. Asenapine for elderly bipolar manic patients. J Affect Disord. 2013;145(1):130–2.
63. Madhusoodanan S, Brenner R, Araujo L, Abaza A. Efficacy of risperidone treatment for psychoses associated with schizophrenia, schizoaffective disorder, bipolar disorder, or senile dementia in 11 geriatric patients: a case series. J Clin Psychiatry. 1995;56(11):514–8.
64. Shulman RW, Singh A, Shulman KI. Treatment of elderly institutionalized bipolar patients with clozapine. Psychopharmacol Bull. 1997;33(1):113–8.
65. Nicolato R, Romano-Silva MA, Correa H, dos Santos RR, Teixeira AL. Stuporous catatonia in an elderly bipolar patient: response to olanzapine. Aust NZ J Psychiatry. 2006;40(5):498.
66. Schneeweiss S, Setoguchi S, Brookhart A, Dormuth C, Wang PS. Risk of death associated with the use of conventional versus atypical antipsychotic drugs among elderly patients. CMAJ. 2007;176(5):627–32.

67. Sajatovic M, Forester BP, Tsai J, Kroger H, Pikalov A, Cucchiaro J, Loebel A. Efficacy of lurasidone in adults aged 55 years and older with bipolar depression: post hoc analysis of 2 double-blind, placebo-controlled studies. J Clin Psychiatry. 2016. (published online August 16).
68. Setoguchi S, Wang PS, Alan Brookhart M, Canning CF, Kaci L, Schneeweiss S. Potential causes of higher mortality in elderly users of conventional and atypical antipsychotic medications. J Am Geriatr Soc. 2008;56(9):1644–50.
69. Konz HW, Meesters PD, Paans NP, van Grootheest DS, Comijs HC, Stek ML, et al. Screening for metabolic syndrome in older patients with severe mental illness. Am J Geriatr Psychiatry Off J Am Assoc Geriatr Psychiatry. 2014;22(11):1116–20.
70. Loo C, Katalinic N, Mitchell PB, Greenberg B. Physical treatments for bipolar disorder: a review of electroconvulsive therapy, stereotactic surgery and other brain stimulation techniques. J Affect Disord. 2010;132(1–2):1–13.
71. Versiani M, Cheniaux E, Landeira-Fernandez J. Efficacy and safety of electroconvulsive therapy in the treatment of bipolar disorder: a systematic review. J ECT. 2010;27(2):153–64.
72. Valenti M, Benabarre A, Garcia-Amador M, Molina O, Bernardo M, Vieta E. Electroconvulsive therapy in the treatment of mixed states in bipolar disorder. Eur Psychiatry. 2008; 23(1):53–6.
73. Sienaert P, Lambrichts L, Dols A, De Fruyt J. Evidence-based treatment strategies for treatment-resistant bipolar depression: a systematic review. Bipolar Disord. 2012;15(1):61–9.
74. (APA) APATFoET. The practice of electroconvulsive therapy. 2nd ed. Washington, DC: APA Press; 2001.
75. (NICE) NifCE. Guidance on the use of electroconvulsive therapy. London: NICE Technology Appraisal Guidance 59; 2003.
76. Stek ML, Wurff van der FFB, Hoogendijk WJG, Beekman ATF. Electroconvulsive therapy for the depressed elderly (review). The Cochrane Library; 2009.
77. van der Wurff FB, Stek ML, Hoogendijk WJ, Beekman AT. The efficacy and safety of ECT in depressed older adults: a literature review. Int J Geriatr Psychiatry. 2003;18(10):894–904.
78. Verwijk E, Comijs HC, Kok RM, Spaans HP, Tielkes CE, Scherder EJ, et al. Short- and long-term neurocognitive functioning after electroconvulsive therapy in depressed elderly: a prospective naturalistic study. Int Psychogeriatr. 2013;26(2):315–24.
79. Tielkes CE, Comijs HC, Verwijk E, Stek ML. The effects of ECT on cognitive functioning in the elderly: a review. Int J Geriatr Psychiatry. 2008;23(8):789–95.
80. Sajatovic M, Strejilevich SA, Gildengers AG, Dols A, Al Jurdi RK, Forester BP, et al. A report on older-age bipolar disorder from the International Society for Bipolar Disorders Task Force. Bipolar Disord. 2015;17(7):689–704.
81. Pacchiarotti I, Bond DJ, Baldessarini RJ, Nolen WA, Grunze H, Licht RW, et al. The International Society for Bipolar Disorders (ISBD) task force report on antidepressant use in bipolar disorders. Am J Psychiatry. 2013;170(11):1249–62.
82. Nemeroff CB, Evans DL, Gyulai L, Sachs GS, Bowden CL, Gergel IP, et al. Double-blind, placebo-controlled comparison of imipramine and paroxetine in the treatment of bipolar depression. Am J Psychiatry. 2001;158(6):906–12.
83. Goodwin GM. The safety of lithium. JAMA Psychiatry. 2015;72(12):1167–9.

Older Age Bipolar Disorder and Substance Use

5

Chaya Bhuvaneswaran, Rita Hargrave and E. Sherwood Brown

5.1 Introduction

The devastating impact of substance use disorders (SUDs) among older adults has only recently attracted the attention of researchers, clinicians, and the general public [1]. Despite the evidence that alcohol and other SUDs affect nearly 1 in 5 older adults, there has been limited examination of these areas in the substance abuse or gerontology literature [2]. There is an even greater paucity of research on the screening, assessment, and treatment protocols for older adults with bipolar disorder and coexisting SUD. Adults with bipolar disorder (compared to other psychiatric disorders) have the highest rate of alcohol use disorder [2]. With the predicted dramatic growth of the aging population, as well as more geriatric patients in outpatient opioid maintenance programs both due to the aging of patients first

C. Bhuvaneswaran
35 Morrill Street, West Newton, MA 02465, USA
e-mail: chayab77@gmail.com

R. Hargrave
4338 Leach St, Oakland, CA 94602, USA
e-mail: ecarenet@yahoo.com

E. Sherwood Brown (✉)
Department of Psychiatry, The University of Texas Southwestern Medical Center,
5323 Harry Hines Blvd, MC 8849, Dallas, TX 75390-8849, USA
e-mail: sherwood.brown@utsouthwestern.edu; esbrow3@gmail.com

S.W. Lehmann and B.P. Forester (eds.), *Bipolar Disorder in Older Age Patients*,
DOI 10.1007/978-3-319-48912-4_5

enrolled in the 1990s and due to patients with prescription opioid misuse in later life, the need and demand for effective, comprehensive mental health services for older adults with psychiatric illness and substance use disorders will continue to grow [3].

Clinical Vignette 5.1

Mr. V, a 67-year-old single man diagnosed with bipolar I disorder in his thirties, presented with manic and psychotic symptoms and intoxicated, has had recurrent, severe depressive episodes not ameliorated by valproic acid, carbamazepine, or antipsychotics. He is inconsistently adherent to a regimen of low-dose lithium—he refuses to allow the dose to be increased to therapeutic blood levels—and insists on continuing a fairly high dose of fluoxetine. Whenever he discontinues lithium, he experiences affective switching and manic episodes. Mr. V has had over twenty lifetime hospitalizations for mood episodes. In between episodes, he lives in an apartment paid for by a sister who manages his care and provides him with income to supplement disability income, but who is herself aging and concerned about her own retirement. He has written moving essays about bipolar disorder and occasionally attends support group meetings, which he calls "talking to the young ones about how it is."

Mr. V recently had an inpatient alcohol detoxification admission where he expressed suicidal ideation while intoxicated. He refused a trial of naltrexone after he was stabilized. When younger, he participated in alcohol residential treatment programs and halfway house communities, but will not consider these options now, commenting that, "I'm too old for all that stuff, it's embarrassing." He has been referred to multiple day treatment and psychosocial groups as well as individual chronotherapy. (Chronotherapy is a therapy to prevent mood episodes in bipolar disorders by regulating exposure to light and darkness as well as manipulating sleep cycle, based on the theory that disrupted circadian rhythms and genetic polymorphisms in suprachiasmatic nucleus underlie sleep disruption in affective disorders.) [4] Mr. V was also enrolled in interpersonal therapy research studies and eventually dropped out of all of these, saying "the only thing that makes me feel better when I'm depressed is a few (vodka) nips." Recently, his physician discussed a trial of an atypical antipsychotic medication for greater mood stability. However, his outpatient psychiatrist and therapist are concerned by the patient's recent neurologic examination that was notable for gait ataxia and neuropsychological testing indicating working memory deficits and confabulation. Furthermore, a toxicology screen was positive for benzodiazepines despite the absence of any current prescription for benzodiazepines after discharge from his recent inpatient detoxification admission.

Learning Points

- Substance abuse should be considered in older patients with bipolar disorder.
- Clinical features—including cognitive changes, medication non-adherence, frequent hospitalization, and suicidal ideation—are all potential indicators of substance use.
- Toxicology screens should be considered in older patients with bipolar disorder with suspected substance use.

In this chapter, we will discuss the following themes highlighted by this clinical vignette: the prevalence and correlates of bipolar disorder and substance use disorders (SUDs); demographic features of older adults with bipolar disorder and SUD; trajectory of illness in older adults with bipolar disorder and SUD; epidemiology, diagnosis, and treatment of specific SUDs in older age bipolar disorder (OABD); and future directions for treatment research among older adults with bipolar disorder.

5.2 Prevalence and Demographic Features of Substance Use Disorder in Older Age Bipolar Disorder

Current epidemiological studies suggest that up to 60 % of adults with bipolar disorder will experience one or more substance use disorders (SUDs) [5–7]. Several studies report that there is a lower prevalence of SUD in elderly bipolar patients compared with younger adults, ranging from 9 to 29 % [8–12]. Although SUD is less common among older than younger adults with bipolar disorder, even low intensity substance use may be particularly harmful for older adults, carrying negative medical and functional consequences [13].

Gender plays a critical role in the clinical presentation and course of bipolar disorder and coexisting SUDs among geriatric patients. Across the life span, women present more often with bipolar disorder later in life, with an average age of diagnosis from 30 to 35 years [14]. In studies of mixed-age populations, the combination of bipolar disorder and SUD is more common in men compared to women [8, 15]. Thus, the increased risk for SUD in men versus women with bipolar disorder follows the pattern observed in the general population. Men are also more likely to have risk factors for SUDs, such as divorced/widowed status, lower level of education, additional primary psychiatric disorders, and higher rates of medical comorbidities [15, 16]. Among women as compared to men with older age bipolar disorder, a coexisting anxiety disorder is more highly associated with SUDs [10]. Although prospective longitudinal studies of bipolar disorder in older adults report that women experience more frequent depressive episodes, older women have a lower prevalence of SUD than older men [17]. Elevated rates of SUD in men with bipolar disorder may be related to gender differences in patterns of substance use. Non-medical prescription opioid use also appears to be more common among men than among women with bipolar disorder [18].

Cross-cultural studies suggest that race/ethnicity exerts a significant influence on the diagnosis, treatment, and prognosis of bipolar disorder in older adults [19]. African American patients have historically been more likely to be diagnosed with psychotic disorders rather than mood disorders, with the true prevalence of bipolar disorder and bipolar disorder with coexisting SUD likely underestimated among older African Americans [19]. Nonwhite race among mixed-age groups has been identified as a risk factor for suicide within bipolar disorder [20]. There is limited research that examines whether this trend persists in the context of older adults, with bipolar disorder and SUD.

Some investigators suggest that ethnicity influences the efficacy of treatment interventions for bipolar disorder and SUD. The STEP-Bipolar Disorder study (after controlling for any SUD) reported 1-year treatment outcomes that were significantly poorer for African Americans compared to Hispanic and non-Hispanic patients [21]. The National Comorbidity Survey Replication (comprised of mixed-age patients) identified healthcare disparities affecting African Americans with bipolar disorder. Controlling for factors such as healthcare utilization, socioeconomic status, or symptom profile, African American patients with bipolar disorder were less likely to receive adequate treatment with mood stabilizer medications, thus placing them at great risk for SUD relapse including a higher rate of inpatient hospitalizations and ED visits [22].

Other factors contributing to reduced treatment response among African American older adults are higher medical burden (e.g., hypertension, diabetes, and obesity) [23] and higher rates of underdiagnosis and misdiagnosis of bipolar disorder [11]. The paucity of cross-cultural research on bipolar disorder and coexisting SUD makes it difficult to ascertain the presence of healthcare disparities among other ethnic minority groups. Native Hawaiians experienced longer and more frequent hospitalizations for bipolar disorder with coexisting SUDs compared to other Asian American groups [24]. Hispanics, Asian Americans, and Native Americans also have higher rates of involuntary commitment for co-occurring SUD and bipolar disorder compared with white counterparts [25]. Fleck et al. [25] postulate that culturally based stigma against seeking or complying with outpatient treatment contributes to greater treatment non-adherence among all ethnic minority patients.

Although ethnicity has been cited as a predictor of high rates of healthcare utilization for older adults, including acute psychiatric care versus outpatient treatment access, socioeconomic status may be a confounding factor [26]. In a study of older African American adults, the elevated rate of acute healthcare utilization was correlated with high rates of homelessness and inadequate insurance coverage (i.e., uninsured or underinsured) [27]. Studies of other cohorts suggest that housing instability (or homelessness) rather than race or ethnicity is predictive of high rates of re-hospitalization and utilization of acute healthcare services [28].

5.3 Trajectory of Illness among Older Adults with Bipolar Disorder and SUD

In general, the presence of bipolar disorder and coexisting SUD predicts more severe course of illness [29]. Of special consideration in older adults is their vulnerability to medication side effects and the physical effects of substances due to age-related changes in pharmacokinetics, multiple medical comorbidities, and polypharmacy [30, 31]. Although there are limited data on the clinical impact of lower severity substance use disorders in older adults, studies of younger populations suggest that even lower intensity substance use patterns could adversely affect the trajectory of bipolar disorder in older adults [32].

The lower rate of SUDs among geriatric bipolar patients may be influenced by underreporting of SUD by older adults due to stigma [33]. Additionally, healthcare professionals are less likely to diagnose bipolar disorder among older adults with SUD. A 2015 study of geriatric hospitalized patients meeting alcohol use disorders (AUDs) criteria found that few of these patients had been evaluated for or diagnosed with bipolar disorder prior to admission [34]. During acute clinical encounters (in emergency departments, medical units, or inpatient psychiatric units), accurate collateral information about current mood symptoms and past psychiatric history may not be available to assist the diagnostic process. Under recognition of SUDs among older adults with bipolar disorder, reflective of lower rates of assessment for SUDs in geriatric populations more generally, likely contributes to delays in diagnosis and treatment [35]. Based on the current rate of substance use among young and middle-aged patients, future cohorts of older adults will probably have higher rates of SUDs than the present cohort [32]. Epidemiological trends suggest that the number of older adults with SUD will increase from 2.5 million people in 1999 to 5.0 million by 2020 [36]. This demographic trend suggests that there will be overall higher rates of older adults with coexisting bipolar disorder and substance use disorder [32]. Studies of mixed-age patients report that bipolar disorder and SUD are associated with increased mood instability [37], greater rates of medication non-adherence [38], and an increased duration of depressive and manic episodes [39]. The SUD–bipolar disorder comorbidity has been associated with higher rates of hospitalizations and suicides [8, 32, 40] and with longer time to symptom remission [41]. Recent studies suggest that among those with bipolar disorder across age groups, even moderate alcohol intake is associated with higher levels of inter-episode sub-syndromal symptoms [42].

Mortality rates may be higher for younger patients with the compared to older patients with bipolar disorder and the comorbidity [43]. Some investigators report that average life expectancy for younger bipolar patients is reduced by 10–12 years [43]. Major causes of the shortened life span are end-stage complications of alcohol dependence, and overdose and toxicity from stimulants and opioids [44]. Alcohol and other substance use disorders have been associated with increased risk of all-cause mortality for both bipolar disorder and depression [44]. The risk of suicide is elevated among bipolar disorder patients and accounts for a 15–20 % rate of suicide-related mortality [45]. Patients with comorbid bipolar disorder and substance use disorders regardless of age or gender are at least twofold more likely to attempt suicide than the general population [46, 47]. SUDs and coexisting bipolar disorder may be associated with aggression, impulsivity, and hostility that increase the propensity to act on suicidal thoughts [48]. Older adults with mood and affective disorders are at highest risk for suicide, and coexisting SUDs further increase their risk of suicide attempts and suicide-related mortality [49].

Research is scarce on resilience factors predictive of long-term remission of bipolar illness in the geriatric bipolar-SUD population; however, potential resilience factors include lower impulsivity, greater number of years of education [50], and earlier age of diagnosis [51]. Vulnerability factors include greater number of depressive episodes and higher scores for impulsivity and risk taking; lifetime trauma exposure [52]; and criminal justice involvement (more common among bipolar disorder patients than those in the general population and most common among bipolar-SUD patients within this group) [53]. Predictors of substance treatment outcome in this population have yet to be identified, though treatment outcome studies are discussed below.

5.4 Epidemiology, Diagnosis, and Treatment for Specific SUDs among Older Age Bipolar Disorder Patients

5.4.1 Alcohol

5.4.1.1 Epidemiology

An estimated 1–2 % of older adults in the general population have alcohol use disorders (AUD) [54]. Specific estimates of geriatric bipolar disorder patients with this SUD range from 13 to 25 %, making it the most common substance use disorder [12]. Research on the relationship between alcohol use disorder severity and suicide risk has produced mixed results [46]. Carra [46] reported that both alcohol dependence and alcohol abuse were associated with increased risk of suicide attempts.

5.4.1.2 Diagnosis

Guidelines for the workup of alcohol use disorders among geriatric bipolar patients are described in *Substance Abuse among Older Adults. Treatment Improvement Protocol (TIP) Series 26* published by SAMHS [55]. Of special note is the Michigan Alcoholism Screening Test-Geriatric Version, which has been adapted for use in this population for other substances and validated for different ethnic groups [56].

5.4.1.3 Treatment

Since patients with comorbid psychiatric disorders are routinely excluded from clinical trials of new treatments for SUD, the safety and efficacy of existing treatments for alcohol use and other SUDs are emerging areas of investigation for patients with bipolar disorder [57]. Given that adults over age 60 are also often excluded from these studies, there is even less information about effective, safe treatment options for older adults with the bipolar disorder–SUD comorbidity. Furthermore, our understanding of psychiatric and medical comorbidity in bipolar disorder derives largely from studies of younger and mixed-age samples [12]. However, it is a clinical priority to identify more effective evidence-based pharmacological [58] and behavioral treatments for comorbid AUD and bipolar disorder across age groups given the role of alcohol dependence in contributing to occupational dysfunction in bipolar disorder through a variety of mechanisms [59] Addressing substance abuse may beneficially impact the course of bipolar disorder. Improved stabilization of bipolar disorder is also likely to aid substance disorder treatment compliance [8].

Patients with AUD and a co-occurring psychiatric disorder have more complex symptoms than patients with either disorder alone, are least likely to engage in psychosocial interventions, and benefit the most from a full arsenal of treatment options including psychotherapy as well as pharmacotherapy [60, 61]. Although the cumulative scope and impact of bipolar disorder with co-occurring alcohol use disorder across age groups have been well documented, there are little data on selection and implementation of optimal treatment strategies [62, 63]. None of the current FDA approved treatments for alcohol use (i.e., disulfiram, naltrexone, and acamprosate) have been demonstrated to be clearly effective among patients with bipolar disorder [57]. Valproate [64] and the combination of lithium and valproate have been shown to improve mood symptoms as well as reduce days of heavy drinking [65]. Several studies suggest that quetiapine lacks efficacy in the treatment of comorbid bipolar disorder and AUD [66, 67]. Other studies of treatment with acamprosate and naltrexone have also failed to show a statistically significant benefit in patients with bipolar disorder and AUD [68, 69].

Several investigators suggest that topiramate is effective in reducing heavy drinking among individuals with alcohol dependence [22, 70]. However, a randomized, placebo-controlled trial of topiramate for mixed-age adults with bipolar disorder and alcohol dependence (compared with a general population of alcohol dependent patients) ($N = 12$) did not support adjunctive use of topiramate [71].

Behavioral therapies for alcohol dependence—including 12-step programs, cognitive behavioral therapy for relapse prevention, and motivational interviewing —merit further exploration, including through randomized controlled studies, for older adults with bipolar disorder. In one mixed methods study of dually diagnosed patients, including OABD patients, the peer support group and peer education emphases of 12-step programs such as Alcoholics Anonymous were identified as helpful even by patients with significant psychiatric symptom burden (i.e., while still experiencing some level of psychosis or mania) [72]. Pilot studies of cognitive behavioral therapy for relapse prevention (including "Third Wave" cognitive behavioral approaches such as mindfulness-based relapse prevention) have shown significant benefit for older adults, including veterans, though have not been specifically tested in older adults with bipolar disorder and comorbid alcohol dependence [73]. Similarly, while case series reports on using integrated motivational interviewing and cognitive behavioral therapies have demonstrated promise among bipolar disorder patients (across age groups) with comorbid AUDs, there is a lack of randomized controlled trials of these psychosocial treatments for OABD patients. Potential future randomized clinical trials could apply existing knowledge to the OABD population, such as from protocols developed by Schmitz and Grillion [74] and Weiss et al. [75], including in integrated community-based group therapy.

5.4.2 Sedative-Hypnotics

5.4.2.1 Epidemiology

Substance use disorders involving benzodiazepines as well as other sedative-hypnotics (such as zolpidem, eszopiclone, and zaleplon) are common despite the well-known adverse effects of these medications among elderly patients (including increased fall risk and cognitive impairment). The estimated prevalence of benzodiazepine use in the general geriatric patient population is 11 % based on limited studies [76], making this SUD in some settings (e.g., outpatient psychiatry) nearly as common as alcohol use disorders. The risk of long-term continuous sedative-hypnotic use (not recommended by most prescribing guidelines) is greater among elderly patients, reflecting greater rates of anxiety and insomnia within this group [77]. It is not yet clear what role gender and ethnicity may play in prevalence. However, Petrovic et al. [78] and colleagues found that female gender, widowed status, borderline personality disorder, and anxiety disorders were risk factors for benzodiazepine dependence, and immigrant patients from developing countries may be at particular risk given high population-wide use (up to 26.7 % among women over age 60 and 14 % among males) of long-acting benzodiazepines for extended duration in Latin America, for example [79]. While studies to identify risk factors within older adults with bipolar disorder are still lacking, bipolar disorder is a known risk factor for benzodiazepine dependence in general due to the high rate of anxiety disorder comorbidity, with nearly 50 % of adults with BD meeting anxiety disorders criteria per lifetime. Further, some raise the possibility that anxiety symptoms, which are often treated and self-treated with sedative-hypnotics, may be primary features of bipolar illness rather than a comorbidity [80].

5.4.2.2 Diagnosis

In addition to the SAMHSA guidelines referenced above, tools such as the A-FRAMES (Assessment, Feedback, Responsibility, Advice, Menu, Empathy, and Self-efficacy) Questionnaire modify existing motivational interviewing tools to address geriatric issues [81]. Other tools are being developed for home evaluations, for more sensitive detection, and for use among prescribers (e.g., STOPP—Screening Tool of Older Person's Potentially Inappropriate Prescriptions) in inpatient and outpatient settings [82].

5.4.2.3 Treatment

Pharmacotherapy rests on use of benzodiazepines in detoxification taper protocol, with potential adjunctive medications proposed such as acetylcholinesterase inhibitors [83], phenobarbital [84], and oxcarbazepine [85]. These medications have yet to be tested among geriatric bipolar disorder patients in treatment for chronic benzodiazepine or other sedative-hypnotic use but hold relevant potential given wide baseline use for mood and cognition within the population. As for other older adults or other groups of patients with advanced liver disease, including cirrhosis, benzodiazepines that do not get oxidized by the liver (oxazepam and lorazepam) are preferable to chlordiazepoxide to minimize the risk of oversedation, accumulation, or toxicity, also given that oxazepam and lorazepam are shorter acting [86]. It is also worth noting that, contrary to the practice (in the 1980s) of "only using alprazolam to detoxify patients from alprazolam," this motto is not supported by clinical evidence, and the recommendation is to use either oxazepam or lorazepam among elderly patients, with phenobarbital substitution also a possibility. Falls, myocardial infarctions, and delirium without signs of autonomic hyperactivity are risks of benzodiazepine withdrawal in the elderly general population, to which dually diagnosed patients may be particularly vulnerable given polypharmacy; thus, medically supervised benzodiazepine withdrawal among OABD patients is critical [87].

5.4.3 Cocaine

5.4.3.1 Epidemiology

Stimulant-induced psychosis or mania can mimic affective disorder-induced episodes in those without bipolar disorder. Among dual diagnosis patients, stimulants may also exacerbate actual mood episodes. Thus, it is critical to consider these substance use disorders (SUDs) on the differential diagnosis given high medical sequelae potentially more severe in elderly populations: primarily cardiovascular and neurologic, including tachycardia and other arrhythmias, cerebrovascular accidents (CVA), seizures (for which elderly patients may be at additional risk already due to polypharmacy), cocaine- and amphetamine-induced myocardial ischemia and infarction, and infectious diseases [88].

Notably, over 80 % of cocaine users, even those without comorbid bipolar disorder as a risk factor, experience paranoia. Further, upwards of 55 % in one cohort reported cocaine-related violent behaviors [89]. Both homicide and suicide risk are elevated in relation to the length and severity of cocaine use. Psychiatric symptoms are more pronounced among crack cocaine users than those dependent on other forms of cocaine (i.e., intranasal powdered cocaine) [89]. Male gender appears to be predictive of cocaine use in the elderly population, though studies specific to geriatric bipolar patients are still lacking. One emergency department study, conducted over a 6-month period of ED visits made by persons above the age of 60, demonstrated that 2 % of these individuals had cocaine-positive urines, with an average age of 66 and 90 % male [90].

5.4.3.2 Diagnosis

Diagnosis by routine toxicology may prove difficult given the short half-life of cocaine (remaining in urine 4–8 h after the dose, with benzoylecgonine (the psychoactive metabolite of cocaine) potentially remaining in urine for up to 60 h after use) and trends toward episodic or binge rather than daily use [91]. Specialized screening tools are under investigation, including adaptation of the Decision Balance Questionnaire for assessing vulnerability to cocaine relapse [92], although none have been validated for geriatric bipolar patients to date.

5.4.3.3 Treatment

Pharmacological studies designed for bipolar disorder patients with coexisting cocaine use disorder have shown initial promising results, including for citicoline, lamotrigine, and quetiapine in recent trials. Other drugs that have been considered in case reports, but not yet tested in randomized clinical studies, include gabapentin, mifepristone, valproate, and pramipexole. A randomized placebo-controlled trial of the cognitive enhancer citicoline, a moderator of phospholipid metabolism that increases acetylcholine levels, demonstrated improved declarative memory and an increased abstinence rate from cocaine, although citicoline did not improve mood [93]. In a 10-week randomized controlled trial of lamotrigine among bipolar disorder patients (depressed or in a mixed episode) with cocaine dependence, self-reported cocaine use (measured by dollars spent) decreased significantly. A follow-up uncontrolled replication study showed improvements in measures of cocaine craving, mood, and drug use [94], while an earlier open-label study also showed a significant decrease in craving [95]. A more recent study showed a similar reduction in cocaine use with benefits occurring earlier in treatment and attenuating over time [96]. Notably, drug dreams, predictors of use and correlated with research study treatment survival among patients with SUDs, also appeared to decrease in other larger studies of lamotrigine [97]. There is less evidence of quetiapine's efficacy for the bipolar cocaine dependence comorbidity, with additional concerns of the possible abuse liability of this drug, though an open-label study ($N = 17$) showed good tolerability and improvement of psychiatric symptoms [98].

5.4.4 Amphetamines

5.4.4.1 Epidemiology

The rates of amphetamine use disorders (including prescribed psychostimulants, as well as illicit drugs such as methamphetamine) are unknown for geriatric bipolar patients specifically. However, given overlap between core affective disorder symptoms (such as impulsivity, risk taking, and euphoria) and the intoxication syndrome for amphetamines, as well as elevated rates of attention-deficit–hyperactivity disorders (ADHD) within the population, bipolar disorder patients in general are at particular risk [99]. Of the estimated 5 % of adults in the general population, over 20 % may have comorbid bipolar disorder [100].

While use of stimulants within the population carries a risk of mania, as well as the medical complications discussed above for cocaine (including cardiovascular and neurologic), studies are also underway of stimulant augmentation of mood stabilizers to address bipolar depression, with preliminary promising results [101, 102].

Prevalence of stimulant dependence estimated from a voluntary bipolar disorder patient registry ($N = 100$) was 2.8 % among those with bipolar I patients, with an age range of 18–65 and a specific prevalence unavailable for patients over age 60 [103]. While specific trends by ethnicity or gender are not known for geriatric bipolar patients, it is notable that bipolar disorder (along with anxiety disorders) was highly correlated with stimulant dependence in a group of gay and transgendered (GBT) men seeking outpatient psychiatric treatment, making elderly LGBT populations a potential priority for outreach and assessment [104].

5.4.4.2 Diagnosis

In addition to a thorough medical workup, including electrocardiogram and urine drug screen (which remain positive for amphetamines for 1–2 days after use), screening through Physical Symptom Screening Triggers checklists (as described in the SAMHSA Tip 26) that assess sleep changes, anxiety, agitation, and availability of stimulants in the household (i.e., prescribed to a family member) may be of particular relevance [1].

5.4.4.3 Treatment

A limited evidence base exists for adjunctive treatments of stimulant dependence among older adults with bipolar disorder. Nevertheless, effective mood stabilization remains the central strategy, and lithium's neuroprotective benefits may ameliorate stimulant-induced reduction in brain choline levels [105]. Among behavioral treatments, in addition to those based on motivational interviewing, 12-step programs, and dual diagnosis models, recent research on contingency management (where participants earn vouchers or other compensation for continued program participation and/or continued verified negative urine screens) has been shown to decrease stimulant use among both younger and older bipolar disorder patients in community health settings [106]. Pharmacotherapy showing initial promise includes citicoline [107] (a randomized controlled trial demonstrating improved mood symptoms among mixed-age patients) and atypical antipsychotic medications. In a trial of quetiapine and risperidone among bipolar disorder patients of age 20–50, patients reported decreased drug craving related to decreased drug use [108]. Research among older adults with BD and psychostimulant use is warranted.

5.4.5 Prescription Opioids

5.4.5.1 Epidemiology

The most commonly abused prescription opioids by general population adults (across age group) are hydrocodone and oxycodone, although both have less abuse potential than the more potent mu agonists, morphine or fentanyl [109]. In large epidemiologic studies such as the National Epidemiologic Study on Alcohol and Related Conditions, there is evidence for bidirectional relationships between bipolar disorder and non-medical use of prescription opioids. Prescription opioid use appears to be a precipitating factor in bipolar mood episodes, the presentation of bipolar disorder, as well as a frequent complication of previously diagnosed bipolar disorder [110]. Male gender and young age are risk factors for prescription opioid use in the population [111], with a 28 % prevalence of bipolar disorder among male patients in one inpatient cohort, and mania a key risk of opioid detoxification [112, 113]. While men appear to be more likely to misuse prescription opioids, women are more likely to receive combination regimens of prescription opioids and sedative-hypnotics, placing them at possibly greater risk of overdose [114]. Other risk factors for prescription opioid use disorders include a positive family history of substance use, as well as personal exposure to violence and sexual assault, with some studies confirming that the diagnosis of bipolar illness constitutes a risk factor for subsequent trauma exposure for both men and women [115]. While comorbidity studies in older adults with bipolar disorder have been limited, rates of prescription opioid overdose deaths increased between 2000 and 2014 for patients over age 55 [116], with polypharmacy, medical comorbidities, and treatment refractory pain among the risk factors for mortality [117]. Up to 10 % of geriatric medical outpatients screen positive for bipolar disorder, type I or II, in cohorts receiving some form of an opioid pain regimen. Therefore, the increased risk of suicide and impulsive or accidental overdose that may be associated with bipolar illness merits thorough assessment for prescription opioid misuse among older adults with bipolar disorder [118].

5.4.5.2 Diagnosis

In addition to standard toxicology screening, physical examination findings (such as pupillary size changes with intoxication versus withdrawal), and workup for medical presentations of prescription opioid misuse (such as chronic pain, new onset weakness, daytime somnolence, or altered mental status), strategies such as Prescription Monitoring Database screening for multiple overlapping opioid prescriptions and other behaviors suggestive of misuse (such as running out of prescriptions early; reports of sharing prescriptions with friends; and hostile or abusive speech directed at providers when requests for early refills are not granted) are recommended [119]. The "opioid epidemic," which as of 2012 includes 2.1 million Americans who misuse prescription drugs, has led to the development and validation of multiple screening tools, including the Opioid Risk Tool, SOAPP-R (Screener and Opioid Assessment for Pain), DIRE (Diagnosis, Intractability, Risk Efficacy), Hospital Misuse Checklist, and Brief Risk Questionnaire. However, these are still pending validation among older adults in the general population and older adults with bipolar disorder who may be at greater risk for prescription opioid misuse [120].

5.4.5.3 Treatment

The current standard of care for all age groups, including geriatric patients, is opioid detoxification followed by aftercare. Such aftercare may take the form of a residential, partial hospital or intensive outpatient level of care that follows 12-step program guidelines. Outpatient supervision is still recommended (including scheduled and random urine drug screens, narcotics contracts around safe use, and, where necessary, visiting nurse services or other in-home monitoring of use) [121]. Dual diagnosis inpatient admission during initial opioid detoxification is critical for older adults with bipolar disorder given the risk of mania during the withdrawal period. In the outpatient context, office-based opioid treatment (OBOT) and methadone maintenance treatment (MMT) referral offer not only safe long-term treatment options, but also possible additional benefit for bipolar disorder patients given mood-stabilizing and antidepressant properties of methadone and buprenorphine [122]. Additionally, gabapentin may play a unique adjunctive mood stabilization and palliative role, with clinical trials evidence still lacking [123].

5.4.6 Illicit Opioids

5.4.6.1 Epidemiology

Illicit opioid use appears to be less common among bipolar disorder patients than alcohol, cocaine, or cannabis. McElroy et al. [101] found an 8 % opioid dependence prevalence in a sample of 288 bipolar disorder patients, while Chengappa et al. [98] detected a 5.6 % prevalence from a voluntary bipolar disorder patient registry. Heroin use appears to be more common than fentanyl or methadone dependence, although combination opioid disorders are common and carry higher overdose risk, with the major risk factor for illicit opioid dependence among geriatric patients being historic use (i.e., use initiated during younger years) [54]. It is not known whether there is a group of older adults with bipolar disorder who initiate illicit heroin or fentanyl use in later life, reflective of the larger need for expanding the knowledge base about substance disorders generally among older adults. Older adults, in particular, experience medical complications from illicit opioid use such as infections from intravenous drug use, pulmonary disease, and cardiovascular illness, with opioids increasing the risk of ventricular arrhythmias. In the general US population, risk factors that predispose to heroin dependence include early age of initiation (with over half those individuals who "ever used" progressing to physiologic and psychological dependence), reduced cost and chemical purity in certain geographic regions (i.e., the Northeastern USA), low socioeconomic status (including homelessness), and positive family history of any psychopathology [124].

5.4.6.2 Diagnosis

Diagnostic assessment of illicit opioid use is similar to the assessment of prescription opioid misuse. Specific physical examination findings include needle marks in skin and septal perforation and epistaxis given increased rates of snorting versus injecting due to increased purity of available heroin trafficked since the 1990s in the USA [125]. Hair testing remains positive for heroin up to 90 days after use.

5.4.6.3 Treatment

Although either buprenorphine or methadone treatment offers standard of care options for those in recovery from heroin dependence, preliminary evidence exists for advantages to methadone clinic management for older adults, including the management of medical comorbidities such as diabetes mellitus, hepatitis C, and gastrointestinal cancers given the highly structured and regulated environment of the methadone clinic, analogous to other directly observed therapies such as for the treatment of infectious diseases [126]. The aging of long-standing opioid dependent patients in maintenance treatment makes treatment research focused on dual diagnosis geriatric patients, including those with bipolar disorder, a public health priority [127].

5.4.7 Cannabis

5.4.7.1 Epidemiology

Among mixed-age populations, SUD rates are reported to be as high as 44 % with cannabis being the lifetime most frequently abused substance (second to alcohol) [128]. Individuals with bipolar disorder and cannabis use disorders may be at increased risk of suicide attempts [129]. Research is lacking on the use of synthetic cannabinoids among bipolar disorder patients including geriatric populations; however, within diverse chronically and severely mentally ill populations, these variants ["K2"; "spice"; and cyclohexylphenols that mimic the effects of Δ9-tetrahydrocannabinol (THC)] have been linked to severe psychosis, treatment refractory mood episodes, and significant functional impairments [130, 131]. Among geriatric patients in the general population, data are limited on patterns of cannabis use; however, novel methods of estimating prevalence—including analyses of registries of medical marijuana clinics and Internet message board analyses—have been explored for other "hidden populations" and could be applicable to elderly users [132, 133].

5.4.7.2 Diagnosis

Marijuana remains positive in the urine for up to 30 days after use. Specific signs, symptoms, and odor are associated with marijuana use such as diaphoresis, scleral injection, and pungent odor resembling skunk, pine, or lemon.

5.4.7.3 Treatment

Persistent cannabis use has been shown to adversely affect long-term treatment outcomes of bipolar disorder, including among patients receiving and compliant with pharmacotherapy regimens that included a mood stabilizer and atypical antipsychotic medication [134]. Effective treatment for those with major mental illness is further complicated by an evolving psychosocial and legal context, in which marijuana is now legal in twenty-four states in the USA, as well as the District of Columbia. Although abstinence is supported as a treatment goal for older adults with bipolar disorder and comorbid cannabis use disorder to help prevent hospitalizations and reduce psychosis-driven violence and suicide, the increasing availability of cannabis through legalization could make this goal even more challenging to achieve [129]. While not a life-threatening syndrome, cannabis withdrawal includes sleep disturbance, gastrointestinal symptoms, and dysphoria and serves as a focus for initial intensive and symptom-targeted treatment including among older adults with bipolar disorder. To date, no pharmacotherapy regimens have been approved specifically for cannabis withdrawal among OABD or adults with bipolar disorder, although lithium showed preliminary efficacy in two recent open-label studies at increasing rates of abstinence, with valproate in conjunction with psychotherapy less well tolerated or effective [135]. Other agents showing initial promise include dronabinol (an FDA-approved cannabinoid agonist), buspirone, *N*-acetylcysteine (thought to reduce drug-seeking behavior through glutamatergic mechanisms), and entacapone (a catechol-*O*-methyl transferase inhibitor affecting dopamine metabolism) [136]. These medications have shown preliminary evidence of tolerability and reduction in cannabis craving. Randomized controlled clinical trials of these medications and also cannabis replacement therapy (CRT) with nabiximols and other candidate molecules [137] among older adults with bipolar disorder are warranted.

5.5 Summary and Future Directions for Treatment Research

Similar to younger and middle-aged individuals with BD, pharmacotherapy remains the mainstay of treatment for older adults with bipolar disorder including those with substance use disorders. Given the critical role of a wide range of behavioral therapies for SUDs, further research on integrated behavioral and pharmacotherapy treatments is warranted, along with more inclusive clinical trials research identifying safe and effective adjunctive drug treatments for older adults with bipolar disorder in recovery.

Clinical Pearls

- Bipolar disorder has the highest rates of substance use disorders of any psychiatric illness.
- A paucity of research has been devoted to substance use disorder among older people with bipolar disorder.
- Patients with bipolar disorder and substance use disorders have more frequent hospitalizations and a more severe and disabling disease course.
- Prescription drug abuse is an emerging major public health concern that warrants attention and research in older people with bipolar disorder.
- Research on the treatment of people with bipolar disorder and substance use disorders, while quite limited, suggests that standard treatments for bipolar disorder (e.g., valproate and lamotrigine) and for substance use disorders (e.g., naltrexone) may be useful in this dual diagnosis population.

References

1. Regler DA, Farmer MD, Rae D et al. Comorbidity of mental disorders with alcohol and drug abuse. JAMA. 1990;264(19):2511–8.
2. Substance abuse among older adults. Treatment Improvement Protocol Series Substance Abuse and Mental Health Services Administration (SAMHA) http://store.samhsa.gov/product/TIP-26-Substance-Abuse-Among-Older-Adults/SMA12-3918.
3. Grey C, Hall PB. Considerations of prescription opioid abuse and misuse among older adults in West Virginia—an under-recognized population at risk. W V Med J. 2016;112(3):42–7.
4. Dallaspezia S, Suzuki M, Benedetti F. Chronobiological therapy for mood disorders. Curr Psychiatry Rep. 2015;17(12):95.
5. Grant BF, Stinson FS, Dawson DA, et al. Prevalence and co-occurrence of substance use disorders and independent mood and anxiety disorder. Results from the National Epidemiologic Survey on Alcohol and Related Conditions. Arch Gen Psychiatry. 2004;61:807–16.
6. Hasin DS, Stinson FS, Ogburn E, et al. Prevalence, correlates, disability, and comorbidity of DSM-IV alcohol abuse and dependence in the United States. Results from the National Epidemiologic Survey on Alcohol and Related Conditions. Arch Gen Psychiatry. 2007;64:830–42.
7. Merikangas KR, Akiskal HS, Angst J, et al. Lifetime and 12-month prevalence of bipolar spectrum disorder in the National Comorbidity Survey Replication. Arch Gen Psychiatry. 2007;64:543–52.
8. Cassidy F, Ahearn EP, Carroll BJ. Substance abuse in bipolar disorder. Bipolar Disord. 2001;3:194–200.
9. Sajatovic M, Blow FC, Ignacio RV. Psychiatric comorbidity in older adults with bipolar disorder. Int J Geriatr Psychiatry. 2006;21:582–7.
10. Goldstein B, Velyvis V, Parkh V. The association between moderate alcohol use and illness severity: a preliminary report. J Clin Psychiatry. 2006;67:102–6.

11. Kilbourne AM, Haas GL, Mulsant BH, Bauer MS, Pincus HA. Concurrent psychiatric diagnoses by age and race among persons with bipolar disorder. Psychiatr Serv. 2004;55(8):931–3.
12. Dols A, Rhebergen D, Beekman A, et al. Psychiatric and medical comorbidities: results from a bipolar elderly cohort study. Am J Geriatr Psychiatry. 2014;22:1066–74.
13. Depp CA, Jeste DV. Bipolar disorder in older adults: a critical review. Bipolar Disord. 2004;6(5):343–67.
14. Marsh WK, Ketter TA, Crawford SL, Johnson JV, Kroll-Desrosiers AR, Rothschild AJ. Progression of female reproductive stages associated with bipolar illness exacerbation. Bipolar Disord. 2012;14(5):515–26.
15. Weiss RD, Ostacher MDJ, Otto M. Does recovery from substance use disorder matter in patients with bipolar disorder? J Clin Psychiatry. 2005;61:361–7.
16. Sonne SC, Brady KT, Morton WA. Substance abuse and bipolar affective disorder. J Nerv Ment Dis. 1994;182:349–52.
17. Altshuler LL, Kupka RW, Hellemann G, Frye MA, Sugar CA, McElroy SL, Nolen WA, Grunze H, Leverich GS, Keck PE, Zermeno M, Post RM, Suppes T. Gender and depressive symptoms in 711 patients with bipolar disorder evaluated prospectively in the Stanley Foundation bipolar treatment outcome network. Am J Psychiatry. 2010;167(6):708–15.
18. Kerridge BT, Saha TD, Chou SP, Zhang H, Jung J, Ruan WJ, Smith SM, Huang B, Hasin DS. Gender and nonmedical prescription opioid use and DSM-5 nonmedical prescription opioid use disorder. Results from the National Epidemiologic Survey on Alcohol and Related Conditions—III. Drug Alcohol Depend. 2015;1(156):47–56.
19. Jarvis GE. Changing psychiatric perception of African-Americans with affective disorders. J Nerv Ment Dis. 2012;200(12):1031–40.
20. Schaffer A, Isometsä ET, Azorin JM, Cassidy F, Goldstein T, Rihmer Z, Sinyor M, Tondo L, Moreno DH, Turecki G, Reis C, Kessing LV, Ha K, Weizman A, Beautrais A, Chou YH, Diazgranados N, Levitt AJ, Zarate CA Jr, Yatham L. A review of factors associated with greater likelihood of suicide attempts and suicide deaths in bipolar disorder: part II of a report of the International Society for Bipolar Disorders Task Force on Suicide in Bipolar Disorder. Aust N Z J Psychiatry. 2015;49(11):1006–20.
21. Gonzalez JM, Bowden CL, Berman N, Frank E, Bauer MS, Kogan JN, Alegría M, Miklowitz DJ. One-year treatment outcomes of African-American and Hispanic patients with bipolar I or II disorder in STEP BD. Psychiatr Serv. 2010;61(2):164–72.
22. Johnson KR, Johnson SL. Inadequate treatment of black Americans with bipolar disorder. Psychiatr Serv. 2014;65(2):255–8.
23. Kemp DE, Sylvia LG, Calabrese JR, Nierenberg AA, Thase ME, Reilly-Harrington NA, Ostacher MJ, Leon AC, Ketter TA, Friedman ES, Bowden CL, Rabideau DJ, Pencina M, Iosifescu DV, LiTMUS Study Group. General medical burden in bipolar disorder: findings from the LiTMUS comparative effectiveness trial. Acta Psychiatr Scand. 2014;129(1):24–34.
24. Sentell T, Unick GJ, Ahn HJ, Braun KL, Miyamura J, Shumway M. Illness severity and psychiatric hospitalization rates among Asian Americans and Pacific Islanders. Psychiatr Serv. 2013;64(11):1095–102.
25. Fleck DE, Keck PE Jr, Corey KB, Strakowski SM. Factors associated with medication adherence in African American and white patients with bipolar disorder. J Clin Psychiatry. 2005;66(5):646–52.
26. Carson NJ, Vesper A, Chen CN, Lê Cook B. Quality of follow-up after hospitalization for mental illness among patients from racial-ethnic minority groups. Psychiatr Serv. 2014;65(7):888–96.
27. Breland JY, Chee CP, Zulman DM. Racial differences in chronic conditions and sociodemographic characteristics among high-utilizing veterans. J Racial Ethn Health Dispar. 2015;2(2):167–75.

28. Hamilton JE, Passos IC, de Azevedo Cardoso T, Jansen K, Allen M, Begley CE, Soares JC, Kapczinski F. Predictors of psychiatric readmission among patients with bipolar disorder at an academic safety-net hospital. Aust N Z J Psychiatry. 2016;50(6):584–93.
29. Lagerberg TV, Andreassen OA, Ringen PA, Berg AO, Larsson S, Agartz I, Sundet K, Melle I. Excessive substance use in bipolar disorder is associated with impaired functioning rather than clinical characteristics: a descriptive study. BMC Psychiatry. 2010;27(10):9.
30. Campbell NL, Boustani MA, Skopelja EN, Gao S, Unverzagt FW, Murray MD. Medication adherence in older adults with cognitive impairment: a systematic evidence-based review. Am J Geriatr Pharmacother. 2012;10(3):165–77.
31. Lala SV, Sajatovic M. Medical and psychiatric comorbidities among elderly individuals with bipolar disorder: a literature review. J Geriatr Psychiatry Neurol. 2012;25(1):20–5.
32. Brennan P, Nichols K, Moos R. Long-term use of VA mental health services by older patient with substance use disorders. Psychiatr Serv. 2002;53:836–41.
33. McGinty EE, Goldman HH, Pescosolido B, Barry CL. Portraying mental illness and drug addiction as treatable health conditions: effects of a randomized experiment on stigma and discrimination. Soc Sci Med. 2015;126:73–85.
34. Bommersbach TJ, Lapid MI, Rummans TA, Morse RM. Geriatric alcohol use disorder: a review for primary care physicians. Mayo Clin Proc. 2015;90(5):659–66.
35. DeMers S, Dinsio K, Carlson W. Psychiatric care of the older adult: an overview for primary care. Med Clin N Am. 2014;98(5):1145–68.
36. Gfroerer M, Penne M, Pemberton M, et al. Substance abuse treatment need among older adults in 2020: the impact of the aging baby-boom cohort. Drug Alcohol Depend. 2002;69:127–35.
37. Ostacher MJ, Perlis R, Nierenberg AA, et al. Impact of substance use disorders on recovery from episodes of depression in bipolar patients: prospective data from the Systematic Treatment Enhancement Program for Bipolar Disorder (STEP-BD). Am J Psychiatry. 2010;167:289–97.
38. Keck PE, McElroy S, Strakowski S, et al. 12-month outcome of patients with bipolar disorder following hospitalization for man or mixed episode. Am J Psychiatry. 1998;155:646–52.
39. Strakowski SM, DelBello MP, Fleck DE, et al. The impact of substance abuse on the course of bipolar disorder. Biol Psychiatry. 2000;48:477–85.
40. Hawton K, Sutton L, Haw C, et al. Suicide and attempted suicide in bipolar disorder: a systematic review or risk factors. J Clin Psychiatry. 2005;66:693–704.
41. Goldberg JF, Garno JL, Leon AC. A history substance abuse complicates remission form acute mania in bipolar disorder. J Clin Psychiatry. 1999;60:733–40.
42. Paykel E, Abbott R, Morriss R. Subsyndromal and syndromal symptoms in the longitudinal course of bipolar disorder Br J Psychiatry. 2006;189:117–23.
43. Kessing LV, Vradi E, Andersen PK. Life expectancy in bipolar disorder. Bipolar Disord. 2015;17(5):543–8.
44. Hjorthøj C, Østergaard ML, Benros ME, Toftdahl NG, Erlangsen A, Andersen JT, Nordentoft M. Association between alcohol and substance use disorders and all-cause and cause-specific mortality in schizophrenia, bipolar disorder, and unipolar depression: a nationwide, prospective, register-based study. Lancet Psychiatry. 2015;2(9):801–8.
45. Miller C, Bauer MS. Excess mortality in bipolar disorders. Curr Psychiatry Rep. 2014;16(11):499.
46. Carra G, Bartoli F, Crocamo C. Attempted suicide in people with co-occurring bipolar and substance use disorders: Systematic review and meta-analysis. J Affect Disord. 2014;167:125–35.
47. Dalton EJ, Cate-Carter TD, Mundo E, Parikh SV, Kennedy JL. Suicide risk in bipolar patients: the role of co-morbid substance use disorders. Bipolar Disord. 2003;5(1):58–61.

48. Watkins HB, Meyer TD. Is there an empirical link between impulsivity and suicidality in bipolar disorders? A review of the current literature and the potential psychological implications of the relationship. Bipolar Disord. 2013;15(5):542–58.
49. Kiosses DN, Szanto K, Alexopoulos GS. Suicide in older adults: the role of emotions and cognition. Curr Psychiatry Rep. 2014;16(11):495.
50. Choi JW, Cha B, Jang J, Park CS, Kim BJ, Lee CS, Lee SJ. Resilience and impulsivity in euthymic patients with bipolar disorder. J Affect Disord. 2015;1(170):172–7.
51. Tse S, Murray G, Chung KF, Davidson L, Ng KL, Yu CH. Exploring the recovery concept in bipolar disorder: a decision tree analysis of psychosocial correlates of recovery stages. Bipolar Disord. 2014;16(4):366–77.
52. Aas M, Henry C, Andreassen OA, Bellivier F, Melle I, Etain B. The role of childhood trauma in bipolar disorders. Int J Bipolar Disord. 2016;4(1):2.
53. Fovet T, Geoffroy PA, Vaiva G, Adins C, Thomas P, Amad A. Individuals with bipolar disorder and their relationship with the criminal justice system: a critical review. Psychiatr Serv. 2015;66(4):348–53.
54. Oslin DW. Evidence-based treatment of geriatric substance abuse. Psychiatr Clin N Am. 2005;28(4):897–911.
55. Substance abuse among older adults. Treatment Improvement Protocol (TIP) Series 26. Rockville, MD: SAMHSA; 2012.
56. Kano MY, Santos MA, Pillon SC. Use of alcohol in the elderly: transcultural validation of the Michigan Alcoholism Screening Test-Geriatric Version (MAST-G). Rev Esc Enferm USP. 2014;48(4):648–55.
57. Tolliver BK, Densantis SM, Brown DG, et al. A randomized, double blind, placebo controlled clinical trial of acamprosate in alcohol dependent individuals with bipolar disorder. A preliminary report. Bipolar Disord. 2012;14:54–63.
58. Vornik LA, Brown ES. Management of comorbid bipolar disorder and substance abuse. J Clin Psychiatry. 2006;67(Suppl 7):24–30.
59. Carroll KM, Onken LS. Behavioral therapies for drug abuse. Am J Psychiatry. 2005;162(8):1452–60.
60. Kelley TM, Daley DC. Integrated treatment of substance use and psychiatric disorder. Soc Work Public Health. 2013;28:388–406.
61. Wenze SJ, Gaudiano BA, Weinstock LM, Tezanos KM, Miller IW. Adjunctive psychosocial intervention following hospital discharge for patients with bipolar disorder and comorbid substance use: a pilot randomized controlled trial. Psychiatry Res. 2015;228(3):516–25.
62. Frye M, Salloum IM. Bipolar disorder and comorbid alcoholism: prevalence rate and treatment considerations. Bipolar Disord. 2006;8:677–85.
63. Singh J, Zarate CA. Pharmacological treatment of psychiatric comorbidity in bipolar disorder: a review of controlled studies. Bipolar Disord. 2006;8:677–85.
64. Salloum IM, Cornelius JR, Daley DC, Kirisci L, Himmelhoch JM, Thase ME. Efficacy of valproate maintenance in patients with bipolar disorder and alcoholism: a double-blind placebo-controlled study. Arch Gen Psychiatry. 2005;62(1):37–45.
65. Kemp D, Gai J, Gabict S, et al. A 6 month double-blind maintenance trial of lithium monotherapy vs the combination of lithium and divalproex for rapid-cycling bipolar disorder and co-occurring substance abuse or dependence. J Clin Psychiatry. 2009;70:113–21.
66. Brown ES, Garza M, Carmody TJ. A randomized double blind, placebo-controlled add on trial of quetiapine in outpatients with bipolar disorder and alcohol use disorders. J Clin Psychiatry. 2008;69:701–4.
67. Stedman M, Pettinati H, Brown ES, et al. A double blind placebo controlled study with quetiapine as adjunctive therapy with lithium or divalproex in bipolar I patients with co-existing alcohol dependence. Alcohol Clin Exp Res. 2010;34:1822–31.
68. Brown ES, Carmody TJ, Schmitz JM, et al. A randomized double blind, placebo-controlled pilot study of naltrexone in outpatients with bipolar disorder and alcohol dependence. Alcohol Clin Exp Res. 2009;33:1863–9.

69. Tolliver B, McRae A, Sonne SC. Safety and tolerability of acamprosate in alcohol dependent individuals with bipolar disorder. Addict Disord Ther Treat. 2009;8:33–8.
70. Litten RZ, Wilford BB, Falk DE, Ryan ML, Fertig JB. Potential medications for the treatment of alcohol use disorder: an evaluation of clinical efficacy and safety. Subst Abus. 2016;37(2):286–98.
71. Sylvia L, Gold A, Stange J. Brief report: a randomized, placebo controlled proof of concept trial of adjunctive topiramate for alcohol use disorders. Am J Addict. 2016;25:94–8.
72. Green CA, Yarborough MT, Polen MR, Janoff SL, Yarborough BJ. Dual recovery among people with serious mental illnesses and substance problems: a qualitative analysis. J Dual Diagn. 2015;11(1):33–41.
73. Schonfeld L, Dupree LW, Dickson-Euhrmann E, Royer CM, McDermott CH, Rosansky JS, Taylor S, Jarvik LF. Cognitive-behavioral treatment of older veterans with substance abuse problems. J Geriatr Psychiatry Neurol. 2000;13(3):124–9.
74. Schmitz A, Grillion C. Assessing fear and anxiety in humans using the threat of predictable and unpredictable aversive events (the NPU-threat test). Nat Protoc. 2012;7(3):527–32.
75. Weiss RD, Griffin ML, Jaffee WB, Bender RE, Graff FS, Gallop RJ, Fitzmaurice GM. A "community-friendly" version of integrated group therapy for patients with bipolar disorder and substance dependence: a randomized controlled trial. Drug Alcohol Depend. 2009;104(3):212–9.
76. Holroyd S, Duryee JJ. Substance use disorders in a geriatric psychiatry outpatient clinic: prevalence and epidemiologic characteristics. J Nerv Ment Dis. 1997;185(10):627–32.
77. Egan M, Moride Y, Wolfson C, Monette J. Long-term continuous use of benzodiazepines by older adults in Quebec: prevalence, incidence and risk factors. J Am Geriatr Soc. 2000;48(7):811–6.
78. Petrovic M, Vandierendonck A, Mariman A, van Maele G, Afschrift M, Pevernagie D. Personality traits and socio-epidemiological status of hospitalized elderly benzodiazepine users. Int J Geriatr Psychiatry. 2002;17(8):733–8.
79. Alvarenga JM, Loyola Filho AI, Firmo JO, Lima-Costa MF, Uchoa E. Prevalence and sociodemographic characteristics associated with benzodiazepines use among community dwelling older adults: the Bambuí Health and Aging Study (BHAS). Rev Bras Psiquiatr. 2008;30(1):7–11.
80. Vázquez GH, Baldessarini RJ, Tondo L. Co-occurrence of anxiety and bipolar disorders: clinical and therapeutic overview. Depress Anxiety. 2014;31(3):196–206.
81. Finfgeld-Connett DL. Treatment of substance misuse in older women: using a brief intervention model. J Gerontol Nurs. 2004;30(8):30–7.
82. Hill-Taylor B, Sketris IS, Gardner DM, Thompson K. Concordance with a STOPP (Screening Tool of Older Persons' Potentially Inappropriate Prescriptions) criterion in Nova Scotia, Canada: benzodiazepine and zoplicone prescription claims by older adults with fall-related hospitalizations. J Popul Ther Clin Pharmacol. 2016;23(1):e1–12.
83. Lin SK. Rapid detoxification of benzodiazepine or Z-drugs dependence using acetylcholinesterase inhibitors. Med Hypotheses. 2014;83(1):108–10.
84. Kawasaki SS, Jacapraro JS, Rastegar DA. Safety and effectiveness of a fixed-dose phenobarbital protocol for inpatient benzodiazepine detoxification. J Subst Abuse Treat. 2012;43(3):331–4.
85. Croissant B, Diehl A, Klein O, Zambrano S, Nakovics H, Heinz A, Mann K. A pilot study of oxcarbazepine versus acamprosate in alcohol-dependent patients. Alcohol Clin Exp Res. 2006;30(4):630–5.
86. Shaw GK. Detoxification: the use of benzodiazepines. Alcohol. 1995;30(6):765–70.
87. Treatment Improvement Protocol (TIP) Series, No. 45. Center for Substance Abuse Treatment. Rockville (MD): Substance Abuse and Mental Health Services Administration (US); 2006.
88. Cregler LL, Mark H. Medical complications of cocaine abuse. N Engl J Med. 1986;315(23):1495–500.

89. Morton WA. Cocaine and psychiatric symptoms. Prim Care Companion J Clin Psychiatry. 1999;1(4):109–13.
90. Rivers E, Shirazi E, Aurora T, Mullen M, Gunnerson K, Sheridan B, Eichhorn L, Tomlanovich M. Cocaine use in elder patients presenting to an inner-city emergency department. Acad Emerg Med. 2004;11(8):874–7.
91. Cameron P, Jellinik G, Kelly AM, Brown A, Little M (eds). Textbook of adult emergency medicine. 4th ed. London: Churchill Livingston; 2014.
92. Prochaska JO, Velicer WF, Rossi JS, Goldstein MG, Marcus BH, Rakowski W, Fiore C, Harlow LL, Redding CA, Rosenbloom D. Stages of change and decisional balance for 12 problem behaviors. Health Psychol. 1994;13(1):39–46.
93. Brown ES, Gorman AR, Hynan LS. A randomized, placebo-controlled trial of citicoline add-on therapy in outpatients with bipolar disorder and cocaine dependence. J Clin Psychopharmacol. 2007;27(5):498–502.
94. Brown ES, Perantie DC, Dhanani N, Beard L, Orsulak P, Rush AJ. Lamotrigine for bipolar disorder and comorbid cocaine dependence: a replication and extension study. J Affect Disord. 2006;93(1–3):219–22.
95. Brown ES, Nejtek VA, Perantie DC, Orsulak PJ, Bobadilla L. Lamotrigine in patients with bipolar disorder and cocaine dependence. J Clin Psychiatry. 2003;64(2):197–201.
96. Brown ES, Todd JP, Hu LT, Schmitz JM, Carmody TJ, Nakamura A, Sunderajan P, Rush AJ, Adinoff B, Bret ME, Holmes T, Lo A. A randomized, double-blind, placebo-controlled trial of citicoline for cocaine dependence in bipolar I disorder. Am J Psychiatry. 2015;172(10):1014–21.
97. Yee T, Perantie DC, Dhanani N, Brown ES. Drug dreams in outpatients with bipolar disorder and cocaine dependence. J Nerv Ment Dis. 2004;192(3):238–42.
98. Brown ES, Nejtek VA, Perantie DC, Bobadilla L. Quetiapine in bipolar disorder and cocaine dependence. Bipolar Disord. 2002;4(6):406–11.
99. Khantzian EJ, Albanese MJ. Self-medication, bipolar disorders, and stimulant dependence. J Clin Psychiatry. 2009;70(6):935–6 (author reply 936-7).
100. Klassen LJ, Katzman MA, Chokka PJ. Adult ADHD and its comorbidities, with a focus on bipolar disorder. J Affect Disord. 2010;124(1–2):1–8.
101. McElroy SL, Martens BE, Mori N, Blom TJ, Casuto LS, Hawkins JM, Keck PE Jr. Adjunctive lisdexamfetamine in bipolar depression: a preliminary randomized, placebo-controlled trial. Int Clin Psychopharmacol. 2015;30(1):6–13.
102. Abbasowa Vinberg M. Psychostimulants in moderate to severe affective disorder: a systematic review of randomized controlled trials. Nord J Psychiatry. 2013;67(6):369–82.
103. Chengappa KN, Levine J, Gershon S, Kupfer DJ. Lifetime prevalence of substance or alcohol abuse and dependence among subjects with bipolar I and II disorders in a voluntary registry. Bipolar Disord. 2000;2(3 Pt 1):191–5.
104. Shoptaw S, Peck J, Reback CJ, Rotheram-Fuller E. Psychiatric and substance dependence comorbidities, sexually transmitted diseases, and risk behaviors among methamphetamine-dependent gay and bisexual men seeking outpatient drug abuse treatment. J Psychoactive Drugs. 2003;35(Suppl 1):161–8.
105. Silverstone PH, Asghar SJ, O'Donnell T, Ulrich M, Hanstock CC. Lithium and valproate protect against dextro-amphetamine induced brain choline concentration changes in bipolar disorder patients. World J Biol Psychiatry. 2004;5(1):38–44.
106. McDonell MG, Srebnik D, Angelo F, McPherson S, Lowe JM, Sugar A, Short RA, Roll JM, Ries RK. Randomized controlled trial of contingency management for stimulant use in community mental health patients with serious mental illness. Am J Psychiatry. 2013;170(1):94–101.
107. Brown ES, Gabrielson B. A randomized, double-blind, placebo-controlled trial of citicoline for bipolar and unipolar depression and methamphetamine dependence. J Affect Disord. 2012;143(1–3):257–60.

108. Nejtek VA, Avila M, Chen LA, Zielinski T, Djokovic M, Podawiltz A, Kaiser K, Bae S, Rush AJ. Do atypical antipsychotics effectively treat co-occurring bipolar disorder and stimulant dependence? A randomized, double-blind trial. J Clin Psychiatry. 2008;69(8):1257–66.
109. Sehgal N, Manchikanti L, Smith HS. Prescription opioid abuse in chronic pain: a review of opioid abuse predictors and strategies to curb opioid abuse. Pain Physician. 2012;15(3 Suppl):ES67–92.
110. Martins SS, Fenton MC, Keyes KM, Blanco C, Zhu H, Storr CL. Mood and anxiety disorders and their association with non-medical prescription opioid use and prescription opioid-use disorder: longitudinal evidence from the National Epidemiologic Study on Alcohol and Related Conditions. Psychol Med. 2012;42(6):1261–72.
111. Shabani A, Jolfaei AG, Vazmalaei HA, Ebrahimi AA, Naserbakht M. Clinical and course indicators of bipolar disorder type I with and without opioid dependence. J Res Med Sci. 2010;15(1):20–6.
112. Albanese MJ, Clodfelter RC Jr, Pardo TB, Ghaemi SN. Underdiagnosis of bipolar disorder in men with substance use disorder. J Psychiatr Pract. 2006;12(2):124–7.
113. Shariat SV, Hosseinifard Z, Taban M, Shabani A. Mania precipitated by opioid withdrawal: a retrospective study. Am J Addict. 2013;22(4):338–43.
114. Back SE, Lawson KM, Singleton LM, Brady KT. Characteristics and correlates of men and women with prescription opioid dependence. Addict Behav. 2011;36(8):829–34.
115. Kolodziej ME, Griffin ML, Najavits LM, Otto MW, Greenfield SF, Weiss RD. Anxiety disorders among patients with co-occurring bipolar and substance use disorders. Drug Alcohol Depend. 2005;80(2):251–7.
116. Rudd RA, Aleshire N, Zibbell JE, Gladden RM. Increases in drug and opioid overdose deaths-United States, 2000–2014. MMWR Morb Mortal Wkly Rep. 2016;64(50–51):1378–82.
117. Zedler B, Xie L, Wang L, Joyce A, Vick C, Kariburyo F, Rajan P, Baser O, Murrelle L. Risk factors for serious prescription opioid-related toxicity or overdose among Veterans Health Administration patients. Pain Med. 2014;15(11):1911–29.
118. Cerimele JM, Chwastiak LA, Dodson S, Katon WJ. The prevalence of bipolar disorder in general primary care samples: a systematic review. Gen Hosp Psychiatry. 2014;36(1):19–25.
119. Ryan R, Santesso N, Lowe D, Hill S, Grimshaw J, Prictor M, Kaufman C, Cowie G, Taylor M. Interventions to improve safe and effective medicines use by consumers: an overview of systematic reviews. Cochrane Database Syst Rev. 2014;4:CD007768.
120. Belgrade MJ, Schamber CD, Lindgren BR. The DIRE score: predicting outcomes of opioid prescribing for chronic pain. J Pain. 2006;7(9):671–81.
121. Just J, Mücke M, Bleckwenn M. Dependence on prescription opioids. Dtsch Arztebl Int. 2016;113(13):213–20.
122. Gold MS, Pottash AC, Sweeney D, Martin D, Extein I. Antimanic, antidepressant, and antipanic effects of opiates: clinical, neuroanatomical, and biochemical evidence. Ann NY Acad Sci. 1982;398:140–50.
123. Olive MF, Cleva RM, Kalivas PW, Malcolm RJ. Glutamatergic medications for the treatment of drug and behavioral addictions. Pharmacol Biochem Behav. 2012;100(4):801–10.
124. Brown R. Heroin dependence. WMJ. 2004;103(4):20–6.
125. Woodcock EA, Lundahl LH, Stoltman JJ, Greenwald MK. Progression to regular heroin use: examination of patterns, predictors, and consequences. Addict Behav. 2015;45:287–93.
126. Fareed A, Casarella J, Amar R, Vayalapalli S, Drexler K. Benefits of retention in methadone maintenance and chronic medical conditions as risk factors for premature death among older heroin addicts. J Psychiatr Pract. 2009;15(3):227–34.
127. Han B, Polydorou S, Ferris R, Blaum CS, Ross S, McNeely J. Demographic trends of adults in New York City opioid treatment programs—an aging population. Subst Use Misuse. 2015;50(13):1660–7.

128. Heffner JL, DelBello MP, Fleck D, et al. Cigarette smoking in the early course of bipolar disorder: association with ages-at onset of alcohol and marijuana use. Bipolar Disord. 2008;10:838–45.
129. Leite RT, Nogueira Sde O, do Nascimento JP, de Lima LS, da Nóbrega TB, Virgínio Mda S, Moreno LM, Sampaio BH, de Matos E, Souza FG. The use of cannabis as a predictor of early onset of bipolar disorder and suicide attempts. Neural Plast. 2015;2015:434127.
130. Fattore L. Synthetic cannabinoids—further evidence supporting the relationship between cannabinoids and psychosis. Biol Psychol. 2016;79(7):539–48.
131. Castaneto M, Gorelick D, Desrosiers N, Hartman T, Pirard S, Huestis M. Synthetic cannabinoids: epidemiology, pharmacodynamics, and clinical implications. Drug Alcohol Depend. 2014;1(144):12–41.
132. Reinarman C, Nunberg H, Lanthier F, Heddleston T. Who are medical marijuana patients? Population characteristics from nine California assessment clinics. J Psychoactive Drugs. 2011;43(2):128–35.
133. Miller PG, Sønderlund AL. Using the internet to research hidden populations of illicit drug users: a review. Addiction. 2010;105(9):1557–67.
134. Kim S, Dodd S, Berk L, Kulkarni J, de Castella A, Fitzgerald PB, Kim JM, Yoon JS, Berk M. Impact of cannabis use on long-term remission in bipolar I and schizoaffective disorder. Psychiatry Investig. 2015;12(3):349–55.
135. Danovitch I, Gorelick DA. State of the art treatments for cannabis dependence. Psychiatr Clin N Am. 2012;35(2):309–26.
136. Marshall K, Gowing L, Ali R, Le Foll B. Pharmacotherapies for cannabis dependence. Cochrane Database Syst Rev. 2014;12:CD008940.
137. Allsop DJ, Lintzeris N, Copeland J, Dunlop A, McGregor IS. Cannabinoid replacement therapy (CRT): nabiximols (Sativex) as a novel treatment for cannabis withdrawal. Clin Pharmacol Ther. 2015;97(6):571–4.

6 Cognitive Impairment and Older Age Bipolar Disorder

Sara Weisenbach and Danielle Carns

Abbreviations

BPD	Bipolar disorder
MoCA	Montreal Cognitive Assessment
IQ-CODE	Informant Questionnaire on Cognitive Decline
WMHs	White matter hyperintensities
AD	Alzheimer's disease
MMSE	Mini-Mental State Examination
MCI	Mild cognitive impairment
SIS	Six-Item Screener
CDT	Clock drawing test
CR	Cognitive rehabilitation
LLD	Late-life depression
PST	Problem-solving therapy

Clinical Vignette 6.1

Ms. R is a 68-year-old, right-handed, Caucasian female with 18 years of education who retired from her professional career as a corporate executive 5 months prior to the admission into our hospital. She was brought to the emergency room after making suicidal gestures and threatening her husband

S. Weisenbach (✉)
Department of Psychiatry, University of Utah School of Medicine,
383 Colorow Road, Salt Lake City, UT 84108, USA
e-mail: sara.weisenbach@hsc.utah.edu

D. Carns
Adler School of Professional Psychology, 17 N. Dearborn St.,
Chicago, IL 60602, USA
e-mail: dcarns36@gmail.com

S.W. Lehmann and B.P. Forester (eds.), *Bipolar Disorder in Older Age Patients*,
DOI 10.1007/978-3-319-48912-4_6

with a knife. The patient had no history of suicidal behaviors, but has a psychiatric history of bipolar disorder (BPD) for which she is taking citalopram, 20 mg, and lamotrigine, 200 mg, daily. Ms. R has a history of hypertension and hyperlipidemia, for which she is prescribed simvastatin, 10 mg, and lisinopril, 20 mg daily. Over the last 2 weeks, she had been presenting as somewhat confused, paranoid, and emotionally labile. She had become perseverative and agitated. Over the past 5 months, she had become markedly fearful of developing dementia because she noticeably became more forgetful during this period, and in the last several months of her work prior to retirement, she became less productive. After an extensive workup of laboratory tests (including thyroid stimulating hormone, B12, and folate) that came back normal during her hospital admission, further assessments were advised. However, due to her manic state at the time of admission, her psychiatrist chose not to assess her cognitive status, but rather to taper her off of the citalopram, in hopes that this would reduce manic symptoms.

Collateral interview with Ms. R's family was conducted during hospital admission. The family reported that throughout her adult life, the patient would have "bursts of energy," typically lasting from several days to 2 weeks, during which she would take on extra work that she would start, but not finish. It was reported that during these times, she did not seem to sleep much and would spend excessive amounts of money planning family trips that they would never take. She was always fairly ostentatious, described by others as "energetic," and "extremely charismatic." Her husband indicated that during periods of "unrest," she would stay at work all night and exhibit hypersexual behaviors that nearly ended their marriage. She also experienced episodes of depression that would typically occur following periods of mania, lasting from weeks to months. While these behaviors were consistent with her diagnosis of BPD I (first recognized when she was age 23), her family was very concerned about the sudden onset of cognitive impairment that had progressively worsened over the past several months. The family reported that she lost her ability to plan, multi-task, and remember to do things, which had profoundly impacted her ability to keep up with daily routines.

During her hospitalization, with tapering of citalopram, Ms. R reached a more stable euthymic state, after which cognitive screening was performed using the Montreal Cognitive Assessment (MoCA) and the Informant Questionnaire on Cognitive Decline (IQ-CODE). Her performance of 23 on the MoCA was below the cutoff score for cognitive impairment (i.e., 24), resulting from poor performance on trails (0/1 point), serial subtraction (1/3 points), delayed recall (3/5 points), and clock drawing tasks (1/3 points). Collateral information, including the IQ-CODE completed by her husband, was consistent with her MoCA performance and indicated that her memory and overall cognition compared to 10 years prior is perceived as much worse at the current time with a seemingly insidious onset. The use of the screening measures provided the clinicians with a patient profile that suggested a significant change in Ms. R's functioning and presence of cognitive impairment that warranted further diagnostic evaluation.

One month after Ms. R was released from the hospital, she remained in a stable, euthymic state. She was seen for comprehensive neuropsychological evaluation as an outpatient. Results of this evaluation revealed preserved general intellectual abilities, which were estimated to be in the high-average range at baseline. Sustained attention, processing speed, and executive functions were areas of weakness, falling in the borderline impaired to low-average range. Her pattern of performance on memory measures was suggestive of limited encoding skills, likely due to difficulty organizing new material into memory, but adequate retrieval of information that was originally encoded. Attentional difficulties were thought to also likely contribute to encoding weakness. Orientation, confrontation naming, psychomotor skills, visuospatial skills, and working memory were within normal limits and similar to estimated baseline functioning. Performance on a functional measure of independent living skills was also within normal limits. Ms. R's cognitive weaknesses were attributed to cognitive effects of OABD and were not thought to be consistent with dementia. Ms. R was referred for therapy to assist with compensating for cognitive weaknesses, and for assistance in solving common everyday problems.

Learning Points

- When patients are being seen in a non-euthymic state, collateral interviews should be conducted to validate information.
- Screening measures for cognitive impairment, medical history, and psychiatric history should be reviewed in great detail together to help guide referrals.
- Assess patients for diagnostic purposes in a euthymic state to ensure valid representation of their current functioning.

6.1 Introduction

Many older adult patients seen in psychiatric settings, such as the vignette of Ms. R, exhibit a clinical presentation that involves mixed affective and cognitive disturbances. These disruptions typically take one of two forms: either a primary mood disturbance with secondary cognitive impairment, or a primary neurodegenerative illness with secondary mood disorder, such as depression. The former pattern, also known as cognitive impairment with depression, involves cognitive impairment that may improve with adequate treatment of depression, while the latter does not [1].

This differentiation highlights the importance of accurate and quick diagnosis, which is a process that begins with being able to effectively screen for impairments and knowing when to refer for neuropsychological evaluation. Screening and referral are discussed in greater detail later in this chapter.

6.2 Cognitive Aging Changes in Bipolar Disorder

Normal aging is associated with changes in a number of cognitive domains [2] most prominently in the areas of processing speed, executive functioning, and episodic memory [3]. Early onset of BPD may confer even greater changes in cognition than what would be seen with normal aging alone. Weisenbach et al. [4] propose that brain changes occurring in the context of normal aging may increase vulnerability to the development of cognitive and functional problems. This may be most evident in cognitive domains for which decrements are already differentially impacted in mood disorder. Moreover, domains impacted even early during the course of disease may demonstrate accelerated decline during aging as a result of increased vulnerability. (For example, Fig. 6.1 displays a model of how to study interactive and non-interactive effects of age and disease on cognitive functioning.) This proposition is in line with Post's [5] argument that proposed that when the central nervous system is subjected to multiple insults over a long period of time,

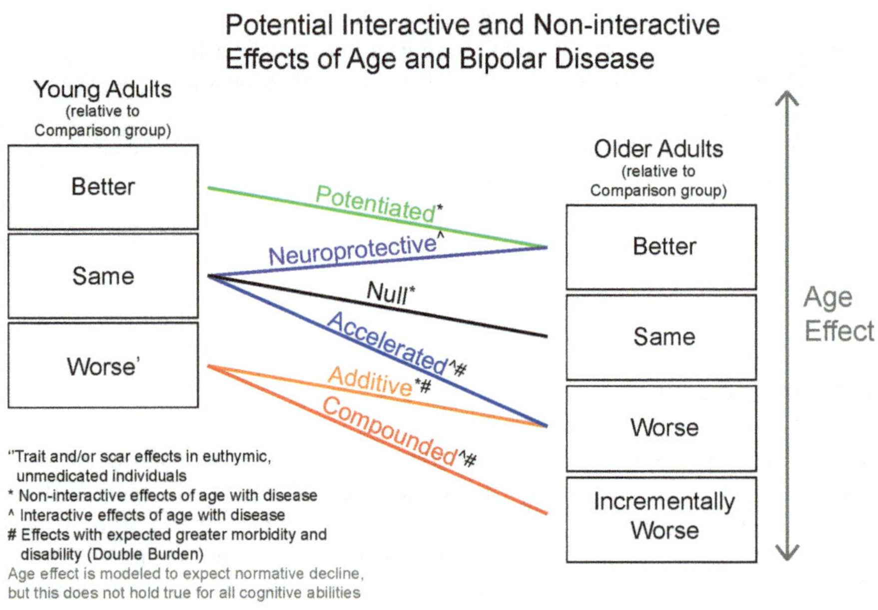

Fig. 6.1 Potential interactive and non-interactive effects of age and bipolar disease (used with permission from Weisenbach et al. [4])

such as occurring during active episodes of mania and depression in the case of BPD, neuronal activity may be permanently altered. Changes in gene expression may underlie these neuronal alterations, which predispose individuals to higher relapse rates and poorer response to treatment with aging, in addition to greater severity of behavioral manifestations of the disease over time, including cognition.

In their cross-sectional study of young and late middle-aged patients with BPD (in the euthymic state) and healthy controls, Weisenbach et al. [4] demonstrated that late middle-aged adults with BPD have especially poor performance (relative to young adults and same-age healthy peers) in the domains of emotion processing, processing speed, and aspects of executive functioning (i.e., verbal fluency, attentional shifting, and interference resolution), with some effects demonstrating an acceleration of the aging process in BPD (similar performance between the two young groups, but poorer performance in the older BPD group relative to same-age controls), and others suggesting a compounded effect of BPD during aging (poorer performance in the young BPD group relative to same-age controls, but incrementally poorer performance in the older BPD group relative to same-age controls). At the same time, verbal memory and other aspects of executive functioning, such as inhibitory control, conceptual reasoning, and set shifting were impacted only by age, regardless of disease status, while fine motor skills and visual memory skills were affected by aging and disease independently. It is important to consider that the older groups in this study were in their mid-50s. Given that more severe cognitive changes are seen in the oldest old during the normal aging process (i.e., a nonlinear trajectory of age-related cognitive changes, [3]) and cognitive changes in BPD have been shown to accelerate after age 65 [6], it is not clear whether these findings would extend to the oldest old with BPD. Other case–control studies of older euthymic BPD patients also demonstrate poorer performance relative to healthy, similarly aged peers across multiple cognitive domains, including processing speed, language, visuomotor skills, episodic memory, working memory, and processing speed [7–10]. At the same time, a study by Sajatovic et al. [11] found no differences in performance among young (40 years and younger) versus older (60 years and older) patients with BPD, when using age-corrected normative scores.

Longitudinal studies of BPD in middle and late life have demonstrated somewhat variable findings. Delaloye et al. [12] found no differences in the trajectory of cognitive changes over two years between BPD and controls. In a different sample, Depp et al. [13] followed patients and controls for up to 3 years and demonstrated greater variability on a measure of global cognition in the BPD patients. Gildengers et al. [14] found that global cognition was poorer at baseline in BPD, relative to controls, and declined more rapidly over 3 years. In a separate study, with a different sample and a more comprehensive neuropsychological battery, Gildengers et al. [15] found poorer cognitive function across all domains, as well as worse performance on instrumental activities of daily living among BPD patients relative to controls at baseline and at 2-year follow-up. However, there was no evidence for accelerated decline in the BPD group across the 2-year period. In summary, studies demonstrate cognitive problems across a multitude of domains in BPD that can occur early during the disease course and may be compounded by and/or accelerated with the aging process, although findings are mixed in this regard.

Clinical characteristics of OABD may also moderate the extent of cognitive impairment observed. First, disease state and greater symptom severity have been shown to impact the severity of cognitive problems, with poorer cognition occurring during manic and depressive, relative to euthymic phases. Having a later onset of BPD may also confer greater risk of cognitive difficulties [16]. After controlling for age, years of illness was not found to be associated with cognition in the study by Weisenbach et al. [4], though there have been studies demonstrating a significant relationship between cognition and number of episodes in patient groups of a wide age range [17, 18] particularly when comparing those with one or two episodes to those with three or more episodes [19].

6.3 Potential Mediators of Cognitive Impairment in OABD

There are likely a number of factors that contribute to cognitive problems in BPD and OABD. While a comprehensive discussion of these variables as they relate to BPD, in general, is covered elsewhere in this volume, we will briefly discuss some of the primary areas currently under investigation in the field. We also refer the reader to a recent manuscript by Sajatovic et al. [11] that provides an excellent overview of possible mediators of cognitive impairment in OABD.

First, medical comorbidities are more common among individuals with BPD than in the general population, including cardiovascular disease, respiratory disorders, type II diabetes mellitus, hypertension, and coronary artery disease, among others, with the majority of patients having three to four comorbid medical conditions [20]. Lifestyle factors, including substance abuse, smoking, poor diet, and metabolic dysregulation as a consequence of psychotropic medication use, contribute to the high prevalence of medical comorbidities in this population [21]. Cognitive impairment has been associated with the presence of medical comorbidities in OABD. A recent study found that hypertension, metabolic syndrome, abdominal obesity, and hyperglycemia were nominally associated with poorer performance in a multitude of cognitive domains, though only hypertension was statistically significant. In at least two studies, greater medical comorbidities have been associated with poorer daily functioning [15, 22], though this is partially accounted for by poorer cognitive functioning [15].

Second, acute side effects of psychotropic medications, in addition to effects of long-term use of psychotropic medications, are thought to contribute to cognitive dysfunction in OABD. With regard to more acute effects, sedating properties of GABA-ergic medications, such as benzodiazepines, are associated with cognitive blunting [23]. Anticholinergic medications also impact cognition to a greater extent than medications without anticholinergic effects [24, 25]. Lithium is known to have anticholinergic properties, for instance, which may explain initial adverse impact on cognition [26]. The longer-term impact of lithium on cognitive functioning is less clear. There have been a handful of longitudinal studies (all limited to 10 years or less) on the effects of long-term lithium use on cognition, though none have revealed findings suggesting that lithium accelerates cognitive decline in BPD [27–30]. In fact, lithium may have neurotrophic/neuroprotective effects [31–33] that can preserve cognition [34, 35] and even prevent or delay the onset of dementia [36].

Third, there have been a number of neuroimaging studies investigating the role of white matter degeneration and gray matter atrophy in BPD, which could underlie cognitive deficits in OABD. Haller et al. [37] found decreased white matter integrity in the ventral portion of the corpus callosum, as well as reduced gray matter density in limbic, subcortical, and prefrontal regions among 19 older BPD patients relative to 47 controls. Findings have been mixed, however. For example, Rej et al. [9] reported increased white matter hyperintensities (WMHs) among controls, relative to OABD, and no differences in total gray matter or hippocampal volume. WMHs were not correlated with cognitive performance in the BPD group. Delaloye et al. [12] found no differences between OABD and controls in the trajectory of changes of gray and white matters over two years. Neuroimaging studies of OABD are limited, and sample sizes are small; thus, more research in this area is needed before making any firm conclusions about the relationship between neurodegeneration and cognitive difficulties in OABD.

Other mechanisms underlying neurocognitive decline in OABD include neurochemical dysregulation, oxidative stress, neuroinflammatory processes, mitochondrial dysfunction, and neurotrophic factors. Dysregulation of the dopaminergic and glutamatergic systems, such as occurring in BPD, can lead to oxidative stress [38, 39], which has been associated with cognitive decline during normal aging [40]. Neuroinflammatory processes are also likely implicated in cognitive decline in the context of BPD. Increased levels of pro-inflammatory cytokines have been demonstrated in BPD [41] and have been associated with cognitive decline both in animal and in human models [42, 43]. Mitochondrial dysfunction, which impairs oxidative energy generation, is increasingly being recognized as relevant to BPD [11] and may also be responsible, at least in part, for the cognitive decline observed in BPD. Finally, neurotrophic factors (i.e., BDNF) have been shown to be decreased, particularly during active episodes [44, 45], and may be reduced more chronically in the later stages of BPD [46]. A recent meta-analysis of ten studies found that low levels of BDNF in BPD were negatively associated with cognitive performance [42]. Figure 6.2 illustrates possible sources of cognitive impairment in OABD.

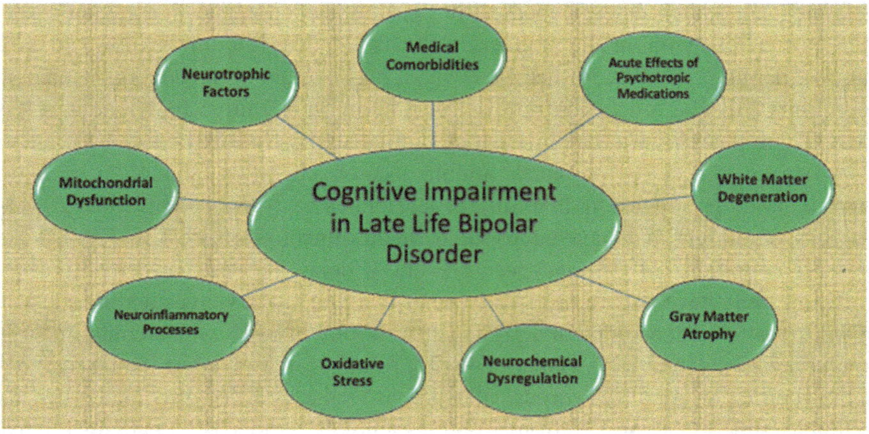

Fig. 6.2 Cognitive impairment in late-life bipolar disorder. Displays possible sources of cognitive impairment in OABD

6.4 Management of Cognitive Impairment in OABD

6.4.1 Screening

Because neuropsychological evaluations are time-consuming and costly and require the expertise of a clinical neuropsychologist, the use of screening methods for populations at high risk of cognitive impairment/decline is imperative. In fact, a combination of poor sensitivity and specificity of screening tests, along with the difficulty acquiring a test that comprehensively assesses cognitive domains, impedes identification of cognitive decline in the early stages [47]. In an effort to prevent delays in detecting cognitive decline, many researchers have conducted investigations as to the sensitivity and specificity of neuropsychological measures, both direct and indirect, for the detection of cognitive impairment (Tables 6.1 and 6.2). Thus, cognitive screening measures need to be easily administered independent of language, culture, and education and must be well tolerated by patients. Cognitive screening instruments can detect the presence of cognitive decline that should be further evaluated through comprehensive neuropsychological evaluation. Ideal cognitive screeners have high sensitivity and specificity, high concurrent and predictive validity, as well as ease of scoring and good inter-rater and test–retest reliability [47]. It is important to keep in mind that cognitive screening should not be used to diagnose mild or major neurocognitive disorders, as they are designed to indicate the presence/absence of cognitive impairment, as opposed to provide the kind of comprehensive evaluation that is necessary for arriving at specific diagnoses.

Direct screening measures are those administered by the clinician. These measures need to be able to quickly assess patients in a clinic and at bedside, and must

Table 6.1 Direct screening measures

Test	Sensitivity	Specificity	Cost	Location
MMSE	63–69 %[a] (dementia)	90–96 %[a] (dementia)	$68.00/pkg 50	http://www4.parinc.com/Products
Six-Item Screener (≥1 error)	100 %[b] (dementia)	38.4 %[b] (dementia)	FREE	https://www.scanhealthplan.com/…/6-item-recall.pdf
Mini-Cog	76–99 %[c] (dementia)	83–93 %[c] (dementia)	FREE	www.alz.org/documents
Clock drawing task (CLOX-I)	90 % (AD)[d] 75 % (MCI)[d]	75 %(AD)[d] 50 %(MCI)[d]	FREE	http://geriatrics.uthscsa.edu/tools/CLOX.pdf
Category fluency	88 %[e] (AD)	96 %[e](AD)	FREE	N/A
MoCA	90 % (MCI)[f] 100 % (AD)[f]	87 %[f]	FREE	http://www.mocatest.org

Notes [a]See [82]
[b]See [57]
[c]See [55]
[d]See [83]
[e]See [84]
[f]See [49]

Table 6.2 Indirect screening measures

Test	Sensitivity	Specificity	Cost	Location
Informant Questionnaire	80–90 %[a] (dementia)	80–90 %[a] (dementia)	FREE	www.alz.org/documents
AD8	84 %[b] (dementia)	80 %[b] (dementia)	FREE	http://knightadrc.wustl.edu/About_Us/PDFs/AD8form2005.pdf

Notes [a]See [85]
[b]See [68]

be sensitive, specific, and efficient [47]. The measures included below are some of the more widely used and popular screening measures, but by no means represent an exhaustive list.

6.4.1.1 Mini-Mental State Examination

The Mini-Mental State Examination [48] (MMSE) is a 30-point measure of global cognitive functioning that takes roughly 5–10 min to administer and is commonly used to track the cognitive changes. The MMSE has been shown to be sensitive for screening of dementia, but is less sensitive for detection of mild neurocognitive disorder (MND), formerly known as mild cognitive impairment. Approximately 80 % of individuals with MCI score above 26 points, which is higher than the most typically used cutoff of 24 points [49]. Relatedly, Spering et al. [50] found that the MMSE does not adequately discriminate between patients with normal versus impaired memory, or visuospatial performance. In addition, while the MMSE includes items assessing orientation, attention, memory, language, and visuospatial skills, it does not formally evaluate executive functions, which are commonly affected in late-life mood disorder [49]. It is also important to consider that MMSE scores are positively associated with education level and negatively correlated with age. Low education and ethnicity, which often co-occur, lead to a trend of scores among Caucasians to be typically higher than scores of other ethnic groups [50]. Normative data for age and educational level are available [51], and while the MMSE is limited in its ability to detect MCI, when used in conjunction with tests that measure executive functioning, such as the clock drawing test (CDT), it yields a better representation of the individual's cognitive status [52].

6.4.1.2 Montreal Cognitive Assessment

The Montreal Cognitive Assessment [49] (MoCA) is a 30-point screening measure assessing visuospatial skills, executive functioning, memory, naming, attention, language, delayed recall, abstraction, and orientation and was developed to address the limitations of the MMSE for accurate detection of MCI and dementia [53]. To account for the impact of education on performance, the MoCA adds one point if education is 12 years or less. Additionally, the MoCA, when compared to the MMSE, places more emphasis on tasks of frontal executive functioning and attention deficits found in the beginning stages of many non-AD dementias and in non-amnestic MCI, in addition to late-life mood disorders. This may account for its higher sensitivity for detecting non-AD dementias and non-amnesic MCI [54]. The suggested cutoff score for cognitive impairment on the MoCA is <26. In cases where the MMSE has been given as an initial screen and yielded normal results when functional impairments are evident, the MoCA should be administered because 100 % of individuals with mild AD had an abnormal MoCA score. When patients present with no functional impairments but complain of cognitive impairment, one should begin the screening with a MoCA because in this case the MMSE would likely yield a normal result [49].

6.4.1.3 Mini-Cog

The Mini-Cog [55] is a 3–5 min cognitive screener comprised of two parts, a delayed three-word recall task and the CDT. This screener was designed to eliminate the effects of educational, linguistic, or cultural biases due to the brief memory task and clock drawing task that are not highly affected by the same biases that are commonly observed with use of screeners such as the MMSE, where common language, culture, and education impact ability [56]. Patients with cognitive impairment will draw an abnormal clock and recall only 1 or 2 of the 3 words after a delay, or will recall no words and have a normal clock (i.e., a positive result [55]). Individuals with a positive result should be evaluated further.

6.4.1.4 Six-Item Screener

The Six-Item Screener [57] (SIS) was developed for use in research to examine large numbers of individuals in a short amount of time and assesses orientation to date and 3-item short-delayed recall. The measure takes 1–2 min to administer in comparison with others, whose administration time is usually 7 min or longer, and can be administered over the phone. The test is scored based on the number of errors made with the sensitivity for dementia being 96.8 % and specificity being 53.3 % for one or more errors, with lower sensitivity (89.6 %) but higher specificity (79.4) for two or more errors [57]. The SIS sensitivity is comparable to the MMSE for the detection of possible dementia and could be used as a first-stage screen for cognitive impairment.

6.4.1.5 Clock Drawing Test

The clock drawing test (CDT) provides a simple and reliable screening measure for cognitive impairment when patients are asked to draw a clock with the hands at 10 past 11. Correctly placing the perceptual features of the clock requires intact frontal executive activity in order to inhibit the tendency to be swayed by placing the hands at the "10" as opposed to 10 min after. In addition to inhibition, it requires (a) auditory comprehension, (b) planning, (c) visual memory and reconstruction, (d) motor programming, (e) numerical knowledge, (f) abstract thinking, and (g) concentration [47]. Practical limitations of CDTs are that there is not one way to administer and score this task. Regarding psychometric properties, the CDT has been shown to have a mean sensitivity of 85 % as well as good inter-rater reliability and good predictive and concurrent validity [58]. Different versions of administration and scoring of CDTs are available. Table 6.1 lists information for CLOX-I [52]. Unfortunately, while CDTs are widely accepted and used, they are traditionally seen as visuospatial and executive functioning tasks, which would not be as useful for detecting amnestic cognitive impairment, for example [52]. While the test is sensitive to detecting cognitive change, it is best used in conjunction with other screening measures, such as the MoCA, and should not be used alone for diagnostic purposes.

6.4.1.6 Category Fluency

Category fluency tasks are comprised of both semantic and phonemic tests of verbal fluency. These measures assess both language and executive functioning and are ideal for bedside administration, as they take roughly 3 min to administer (with some variation depending upon versions used). With regard to screening for cognitive impairment, research has shown that patients' abilities on semantic fluency tasks decline as cognitive impairments worsen [59]. An individual's semantic fluency score is typically lower than the phonemic fluency in the case of amnestic MCI compared to controls and is positively correlated with memory performance [60]. This research suggests that clinicians should be cognizant of the differences in performance between fluency tasks to help determine whether further neuropsychological evaluation for cognitive impairment is warranted. Because fluency measures are limited in the cognitive abilities upon which they draw, they should be used in conjunction with other more comprehensive screening measures.

When assessing individuals with cognitive impairments, it can be helpful to gather collateral information, which can be done quickly using informant questionnaires. Such information can indicate whether the cognitive problems observed currently are long-standing in nature, or represent a significant change for the individual, possibly reflecting a neurodegenerative process. Individuals who have frequent exposure to the patient, including the patient's spouse and child, etc., have been shown to consistently and accurately report symptoms regarding orientation, memory, problem solving, and judgment when correlated to the performance on semi-structured interviews. Collateral information has shown to assist in delineating normal aging from dementia, since it can provide an indication of the patient's baseline level of functioning [61]. Furthermore, subjective reports of mild cognitive impairments often lead to an underreporting of deficits [62]. With this in mind, informant measures such as the IQ-CODE [62] and the AD8 [63] can promote accurate screening for referrals and ultimately diagnosis. Unfortunately, many caregivers of individuals with cognitive impairments have difficulty coping with lifestyle changes and can be at risk of developing depression due to feeling over-burdened [64]. Pressure to keep patients safe, healthy, and well places many under immense amounts of stress due to caring for an individual with cognitive impairment, causing subjective feelings and mood to negatively impact the reporting of deficits the patient has incurred, contributing to possible over-reporting of symptoms [65]. Informant questionnaires should be used in conjunction with performance-based screening measures, such as those described above. While we discuss informant measures below in further detail, there are many other measures that can be utilized to collect data, such as the Measurement of Everyday Cognition Scale (E-Cog); [66] that are not discussed here.

6.4.1.7 Informant Questionnaire on Cognitive Decline

The Informant Questionnaire on Cognitive Decline in the Elderly (IQCODE) is a 26-item informant interview used as a measure of functional change [62]. Total scores range from 26 to 130 and are achieved from summing scores ranging from 1 (has become much better) to 5 (has become much worse), with higher scores representing greater decline in cognitive functioning [67]. This measure has high internal consistency and high test–retest reliability and has been shown to be sensitive in the detection of dementia [62].

6.4.1.8 AD8

The AD8 is a 3-min assessment used to determine intra-individual cognitive changes. It consists of eight questions that are summed (i.e., plus one) if the informant endorses "yes, there has been a change in cognitive functioning," and yields a maximum score of 8 that indicates over the past several years there has been a noticeable decline in thinking and memory problems [68]. This screening measure is sensitive for detecting early cognitive decline, as well as differentiating between amnesic and non-amnesic forms of dementia, and performs well independently of age, race, education level, sex, and MMSE scores. The AD8 functions as an accurate brief screening measure that has strong internal consistency, concurrent validity, construct validity, and inter-rater and intermodal reliability [68] and can be used to assist in detecting changes in individuals' cognitive impairment.

6.4.2 Referring for Neuropsychological Assessment

Referral for comprehensive neuropsychological evaluation should be made when reversible causes of cognitive impairment, such as metabolic changes causing delirium, have been ruled out, and a positive result is indicated on cognitive screen. The screening measure(s) that the clinician chooses should be first based upon its sensitivity and specificity in detecting cognitive impairment, as described in the sections above, but is also realistically based upon how much time is available to administer the measure. While the MoCA, for example, is a comprehensive screening measure and can detect milder forms of cognitive impairment than the MMSE or Mini-Cog, it can take up to 20 min to administer. The Mini-Cog was developed to be a much briefer screen that is often feasible to administer in a busy office environment. One strategy would be to administer lengthier screens, such as the MoCA, when families (via informant screens completed in the waiting room) and/or patients are complaining of cognitive changes but pass a briefer screen, such as the Mini-Cog.

When writing referral questions, it is helpful to the neuropsychologist to have some context for why the patient is being referred for further evaluation, for example, how long have (newer onset) cognitive problems been present, what was the performance on a cognitive screen, and what tests have been performed to rule out reversible causes of cognitive impairment. It is also helpful to know how the referring physician is hopeful the evaluation will guide treatment planning. For example, are there concerns about driving, financial decision making, medication regimen, etc.

6.4.3 Treatment

Effective management of cognitive problems in OABD has received very little attention in the literature to date, although some recent investigations have taken place on this topic. Gildengers et al. [69] conducted a 12-week open-label pilot study of treatment of cognitive problems with donepezil in 12 older adults with BPD I or II. All patients evidenced mild cognitive problems on screening (using the MMSE, Dementia Rating Scale (DRS), or the Executive Interview (EXIT)) and received 5–10 mg of donepezil daily for three months. Nine participants remained in the trial for its duration. No improvement was detected in cognitive performance neither on measures of attention, processing speed, or executive functions, nor on a measure of instrumental activities of daily living. Seven of the nine participants chose to continue treatment with donepezil following the completion of the study due to the subjective perception of improved attention, concentration, and performance on instrumental activities of daily living. To date, this is the only known study of treatment with acetylcholinesterase inhibitors among OABD. It was underpowered to achieve significant effects and was not randomized or blinded. Additionally, cognitive problems in the sample were quite mild; thus, it is unknown whether medication for more advanced cognitive problems in OABD would be efficacious.

Another possible treatment option for cognitive problems in OABD is that of cognitive rehabilitation (CR). The theory behind CR is that with training, practice, and/or learning, the brain has the capacity to change as a result of neural plasticity [70, 71]. While methods vary widely, programs generally focus on enhancing cognition and daily functioning through training of specific skills, such as memory, attention, and social cognition. The psychosis literature is replete with studies demonstrating the beneficial effects of CR programs on the improvement of cognition and daily function [72]. However, when these programs have been applied to patients with BPD, they have not been effective, which has been attributed to the sessions being too easy, and patients reacting with boredom and withdrawal [73]. A systematic review by Kluwe-Schiavon et al. [74] identified only four controlled CR studies in the BPD literature. Rehabilitation strategies were highly variable, but on average entailed 17 h of intervention sessions, at less than 1 h per week. None of the studies demonstrate significant changes on objective cognitive tests/ tasks following the intervention, though the improvement of subjective report of executive functioning was found in three of the four studies. One study that trained social cognition demonstrated some evidence of improvement on an objective social cognitive task. While findings are disappointing, it is important to keep in mind that methodology, including the total hours of intervention, was widely variable across studies. There have been a number of reviews, meta-analyses, and practice guideline recommendations that highlight the key components of successful CR programs [75, 76]. The use of a facilitator or treatment guide, at least initially, is an important part of generalizing gains from practice to everyday challenges and problems and, on average, entails 23 h of training (in Class I studies) [77, 78].

The literature on CR in BPD is still in its infancy, and large, well-designed CR interventions that draw from the literature on development of successful CR programs are needed. It may also be useful to draw from the late-life depression (LLD) literature in developing treatments for cognitive problems in BPD. Problem-solving therapy (PST) is designed to address both the mood and executive dysfunction components that contribute to the significant disability associated with LLD [79]. Alexopoulos et al. [80] compared PST to supportive therapy in improving functional disability and severity of depressive symptoms in a sample of 201 depressed older adults with executive functioning impairments. Participants were assessed at baseline and at 12, 24, and 36 weeks post-treatment. Those who completed PST demonstrated significantly greater reductions in functional disability ratings compared to the supportive therapy group and maintained therapeutic gains made over the supportive therapy group at over the 36 weeks. Interestingly, those with the poorest executive functioning and greatest number of depressive episodes at baseline had the most positive responses to PST, suggesting that difficult-to-treat older adults may especially benefit from this therapeutic approach. A recent study by Morimoto et al. [81] utilized computerized CR of executive functioning in 11 treatment-resistant patients with LLD, finding that it was equally as effective in improving depressive symptoms as was escitalopram (20 mg for

12 weeks), but with faster response rate (4 relative to 12 weeks). Most relevant for this chapter, patients undergoing CR experienced greater improvement on objective executive functioning performance relative to those receiving psychotropic treatment. For patients such as Ms. R, treatments such as PST or CR may be beneficial in improving cognition and daily functioning, though interventions that use gold standard CR or PST treatments and are firmly grounded in the scientific literature of cognitive problems in OABD are desperately needed before clinical practice guidelines in this arena can be developed.

6.5 Summary and Conclusions

Cognitive problems in OABD are relatively common and may represent acceleration or compounded effect of normal aging. Routine screening, followed by referral for neuropsychological evaluation, in the case of positive screen, is essential for accurate prognosis and treatment. A number of mechanisms have been identified that may contribute to cognitive problems, such as effects of medical comorbidities on neural functioning, white matter degeneration, gray matter atrophy, neurochemical dysregulation, oxidative stress, neuroinflammatory processes, mitochondrial dysfunction, and neurotrophic factors. Treatments for compensation and/or enhancement of cognition and functioning in OABD are sorely needed and should be targeted for future clinical trials.

Clinical Pearls

- Older adults with BPD commonly present with mild cognitive impairments across multiple cognitive domains, which may represent acceleration or compounded effect of normal aging.
- Cognitive impairment in OABD may be due to multiple factors, including the effects of medical comorbidities on neural functioning, white matter degeneration, gray matter atrophy, neurochemical dysregulation, oxidative stress, neuroinflammatory processes, mitochondrial dysfunction, and neurotrophic factors.
- Routine cognitive screening should be performed by clinicians to assist with early detection of cognitive impairment.
- A positive screen requires further evaluation and referral to neuropsychology after reversible forms of cognitive impairment have been ruled out, because the specificity of the screening tests is not optimal, nor comprehensive.
- High sensitivity and specificity should be considered when choosing screening instruments, but administration length will also guide decisions. The MoCA should be administered to patients who pass briefer

instruments, such as the Mini-Cog, and who present with self or observant report of cognitive problems that are not long-standing.

- Treatment for cognitive problems in OABD has not been well studied, though therapies such as PST and CR, successfully used in LLD, might be considered.

References

1. Wright SL, Persad C. Distinguishing between depression and dementia in older persons: neuropsychological and neuropathological correlates. J Geriatr Psychiatry Neurol. 2007;20(4):189–98.
2. Park HL, O'Connell JE, Thomson RG. A systematic review of cognitive decline in the general elderly population. Int J Geriatr Psychiatry. 2003;18(12):1121–34.
3. Verhaeghen P, Salthouse TA. Meta-analyses of age-cognition relations in adulthood: estimates of linear and nonlinear age effects and structural models. Psychol Bull. 1997;122(3):231–49.
4. Weisenbach SL, Marshall D, Weldon AL, Ryan KA, Vederman AC, Kamali M, et al. The double burden of age and disease on cognition and quality of life in bipolar disorder. Int J Geriatr Psychiatry. 2014;29(9):952–61.
5. Post RM. Kindling and sensitization as models for affective episode recurrence, cyclicity, and tolerance phenomena. Neurosci Biobehav Rev. 2007;31(6):858–73.
6. Gualtieri CT, Johnson LG. Age-related cognitive decline in patients with mood disorders. Prog Neuropsychopharmacol Biol Psychiatry. 2008;32(4):962–7.
7. Delaloye C, Moy G, Baudois S, De Bilbao F, Remund CD, Hofer F, et al. Cognitive features in euthymic bipolar patients in old age. Bipolar Disord. 2009;11(7):735–43.
8. Gildengers AG, Butters MA, Chisholm D, Anderson SJ, Begley A, Holm M, et al. Cognition in older adults with bipolar disorder versus major depressive disorder. Bipolar Disord. 2012;14(2):198–205.
9. Rej S, Butters MA, Aizenstein HJ, Begley A, Tsay J, Reynolds CF, et al. Neuroimaging and neurocognitive abnormalities associated with bipolar disorder in old age. Int J Geriatr Psychiatry. 2014;29(4):421–7.
10. Schouws SNTM, Comijs HC, Stek ML, Dekker J, Oostervink F, Naarding P, et al. Cognitive impairment in early and late bipolar disorder. Am J Geriatr Psychiatry. 2009;17(6):508–15.
11. Sajatovic M, Forester BP, Gildengers A, Mulsant BH. Aging changes and medical complexity in late-life bipolar disorder: emerging research findings that may help advance care. Neuropsychiatry. 2013;3(6):621.
12. Delaloye C, Moy G, de Bilbao F, Weber K, Baudois S, Haller S, et al. Longitudinal analysis of cognitive performances and structural brain changes in late-life bipolar disorder. Int J Geriatr Psychiatry. 2011;26(12):1309–18.
13. Depp CA, Savla GN, Moore DJ, Palmer BW, Stricker JL, Lebowitz BD, et al. Short-term course of neuropsychological abilities in middle-aged and older adults with bipolar disorder. Bipolar Disord. 2008;10(6):684–90.
14. Gildengers AG, Mulsant BH, Begley A, Mazumdar S, Hyams AV, Reynolds Iii CF, et al. The longitudinal course of cognition in older adults with bipolar disorder. Bipolar Disord. 2009;11(7):744–52.

15. Gildengers AG, Chisholm D, Butters MA, Anderson SJ, Begley A, Holm M, et al. Two-year course of cognitive function and instrumental activities of daily living in older adults with bipolar disorder: evidence for neuroprogression? Psychol Med. 2013;43(04):801–11.
16. Martino DJ, Strejilevich SA, Marengo E, Igoa A, Fassi G, Teitelbaum J, et al. Relationship between neurocognitive functioning and episode recurrences in bipolar disorder. J Affect Disord. 2013;147(1–3):345–51.
17. El-Badri SM, Ashton CH, Moore PB, Marsh VR, Ferrier IN. Electrophysiological and cognitive function in young euthymic patients with bipolar affective disorder. Bipolar Disord. 2001;3(2):79–87.
18. Robinson LJ, Nicol Ferrier I. Evolution of cognitive impairment in bipolar disorder: a systematic review of cross-sectional evidence. Bipolar Disord. 2006;8(2):103–16.
19. López-Jaramillo C, Lopera-Vásquez J, Gallo A, Ospina-Duque J, Bell V, Torrent C, et al. Effects of recurrence on the cognitive performance of patients with bipolar I disorder: implications for relapse prevention and treatment adherence. Bipolar Disord. 2010;12(5): 557–67.
20. Lala SV, Sajatovic M. Medical and psychiatric comorbidities among elderly individuals with bipolar disorder a literature review. J Geriatr Psychiatry Neurol. 2012;25(1):20–5.
21. Kemp DE, Gao K, Chan PK, Ganocy SJ, Findling RL, Calabrese JR. Medical comorbidity in bipolar disorder: relationship between illnesses of the endocrine/metabolic system and treatment outcome: medical comorbidity and treatment outcome. Bipolar Disord. 2010;12 (4):404–13.
22. Epping-Jordan J, Ustun B. The WHODAS II: leveling the playing field for all disorders. WHO Bull Ment Health. 2000;6:5–6.
23. Gualtieri CT, Johnson LG. Comparative neurocognitive effects of 5 psychotropic anticonvulsants and lithium. Medscape Gen Med. 2006;8(3):46.
24. Nebes RD, Pollock BG, Mulsant BH, Kirshner MA, Halligan E, Zmuda M, et al. Low-level serum anticholinergicity as a source of baseline cognitive heterogeneity in geriatric depressed patients. Psychopharmacol Bull. 1997;33(4):715–20.
25. Nebes RD, Pollock BG, Meltzer CC, Saxton JA, Houck PR, Halligan EM, et al. Serum anticholinergic activity, white matter hyperintensities, and cognitive performance. Neurology. 2005;65(9):1487–9.
26. Chew ML, Mulsant BH, Pollock BG, Lehman ME, Greenspan A, Mahmoud RA, et al. Anticholinergic activity of 107 medications commonly used by older adults. J Am Geriatr Soc. 2008;56(7):1333–41.
27. Engelsmann F, Katz J, Ghadirian AM, Schachter D. Lithium and memory: a long-term follow-up study. J Clin Psychopharmacol. 1988;8(3):207–11.
28. Moorhead TWJ, McKirdy J, Sussmann JED, Hall J, Lawrie SM, Johnstone EC, et al. Progressive gray matter loss in patients with bipolar disorder. Biol Psychiatry. 2007;62 (8):894–900.
29. Mur M, Portella MJ, Martínez-Arán A, Pifarré J, Vieta E. Persistent neuropsychological deficit in euthymic bipolar patients: executive function as a core deficit. J Clin Psychiatry. 2007;68(7):1078–86.
30. Mur M, Portella MJ, Martínez-Arán A, Pifarré J, Vieta E. Long-term stability of cognitive impairment in bipolar disorder: a 2-year follow-up study of lithium-treated euthymic bipolar patients. J Clin Psychiatry. 2008;69(5):1478-719.
31. Chiu C-T, Wang Z, Hunsberger JG, Chuang D-M. Therapeutic potential of mood stabilizers lithium and valproic acid: beyond bipolar disorder. Pharmacol Rev. 2013;65(1):105–42.
32. Hunsberger J, Austin DR, Henter ID, Chen G. The neurotrophic and neuroprotective effects of psychotropic agents. Dialogues Clin Neurosci. 2009;11(3):333–48.
33. Malhi GS, Tanious M, Das P, Coulston CM, Berk M. Potential mechanisms of action of lithium in bipolar disorder. Current understanding. CNS Drugs. 2013;27(2):135–53.

34. Bersani G, Quartini A, Zullo D, Iannitelli A. Potential neuroprotective effect of lithium in bipolar patients evaluated by neuropsychological assessment: preliminary results. Hum Psychopharmacol. 2016;31(1):19–28.
35. Rybakowski JK, Permoda-Osip A, Borkowska A. Response to prophylactic lithium in bipolar disorder may be associated with a preservation of executive cognitive functions. Eur Neuropsychopharmacol J Eur Coll Neuropsychopharmacol. 2009;19(11):791–5.
36. Kessing LV, Forman JL, Andersen PK. Does lithium protect against dementia? Bipolar Disord. 2010;12(1):87–94.
37. Haller S, Xekardaki A, Delaloye C, Canuto A, Lövblad KO, Gold G, et al. Combined analysis of grey matter voxel-based morphometry and white matter tract-based spatial statistics in late-life bipolar disorder. J Psychiatry Neurosci JPN. 2011;36(6):391–401.
38. Kulak A, Steullet P, Cabungcal J-H, Werge T, Ingason A, Cuenod M, et al. Redox dysregulation in the pathophysiology of schizophrenia and bipolar disorder: insights from animal models. Antioxid Redox Signal. 2013;18(12):1428–43.
39. Rees JN, Florang VR, Anderson DG, Doorn JA. Lipid peroxidation products inhibit dopamine catabolism yielding aberrant levels of a reactive intermediate. Chem Res Toxicol. 2007;20(10):1536–42.
40. Dröge W, Schipper HM. Oxidative stress and aberrant signaling in aging and cognitive decline. Aging Cell. 2007;6(3):361–70.
41. Goldstein BI, Kemp DE, Soczynska JK, McIntyre RS. Inflammation and the phenomenology, pathophysiology, comorbidity, and treatment of bipolar disorder: a systematic review of the literature. J Clin Psychiatry. 2009;70(8):1078–90.
42. Bauer IE, Pascoe MC, Wollenhaupt-Aguiar B, Kapczinski F, Soares JC. Inflammatory mediators of cognitive impairment in bipolar disorder. J Psychiatr Res. 2014;56:18–27.
43. Brietzke E, Kapczinski F. TNF-alpha as a molecular target in bipolar disorder. Prog Neuropsychopharmacol Biol Psychiatry. 2008;32(6):1355–61.
44. Kapczinski F, Frey BN, Kauer-Sant'Anna M, Grassi-Oliveira R. Brain-derived neurotrophic factor and neuroplasticity in bipolar disorder. Expert Rev Neurother. 2008;8(7):1101–13.
45. Fernandes BS, Molendijk ML, Köhler CA, Soares JC, Leite CMGS, Machado-Vieira R, et al. Peripheral brain-derived neurotrophic factor (BDNF) as a biomarker in bipolar disorder: a meta-analysis of 52 studies. BMC Med. 2015;13:289.
46. Kapczinski F, Vieta E, Andreazza AC, Frey BN, Gomes FA, Tramontina J, et al. Allostatic load in bipolar disorder: implications for pathophysiology and treatment. Neurosci Biobehav Rev. 2008;32(4):675–92.
47. Shulman KI. Clock-drawing: is it the ideal cognitive screening test? Int J Geriatr Psychiatry. 2000;15(6):548–61.
48. Folstein MF, Folstein SE, McHugh PR. "Mini-mental state". A practical method for grading the cognitive state of patients for the clinician. J Psychiatr Res. 1975;12(3):189–98.
49. Nasreddine ZS, Phillips NA, Bédirian V, Charbonneau S, Whitehead V, Collin I, et al. The montreal cognitive assessment, MoCA: a brief screening tool for mild cognitive impairment. J Am Geriatr Soc. 2005;53(4):695–9.
50. Spering CC, Hobson V, Lucas JA, Menon CV, Hall JR, O'Bryant SE. Diagnostic accuracy of the MMSE in detecting probable and possible Alzheimer's disease in ethnically diverse highly educated individuals: an analysis of the NACC database. J Gerontol A Biol Sci Med Sci. 2012;67(8):890–6.
51. Crum RM, Anthony JC, Bassett SS, Folstein MF. Population-based norms for the Mini-Mental State Examination by age and educational level. JAMA. 1993;269(18):2386–91.
52. Royall DR, Cordes JA, Polk M. CLOX: an executive clock drawing task. J Neurol Neurosurg Psychiatry. 1998;64(5):588–94.
53. Hoops S, Nazem S, Siderowf AD, Duda JE, Xie SX, Stern MB, et al. Validity of the MoCA and MMSE in the detection of MCI and dementia in Parkinson disease. Neurology. 2009;73(21):1738–45.

54. Smith T, Gildeh N, Holmes C. The Montreal Cognitive Assessment: validity and utility in a memory clinic setting. Can J Psychiatry Rev Can Psychiatr. 2007;52(5):329–32.
55. Fage BA, Chan CCH, Gill SS, Noel-Storr AH, Herrmann N, Smailagic N, et al. Mini-Cog for the diagnosis of Alzheimer's disease dementia and other dementias within a community setting. Cochrane Database Syst Rev. 2015;2:CD010860.
56. Borson S, Scanlan JM, Watanabe J, Tu S-P, Lessig M. Simplifying detection of cognitive impairment: comparison of the Mini-Cog and Mini-Mental State Examination in a multiethnic sample. J Am Geriatr Soc. 2005;53(5):871–4.
57. Callahan CM, Unverzagt FW, Hui SL, Perkins AJ, Hendrie HC. Six-item screener to identify cognitive impairment among potential subjects for clinical research. Med Care. 2002;40 (9):771–81.
58. Schramm U, Berger G, Müller R, Kratzsch T, Peters J, Frölich L. Psychometric properties of Clock Drawing Test and MMSE or Short Performance Test (SKT) in dementia screening in a memory clinic population. Int J Geriatr Psychiatry. 2002;17(3):254–60.
59. Malek-Ahmadi M, Small BJ, Raj A. The diagnostic value of controlled oral word association test-FAS and category fluency in single-domain amnestic mild cognitive impairment. Dement Geriatr Cogn Disord. 2011;32(4):235–40.
60. Cottingham ME, Hawkins KA. Verbal fluency deficits co-occur with memory deficits in geriatric patients at risk for dementia: implications for the concept of mild cognitive impairment. Behav Neurol. 2010;22(3–4):73–9.
61. Cacchione PZ, Powlishta KK, Grant EA, Buckles VD, Morris JC. Accuracy of collateral source reports in very mild to mild dementia of the Alzheimer type. J Am Geriatr Soc. 2003;51(6):819–23.
62. Farias ST, Mungas D, Jagust W. Degree of discrepancy between self and other-reported everyday functioning by cognitive status: dementia, mild cognitive impairment, and healthy elders. Int J Geriatr Psychiatry. 2005;20(9):827–34.
63. Galvin JE, Roe CM, Coats MA, Morris JC. Patient's rating of cognitive ability: using the AD8, a brief informant interview, as a self-rating tool to detect dementia. Arch Neurol. 2007;64(5):725–30.
64. Papastavrou E, Kalokerinou A, Papacostas SS, Tsangari H, Sourtzi P. Caring for a relative with dementia: family caregiver burden. J Adv Nurs. 2007;58(5):446–57.
65. Donaldson C, Tarrier N, Burns A. The impact of the symptoms of dementia on caregivers. Br J Psychiatry J Ment Sci. 1997;170:62–8.
66. Farias ST, Mungas D, Reed BR, Cahn-Weiner D, Jagust W, Baynes K, DeCarli C. The measurement of everyday cognition (ECog): Scale development and psychometric properties. Neuropsychology. 2008;22(4):531–44.
67. Harrison JK, Fearon P, Noel-Storr AH, McShane R, Stott DJ, Quinn TJ. Informant Questionnaire on Cognitive Decline in the Elderly (IQCODE) for the diagnosis of dementia within a general practice (primary care) setting. Cochrane Database Syst Rev. 2014;7: CD010771.
68. Galvin JE, Roe CM, Xiong C, Morris JC. Validity and reliability of the AD8 informant interview in dementia. Neurology. 2006;67(11):1942–8.
69. Gildengers AG, Butters MA, Chisholm D, Reynolds CF, Mulsant BH. A 12-week open-label pilot study of donepezil for cognitive functioning and instrumental activities of daily living in late-life bipolar disorder. Int J Geriatr Psychiatry. 2008;23(7):693–8.
70. Kolb B, Whishaw IQ. Brain plasticity and behavior. Annu Rev Psychol. 1998;49:43–64.
71. Lövdén M, Bodammer NC, Kühn S, Kaufmann J, Schütze H, Tempelmann C, et al. Experience-dependent plasticity of white-matter microstructure extends into old age. Neuropsychologia. 2010;48(13):3878–83.
72. Revell ER, Neill JC, Harte M, Khan Z, Drake RJ. A systematic review and meta-analysis of cognitive remediation in early schizophrenia. Schizophr Res. 2015;168(1–2):213–22.

73. Fuentes-Durá I, Balanzá-Martínez V, Ruiz-Ruiz JC, Martínez-Arán A, Girón M, Solé B, et al. Neurocognitive training in patients with bipolar disorders: current status and perspectives. Psychother Psychosom. 2012;81(4):250–2.
74. Kluwe-Schiavon B, Viola TW, Levandowski ML, Bortolotto VR, Souza LSAE, Tractenberg SG, et al. A systematic review of cognitive rehabilitation for bipolar disorder. Trends Psychiatry Psychother. 2015;37(4):194–201.
75. Anaya C, Martinez Aran A, Ayuso-Mateos JL, Wykes T, Vieta E, Scott J. A systematic review of cognitive remediation for schizo-affective and affective disorders. J Affect Disord. 2012;142(1–3):13–21.
76. Cicerone KD, Langenbahn DM, Braden C, Malec JF, Kalmar K, Fraas M, et al. Evidence-based cognitive rehabilitation: updated review of the literature from 2003 through 2008. Arch Phys Med Rehabil. 2011;92(4):519–30.
77. Tiersky LA, Anselmi V, Johnston MV, Kurtyka J, Roosen E, Schwartz T, et al. A trial of neuropsychologic rehabilitation in mild-spectrum traumatic brain injury. Arch Phys Med Rehabil. 2005;86(8):1565–74.
78. Westerberg H, Jacobaeus H, Hirvikoski T, Clevberger P, Ostensson M-L, Bartfai A, et al. Computerized working memory training after stroke–a pilot study. Brain Inj. 2007;21(1):21–9.
79. Alexopoulos GS, Raue PJ, Kanellopoulos D, Mackin S, Arean PA. Problem solving therapy for the depression-executive dysfunction syndrome of late life. Int J Geriatr Psychiatry. 2008;23(8):782–8.
80. Alexopoulos GS, Raue PJ, Kiosses DN, Mackin RS, Kanellopoulos D, McCulloch C, et al. Problem-solving therapy and supportive therapy in older adults with major depression and executive dysfunction: effect on disability. Arch Gen Psychiatry. 2011;68(1):33–41.
81. Morimoto SS, Wexler BE, Liu J, Hu W, Seirup J, Alexopoulos GS. Neuroplasticity-based computerized cognitive remediation for treatment-resistant geriatric depression. Nat Commun. 2014;5(5):4579.
82. Lezak MD, Howelson DB, Bigler ED, Tranel D. Neuropsychological assessment. 5th ed. New York: Oxford University Press; 2012.
83. De Jager CA, Hogervorst E, Combrinck M, Budge MM. Sensitivity and specificity of neuropsychological tests for mild cognitive impairment, vascular cognitive impairment and Alzheimer's disease. Psychol Med. 2003;33(6):1039–50.
84. Canning SJD, Leach L, Stuss D, Ngo L, Black SE. Diagnostic utility of abbreviated fluency measures in Alzheimer disease and vascular dementia. Neurology. 2004;62(4):556–62.
85. Jorm AF. The Informant Questionnaire on cognitive decline in the elderly (IQCODE): a review. Int Psychogeriatr IPA. 2004;16(3):275–93.

Lithium in Older Age Bipolar Disorder

7

Soham Rej

7.1 Introduction

Lithium remains the gold-standard medication for bipolar disorder (BD) [1], with 30–40 % of patients responding preferentially to its use [2, 3]. Lithium appears to be superior to alternative existing bipolar pharmacotherapies for mood stability, suicidality, and other mental health outcomes [4–6]. Out of the existing older age bipolar disorder (OABD) pharmacotherapies, lithium currently has the best evidence base in the treatment of all phases of illness: acute mania, acute depression, and maintenance [7]. Although randomized controlled trial (RCT) evidence in OABD is not yet available [8], lithium appears to have a similar therapeutic profile in late life. In the large NIH-funded STEP-BD trial, 42 % of older adults on lithium monotherapy achieved symptomatic recovery [9].

Despite lithium's effectiveness, its use in OABD has declined dramatically in the past two decades [10, 11]. In large part, this is probably due to the emergence of novel therapeutic options in BD such as atypical antipsychotics [11, 12]. Atypical antipsychotics have been felt to be comparatively safe—although this may not necessarily be the case for cardiovascular, neurologic, cognitive, and even renal outcomes [13, 14]. In light of perceived "safer" alternatives and lithium's narrow therapeutic index and risk of toxicity in combination with certain anti-inflammatory and antihypertensive medications [15], clinicians often avoid prescribing lithium in late life [7, 16, 17]. In North America, it is estimated that only 8 % of adult patients and <15 % of older adults with BD are treated with lithium [11, 18].

S. Rej (✉)
Division of Geriatric Psychiatry, Department of Psychiatry, Institute for Community and Family Psychiatry, Jewish General Hospital, 4333 Cote-Ste-Catherine, Room 147, Montreal, QC H3T 1E4, Canada
e-mail: soham.rej@mail.mcgill.ca

S.W. Lehmann and B.P. Forester (eds.), *Bipolar Disorder in Older Age Patients*,
DOI 10.1007/978-3-319-48912-4_7

This chapter will provide an overview of the epidemiology of these effects with an emphasis on geriatric data and potential mechanisms underlying these medical effects, as well as guidance on lithium dosing and other strategies to minimize lithium-associated medical effects in late-life BD.

Clinical Vignette 7.1

Ms. X is a 76-year-old woman who has been chronically using lithium for bipolar disorder, type 1 for over 40 years. She had a strong family history of bipolar disorder (mother and brother had an excellent response to lithium), and she had 2 discrete episodes of depression before developing mania in her mid-20s. She was started on lithium in the 1970s and since then has had a good lithium response. She has been psychiatrically stable for the past 25 years, with few residual symptoms and no recent episodes of mania or depression. She has not had any cognitive difficulties in her day-to-day life. Her most recent lithium levels hovered around 0.7–0.8 mmol/L with a dose of 600 mg every night, while her GFR stayed around 65–75 mL/min/1.73 m^2.

She lives with her son and interacts regularly with a small group of friends. She is physically inactive, but has a relatively small number of medical problems for someone with OABD: diabetes mellitus, dyslipidemia, arthritis, and hypothyroidism. These conditions are well controlled with her medications, which include: metformin, atorvastatin, acetominophen, and levothyroxine.

Five weeks ago, she was diagnosed with hypertension by her family physician and was started on an antihypertensive (hydrochlorothiazide). A week ago, she presented to her psychiatrist's office with new onset mild cognitive deficits, fatigue, and a coarse hand tremor. On laboratory examination, her lithium level was 1.1 mmol/L and her eGFR was 40 mL/min/1.73 m^2, down from her usual 65 mL/min/1.73 m^2. Her psychiatrist reviewed Ms. X's medication list and realized the only medication change had been the addition of hydrochlorothiazide. Hydrochlorothiazide can diminish lithium's elimination from the kidneys which can increase lithium levels by up to 50 %. As a result, Ms. X's psychiatrist suspected hydrochlorothiazide/lithium drug interaction as the cause of Ms. X's current clinical presentation.

The psychiatrist contacted her family physician. It was decided that the Ms. X's hypertension could be managed using non-pharmacological approaches for now, and hydrochlorothiazide was stopped. A week later, the psychiatrist saw the patient again. Now the cognitive deficits, fatigue, and tremor had resolved and her eGFR had improved significantly to 60 mL/min/1.73 m^2, while the lithium level had returned to 0.8 mmol/L.

Ms. X and her psychiatrist had a detailed discussion about what to do if hydrochlorothiazide, or any medication known to increase lithium levels, would need to be started in the future. Since lithium has been very helpful to the stability of bipolar disorder and since lithium responders often have relatively poor response to other medications, all attempts would be to keep her on lithium, if possible.

For example, if a medication known to increase lithium levels was started or that medication's dose was modified, lithium levels would be repeated 5–7 days after the medication change. If the lithium level became high, the lithium dose would be lowered accordingly. Ms. X is considering a trial of lowering her usual lithium level to 0.6 mmol/L to see whether this can give psychiatric stability, while lowering the risk of acute kidney injury and acute neurological toxicity. Ms. X will also continue receiving lithium level and eGFR monitoring every 3 months with her psychiatrist.

Learning Points

- Drug–drug interactions can lead to serum lithium-level elevations and acute lithium toxicity, particularly in older adults. Close monitoring with 5–7 days after medication changes can be helpful in preventing these drug–drug interactions
- Relatively modest lithium-level elevations can have serious acute medical consequences.
- Communication between mental health practitioners, primary care clinicians, and medical specialists can help ensure optimal physical and mental health in older lithium users.

7.2 Overview of Lithium-Related Medical Comorbidity in Older Age Bipolar Disorder

In considering lithium-related medical comorbidity in OABD, it is helpful to examine the association between aging and medical comorbidity, the risk of medical comorbidity associated with BD, and the effects of concurrent pharmacotherapy on medical morbidity.

7.2.1 Aging and Lithium-Related Medical Risk

The McGill Geriatric Lithium-Induced Diabetes Insipidus Clinical Study (McGLIDICS) was the first study to systematically compare medical comorbidity between geriatric and younger adult lithium users [19]. The vast majority of the patients in this study had BD (89.0 %). Among younger patients treated with lithium, rates of hypertension (13.0 %), diabetes mellitus (12.7 %), and hypercholesterolemia (31.5 %) were comparable to other bipolar samples [20], but higher than in non-lithium populations [21]. In older patients treated with lithium, these diseases were much more common compared to younger patients on lithium (44.2, 26.7, and 48.8 %, respectively). Additionally, renal dysfunction became highly prevalent in older age (42.9 %) at approximately the same prevalence as community-dwelling elderly (37.8 %) [22]. Of note, hypercalcemia (5.1 vs. 2.0 %) and hypothyroidism rates (39.5 vs. 33.3 %) were not significantly higher in older lithium users compared to younger lithium users. This may be due to how uncommon hypercalcemia is, or, in the case of hypothyroidism—that aging may have less of a role to play in the prevalence of that particular lithium-associated effect. Other studies have also examined the effects of geriatric lithium use on medical comorbidity and are described in greater detail in subsequent sections of this chapter [23, 24].

Overall, the elevated medical comorbidity rates in geriatric lithium users speaks to the possible misattribution of a substantial percentage of medical effects to lithium, when normal aging may often be the "culprit" [25, 26]. The high prevalence of medical disorders in late-life lithium users also suggests that middle age and early old age may be a potential window to prevent the development of these medical illnesses [27]. Although the medical comorbidity rates in McGLIDICS [19] were higher than those found in general population samples [21], they were still similar to rates found in other older age bipolar samples [20, 28, 29].

7.2.1.1 The Risk of Medical Comorbidity in Older Age Bipolar Disorder

BD is associated with a two-fold increased rate of cardiovascular mortality and >10–15-year decreased life expectancy compared to the general population [30, 31]. A recent large study in the UK (n = 1720, mean age 47) had similar findings across several medical comorbidities [32]. Asthma, diabetes mellitus, hyperlipidemia, epilepsy, hypertension, kidney, and thyroid disease were all more common in patients with BD than in patients with major depression or healthy controls [32].

There is a small, yet growing literature examining medical comorbidity in OABD [11, 19, 20, 28, 29, 33–39]. Even though OABD has often been considered a "survivor cohort" of patients who were physically less ill than patients who died in middle age [7, 20, 40], medical comorbidity remains very common. The average patient with OABD has 3–4 medical conditions, the most common being hypertension (45–69 %), diabetes mellitus (18–31 %), and cardiovascular disease (9–49 %) [20]. Cardiovascular risk and cardiovascular disease appear to be very common in OABD, accounting for many of the chronic medical illnesses (e.g., stroke, chronic kidney disease, and dementia) and excess mortality observed in this disorder.

Additionally, BD patients with more severe BD from a mental health perspective have been found to have higher risk of all-cause medical comorbidity [32]. Taken together, this points to the role of medical comorbidity as an integral component of BD pathophysiology, with more severe BD having more severe psychiatric and physical manifestations [11, 41].

7.2.1.2 Lifestyle Factors and Medical Comorbidity in OABD

Lifestyle factors common in bipolar disorder such as decreased physical activity, unhealthy diet, and substance use (e.g., smoking) can contribute to cardiovascular risk (e.g., by increasing body mass index), and thereby indirectly increasing the burden of medical comorbidity in OABD (e.g., for cerebrovascular, cardiac, renal, and other diseases) [42]. Therefore, lifestyle behaviors often seen in OABD contribute to patients' burden of medical comorbidity.

7.2.1.3 Older Age Bipolar Disorder Pharmacotherapy Effects on Medical Health Service Utilization

A recent study of medical health service utilization in OABD ($n = 1388$) examined patients with bipolar disorder who were prescribed lithium, valproate, and other pharmacotherapy after discharge from psychiatric hospitalization for a year to determine non-psychiatric medical health service utilization rates [11]. The authors found that while the 1-year medical hospitalization and emergency room visit rates were very high at 22 and 39 %, respectively [11], the pharmacotherapy groups (lithium included) did not differ from each other. One explanation could be that if a patient has a predisposition to a medical comorbidity (e.g., diabetes mellitus) but has not shown clinical evidence of this medical comorbidity by a certain age (e.g., age-related factors increase the risk of diabetes mellitus), it is less likely that pharmacotherapy will "push a them over the edge" and lead them to develop the medical comorbidity de novo in late life [40]. As a result, it is possible that pharmacotherapy effects on medical comorbidity are less prominent in OABD compared to younger age bipolar disorder.

In summary, studies indicate that the most medical comorbidity in older age bipolar disorder is due to the effects of aging, the biology of bipolar disorder itself, and lifestyle factors rather than the medications prescribed to treat bipolar disorder. It is with this lens that we will examine specific types of medical comorbidity that may be elevated in lithium users and methods to minimize medical comorbidity.

7.2.2 Lithium-Associated Kidney Disease

Lithium's effects on the kidney have been extensively studied for over 40 years [43, 44]. Lithium use has been associated with nephrogenic diabetes insipidus (NDI), acute kidney injury (AKI), and chronic kidney disease (CKD). Management approaches for kidney disease and other medical comorbidities will be discussed broadly under "Lithium Dosing" and "Clinical Pearls" sections.

7.2.2.1 Nephrogenic Diabetes Insipidus (NDI)

Nephrogenic diabetes insipidus (NDI) is a condition involving excessive thirst (polydipsia) due to excessive dilute urine (polyuria). NDI can be defined either by decreased water-restriction urine osmolality (UOsm; UOsm <300 mOsm/Kg) or polyuria (>3 L/24 h). NDI occurs commonly in geriatric lithium users: 12–19 % have decreased 10-h-water-restriction urine osmolality (UOsm) [19, 45], while

33 % have polyuria (defined as >3 L/day) [45]. NDI risk factors include: older age [46–48], non-response to lithium [49, 50], concomitant antipsychotic use [51–55] or other psychotropic use in addition to lithium [56], slow-release lithium formulation [47, 57], twice-daily lithium dosing [50, 58–60], increased lithium level [48, 54, 57], and longer duration of lithium use [45–47, 61–64]. Since 24-h water restriction or 24-h urine volume is not well tolerated by patients [65], UOsm measured after 10-h water restriction can be a useful practical approach to assessing NDI. In this type of test, patients are instructed not eat or drink anything in the 10 h preceding the urine test (e.g., overnight) and can take morning medications, food, and fluids after the test. Some patients complain of significant polydipsia (thirst) and for those patients a teaspoon or two of water to hydrate the mouth over the 10-h-water-restriction period can be a pragmatic strategy. Recent studies suggest that 10-h-water-restriction UOsm <300 or urine specific gravity <1.010 may be a sufficient clinical screen for NDI [19, 65, 66].

The development of NDI in a patient treated with lithium should be a cause of concern for the clinician. After controlling for age, diabetes mellitus, and hypertension (the main risk factors for chronic kidney disease (CKD), NDI increases the risk of CKD threefold [11, 67–69]. In effect, in patients with proper lithium dosing and monitoring, NDI is the main lithium-related pathway to CKD. Moreover, NDI increases the risk of AKI and dangerous hypernatremia [66, 70]. The only randomized controlled trial-supported treatment for NDI (or any renal effect of lithium) is amiloride at 5–20 mg/day [71, 72]. If this treatment is pursued, it should be performed with close monitoring by a nephrologist, given the potential risk for AKI with potassium-sparing diuretics [43]. In the early phases of NDI (first 5–10 years of lithium use), lithium dose reduction or discontinuation can also be effective [73]. Although it has long been hypothesized that NDI may represent the early phase of CKD in lithium users [73], this is not completely clear since, even though NDI is a risk factor for CKD, many patients with NDI may not necessarily develop severe CKD [74]. Ongoing studies are now evaluating the potential role of statins in the prevention/treatment of lithium-induced NDI [75].

7.2.2.2 Acute Kidney Injury (AKI)

Acute kidney injury (AKI) occurs with a 5-year prevalence of 1.3–7 % in geriatric lithium users [15, 69, 76]. AKI has been defined as an acute reduction in eGFR by 50 % from baseline (severe) or by smaller 20–25 % increments (mild) [77]. Risk factors for AKI in older lithium users include increased age [78–80], previous episode of lithium toxicity [78, 79, 81], NDI [79], and the use of angiotensin converting enzyme (ACE) inhibitors, loop diuretics [15], nonsteroidal anti-inflammatory drugs [82, 83], cyclo-oxygenase 2 (COX2) inhibitors [84], and diuretics [85].

Despite recent data indicating that lithium-associated AKI tends to resolve within 3 months with usual clinical care [86], there is considerable evidence suggesting that AKI significantly increases the risk of CKD [67, 69]. AKI also promotes a cascade of events which can lead to marked lithium-level elevations, NDI, dehydration, and further progression of AKI and lithium level elevations, which can cause acute damage to other organ systems (e.g., acute neurological toxicity) [87].

7.2.2.3 Chronic Kidney Disease (CKD)

Chronic kidney disease (CKD) is defined as a chronic reduction of renal function as determined by at least two measurements separated by at least 3 months [88]. There are several stages of CKD, ranging from moderate CKD (estimated glomerular filtration rate (eGFR) <60 mL/min/1.73 m^2) to end-stage renal disease (ESRD; eGFR <15 mL/min/1.73 m^2 or requiring chronic hemodialysis). CKD is associated with poor quality of life, as well as increased health service utilization, disability, and mortality [89, 90]. Despite the association between lithium use and increased risk for AKI, the association between lithium and CKD remains unclear and controversial [26, 44, 69, 91–93]. When larger population-based studies have controlled for age, diabetes mellitus, hypertension, atypical antipsychotic use (recent data suggest antipsychotics can increase CKD risk twofold [13, 69]), and bipolar diagnosis, the relationship between lithium levels and lithium treatment duration with CKD and renal function often appears to be negligible [26, 69, 91, 92]. However, more definitive research is needed. The prevalence of moderate CKD in older lithium users is roughly 42–50 % [19, 45, 69], which is not very different from the general geriatric population (37 %) [22].

A number of strategies have been identified that may be helpful in preventing CKD in older lithium users. These include preventing and treating NDI and AKI which can contribute to CKD [73]. Similarly, preventing and managing cardiovascular risk factors as well as ensuring good primary care/specialist follow-up can also be helpful. Lifestyle interventions such as exercise, healthy diet, and smoking cessation can be effective in lowering cardiovascular risk. The International Society for Bipolar Disorders' guidelines have recommended monitoring lithium levels, electrolytes, and renal function every 3 months [86] and within 1 week of adjusting the dose of diuretics, NSAIDs, angiotensin II receptor blockers (ARBs), or ACE inhibitors [15, 69] (Box 7.1). Lithium dosing regimens can affect CKD risk: Using once-daily lithium dosing and avoiding slow-release formulations may be protective against CKD [94, 95]. Close monitoring of lithium levels and eGFR every 3 months or less in geriatric patients with premorbid CKD (premorbid CKD = eGFR <60 mL/min/1.73 m^2) may be beneficial [96, 97]. Finally, consulting nephrology specialists can be useful and is indicated if: (1) eGFR <30 mL/min/1.73 m^2, or (2) decline in eGFR faster than 5 mL/min/1.73 m^2 in 1 year or 10 mL/min/1.73 m^2 in 5 years [88].

Box 7.1 Principles of clinical management

- Monitor lithium levels, electrolytes, and renal function (eGFR) every 3 months.
- Monitor ionized calcium, thyroid function, fasting glucose, glycosylated hemoglobin (HbA1c), lipid profile, body mass index, 10-h water-restriction urine osmolality, every year.

- Use serum lithium levels <0.8 mmol/L, if clinically possible. Often 0.4–0.6 mmol/L is sufficient if a patient has predominantly bipolar depression.
- Lithium level "cut-offs" (e.g., <0.8 mmol/L) are guides, but if renal function declines or neurological/cognitive effects (e.g., cognitive dulling, unexplained fatigue, delirium, significant coarse tremor, Parkinsonism, or acute gait disturbance) are clinically observed, dose reductions may be necessary.
- Frequent laboratory monitoring is especially important in geriatric patients with pre-morbid chronic CKD (eGFR <60 mL/min/1.73 m^2)—this includes eGFR and lithium level monitoring.
- Consult nephrology if: (1) the eGFR is <30 mL/min/1.73 m^2, or (2) the decline in eGFR faster than 5 mL/min/1.73 m^2 in 1 year or 10 mL/min/1.73 m^2 in 5 years.
- Use concurrent medication cautiously, particularly those associated with lithium level elevations: loop diuretics, hydrochlorothiazide and other diuretics, ACE inhibitors/ARBs, NSAIDS.
- Prevent and/or treat other renal disorders (AKI, NDI), which can otherwise increase the risk of CKD.
- Cardiovascular risk underlies most of the medical comorbidity observed in late-life bipolar disorder.
- Prevent and treat cardiovascular and metabolic risk factors: especially hypertension, diabetes mellitus, and ischemic coronary disease, but also smoking, dyslipidemia, and obesity.
- Maintain good communication with primary care and medical specialists
- Consultation with an endocrinologist should be obtained for patients with cardiovascular/metabolic risk factors or hypothyroidism which are not manageable by the patient's primary care team.
- For patients with symptomatic hypercalcemia or who have an elevated PTH level, consultation with an endocrinologist may be helpful.
- Carefully weigh psychiatric benefits and medical risks before lithium discontinuation in this population: the risk of affective relapse is very high [139].
- Be aware that most medical comorbidity in late-life bipolar disorder is due to aging, the biology of bipolar disorder itself, and lifestyle factors—NOT the medications we prescribe.

7.2.3 Lithium-Associated Endocrine Disease

7.2.3.1 Hyperparathyroidism

Parathyroid hormone (PTH) elevations have been identified in up to 23 % of patients with chronic lithium exposure [23, 98]. Hypercalcemia in older lithium users, though, appears to be relatively low in adequately powered studies. In the McGLIDICS sample ($n = 100$), hypercalcemia was uncommon in both geriatric and non-geriatric adult lithium users (5.1 vs. 2.0 %, $p = 0.53$) [19]. Other more recent geriatric lithium studies ($n = 333$) using a similar hypercalcemia definition (>2.62 mmol/L) [99] also found rates <5 % [100]. Since hypercalcemia itself is relatively uncommon in older lithium users, and studies in this area are few, it remains unclear how frequently older lithium users experience usual clinical symptoms of hypercalcemia, such as fatigue, constipation, nephrolithiasis, and bone pain [23].

The etiology and clinical features of lithium-associated hyperparathyroidism may differ from other forms of hyperparathyroidism since lithium alters the set point of the calcium-sensing receptor in the parathyroid gland. Along similar lines, the classic clinical picture of hyperparathyroidism of "bones, stones, groans, and moans" is not usually seen with lithium-associated hyperparathyroidism [23]. Some caution should be undertaken if hypercalcemia is observed in the context of chronic kidney disease, which can increase hyperparathyroidism risk and complicate treatment [23]. The best measure of hypercalcemia is ionized calcium rather than total serum calcium, and so studies only examining total calcium may potentially underestimate hypercalcemia rates [101]. The reference range for ionized calcium has been 1.1–1.35 mmol/L [101]. If there is symptomatic hypercalcemia or there is associated elevations in PTH (e.g., >65 ng/L), endocrinology consultation should be obtained. Treatment with cincalcet may be recommended by the endocrinologist to reduce the calcium level. Even symptomatic hypercalcemia may not necessarily require lithium discontinuation, especially if lithium has been very effective in a patient, but does require close monitoring.

To summarize, lithium is associated with hyperparathyroidism and hypercalcemia, and merits annual serum calcium monitoring [23, 102]. However, it is worth remembering that clinically important hypercalcemia is not common in chronic lithium users, even in late life. In those cases where hypercalcemia is symptomatic or associated with increased PTH, an endocrinology consultation should be obtained to initiate treatment and determine whether lithium can be continued.

7.2.3.2 Hypothyroidism

Lithium users have a twofold increased risk of hypothyroidism compared to the general population [93]. In the McGLIDICS sample, hypothyroidism was common in both geriatric and adult patients (39.5 and 33.3 % alike), similar to the 32 % prevalence reported in other old age lithium samples [103, 104]. A 6 % incidence of hypothyroidism has been reported in the first 18 months of geriatric lithium use, compared to a 3 % incidence in nonusers [103]. There does not appear to be a lithium duration/dose–response relationship with thyroid function [105]. The evidence suggests that hypothyroidism is clearly associated with lithium use and that this can occur early during treatment regardless of age. Lithium-associated hypothyroidism appears to involve the accumulation of lithium in the thyroid gland, and through immune-related processes, this leads to thyroid stimulating hormone (TSH) suppression and concomitant hypothyroidism [106, 107]. Hypothyroidism in late life has some unique aspects: Hypothyroidism is generally more prevalent with increasing age and symptoms (e.g., fatigue, weight gain, and hair loss) are often subtle, so the presence of a TSH >10 mU/L is often enough to make a diagnosis [107].

In terms of management, synthetic thyroid hormone (thyroxine; T4) supplementation is usually sufficient and lithium discontinuation is rarely, if ever, indicated. It is controversial whether subclinical hypothyroidism, (TSH >5 mU/L), should be treated in the absence of symptoms. Given the high risk of hypothyroidism in lithium users and its clinical importance, the International Society for Bipolar Disorders and similar groups have suggested that thyroid function should be monitored using TSH at least annually, and perhaps more often during the early phase of treatment (e.g., every 3 months), when it is more likely to occur [102].

7.2.4 Cardiovascular Risk Factors

Metabolic syndrome is very common in bipolar disorder 43–45 % [20, 29], as are dyslipidemia 23–50 % [19, 28], hypertension 30–80 % [19, 20, 28, 69], and diabetes mellitus 15–26.7 % [19, 20, 69]. Much of this is attributable to massive obesity rates (up to 50 %) [39], BD biology (e.g., inflammation, oxidative stress, and endothelial dysfunction [108]), and lifestyle factors (e.g., low physical activity, poor diet, cigarette smoking, and other substance abuse) in aging BD patients. Combined with high smoking rates (>30 %) [29], these facts help explain the high rates of coronary disease, cerebrovascular disease, renal disease, and dementia in OABD [11].

Is there a relationship between lithium use and cardiovascular disease? On the one hand, lithium is associated with weight gain, but perhaps no more than other alternative bipolar pharmacotherapies [109]. Based on epidemiologic and basic science research, lithium has been reported to have protective effects on endothelial vessels [110], and may be protective against diabetes mellitus compared to other BD medications [111]. Future clinical trials will be needed to confirm these potential effects.

7.2.5 Neurological Disease

7.2.5.1 Acute Neurological Toxicity

The acute neurological toxicity of lithium due to acute elevations in lithium levels (e.g., due to dehydration, drug interactions, AKI, or lithium overdose) was described in 1968 by Professor Mogen Schou, whose pioneering research led to lithium's widespread utilization in bipolar disorder. The clinical presentation of acute neurological toxicity due to lithium includes confusion, sluggishness, coarse tremor, muscle twitching, gait disturbances, and sometimes even seizures [112]. As with acute renal toxicity, the standard of management is conservative measures/hydration for mild cases and hemodialysis for severe cases [43]. In older adults, the incidence of acute lithium toxicity in a large population-based study was 1.5 % per person year [15]. It is worth noting that serum lithium levels are poor predictors of brain lithium levels in older people; therefore, serum levels may not necessarily correlate with clinical evidence of neurotoxicity [113].

Recent studies are beginning to demonstrate that the neurological toxicity associated with lithium's usual use in older adults may not be worse than alternative medications. Delirium rates in geriatric lithium users did not differ from valproate-exposed patients [114]. Similarly, although a syndrome of tremor and rigidity has been described with lithium neurotoxicity [115, 116] and intention tremor can occur at low lithium levels in older adults, new data suggest that lithium may not increase the risk of parkinsonism or L-Dopa use compared to alternative bipolar pharmacotherapies (valproate or antipsychotics) [117]. Clinically, L-Dopa prescribing may not be appropriate in lithium users without true Parkinsonism or Parkinson's disease (e.g., lithium tremor without other aspects of Parkinsonism such as cogwheel rigidity, bradykinesia, or postural instability) and for whom a trial of lithium dose reduction may be safe from a mental health perspective.

7.2.5.2 Cognition and Dementia

Emerging data from population-based studies and clinical trials are starting to show that lithium may have preventive effects in dementia. Bipolar disorder is associated with a twofold higher risk of being diagnosed with dementia; however, dementia rates appear to be much lower in chronic lithium users compared to nonusers. Chronic lithium users with bipolar disorder have a similar dementia risk as people without bipolar disorder [118, 119]. Previously, it was believed that lithium predisposes to poor cognitive outcomes in older adults, but this appears to be only at neurotoxic doses [113]. New geriatric data suggest that lithium exposure may be associated with improved white matter integrity and cognition [7]. Ongoing research is confirming whether lithium can actually be used to prevent/treat dementia and expanding investigation of lithium's neuroprotective effects in several neurological conditions [120, 121].

7.2.5.3 Cerebrovascular Accidents (CVAs)

Bipolar disorder is known to be associated with cerebrovascular accidents (CVAs), particularly late-onset bipolar disorder beginning after age 50 [7]. A recent population-based study of older age bipolar inpatients suggests an overall 5-year prevalence of CVA of 3.5 % [11]. In general, evidence of CVA or cerebrovascular burden has been associated with poorer bipolar outcome and worse lithium response [7].

Emerging data reveal that lithium may be associated with a more than 50 % reduction in CVA risk among bipolar patients [122], although this has yet to be confirmed in an RCT (randomized controlled trial). Basic science research is demonstrating that lithium's anti-inflammatory, antioxidant, and endothelial effects may contribute to its potential protective role in CVA [110, 123].

7.2.6 Other Effects

7.2.6.1 Dermatological Effects

There do not appear to be any geriatric studies examining the dermatological effects of lithium. The adult literature on dermatological effects has reported a broad prevalence range for dermatological effects ranging from 3 to 45 % (acne, alopecia, or psoriasis), with a 2–6 % rate of psoriasis [109]. A recent meta-analysis, however, did not find a statistically significant difference in risk of developing these dermatological conditions in people exposed to and unexposed to lithium [44]. Topical lithium has even been helpful in one dermatological condition, seborrhoeic dermatitis, with RCT-level evidence [124]. However, topical lithium is not been used in the treatment of psychiatric disorders.

Overall, it seems that lithium does not appear to be associated with an increased risk of dermatological conditions at a population level, although such conditions do occur in individual patients. The general management of lithium-associated dermatological conditions is to use conventional condition-specific dermatological treatments, and to lower dosing/discontinue lithium, if possible [125].

7.3 Potential Biological Mechanisms Underlying Lithium-Associated Medical Effects

Nephrogenic diabetes insipidus (NDI) may be the adverse effect of lithium treatment whose physiologic basis is best understood [126]. NDI has the most robust and most replicated dose–response association with longer lithium duration and higher lithium levels across decades of research [23, 67, 73]. Emerging data suggest that NDI predicts the occurrence of several other medical conditions such as CKD, diabetes mellitus, and hypothyroidism [127]. This suggests that lithium-associated medical illnesses may share similar biological mechanisms. This would not be surprising since most of lithium's biological actions are thought to be inside the cell or in the intracellular matrix [126].

While the precise mechanism underlying lithium's therapeutic effects is unclear, lithium is believed to interact with inositol monophosphate [126] and protein kinase C [128] pathways, consequently modulating calcium-related intracellular signaling, cyclic AMP (cAMP), protein kinase A, protein kinase B (AKt), and inhibition of glycogen synthase kinase-3 Beta (GSK3Beta) [129], leading to many downstream effects. Recently, phosphodiesterases (which hydrolyze cAMP) [130], mTOR [131], G-protein couple receptors, epithelial sodium channel (ENaC) [130], and the mitogen-activated protein kinases (ERK1/2, p38) have also been implicated [132] in lithium's mechanism of action.

7.4 Lithium Dosing

What is the ideal serum lithium level for older adults? There currently are no specific guidelines for clinical management.

While many experts have recommended using levels as low as <0.5–0.6 mmol/L in older age BD to avoid toxicity [7, 133], the levels required for the therapeutic effects in late life for acute mania may be somewhat similar to those used in younger adult BD at approximately 0.6–1.0 mmol/L for maintenance [9]. The optimum lithium serum level for bipolar depression and maintenance, however, may be as low as 0.4–0.6 mmol/L [1, 134]. Since the most difficult-to-treat mood aspects of late-life bipolar disorder are acute depression and maintaining euthymia [7] and higher lithium levels even in the 0.8 mmol/L range can be associated with cognitive dulling and a mild depressive/fatigued phenotype [113], it can be useful to aim for 0.4 mmol/L for acute bipolar depression and 0.6 mmol/L in acute mania. Then, only if necessary, the dosage can be uptitrated as is safely tolerated and as is effective.

Long-term renal and neurological tolerability in older adults appear to be acceptable at lithium levels <0.8 mmol/L for most patients, although lower doses are preferable if possible. A recent 4-year RCT demonstrated that compared to placebo, lithium levels 0.25–0.5 mmol/L are not associated with deteriorations in renal function [135]. Observational data corroborate the relative long-term safety of levels <0.8 mmol/L in older adults [86, 91, 136]. Although neurological manifestations of lithium toxicity are also not commonly observed at levels <0.8 mmol/L, there appears to be a poor correlation between serum and brain lithium levels [113], particularly in later life [137]. Serum lithium level "cutoffs" (e.g., <0.8 mmol/L) are helpful as clinical guidance, but if renal function declines or neurological/cognitive effects are clinically observed, dose reductions may still be necessary. If a therapeutic effect is observed at 0.4–0.6 mmol/L (e.g., for bipolar depression), this may be a sufficient and well-tolerated dose.

Because of the increased risk of toxicity in older patients, it is best practice to begin lithium therapy at a dose of 150 mg qhs, and then titrate the dose upward based on lithium-level results (checking 5–7 days after each dose adjustment). Nightly (qhs) dosing is often preferred by patients because it can be helpful to sleep and minimize potential daytime sleepiness or cognitive dulling. Sometimes using alternate day dosing (e.g., alternating between 150 mg and 300 mg every second day) can be a useful strategy to achieve certain lithium levels. Often, a small adjustment using alternate day dosing can allow a patient to experience a therapeutic effect while avoiding a medical effect (e.g., renal decline). However, this approach can be confusing and may be difficult for many outpatients to maintain, so using a dosette box and having good communication with the pharmacy can be very helpful. Finding the "right dose for the right level" is difficult, since the dose required to achieve a certain level can decrease by threefold over the life span (and is mostly dictated by a person's renal function) [94, 138]. Table 7.1 shows geriatric lithium dosing based on the available literature [9, 43, 59, 94, 133, 138].

Table 7.1 Approximate geriatric lithium dosing guidance

Age category (years)	Target lithium level[a] (mmol/L)	Approximate lithium daily dose[b] (mg/day)	Starting dose[b] (mg/day)
45–59	0.4–0.8	600–1200	300–450
60–79	0.4–0.8	300–600	150
80–95	0.4–0.6	150–300	150

[a]The target lithium level is a compromise between effectiveness and safety, keeping in mind that some patients will tolerate a lower lithium level than listed, as evidenced by clinical assessment of impairment in renal, neurological, or cognitive function

[b]Approximate lithium daily dose is based on a modest number of small-to-moderately sized studies [9, 94, 133, 138]. These doses are approximate guides. The key principle is to start low, increase slowly, and titrate based on lithium levels and clinical effectiveness/tolerability. The relationship between serum lithium level and dose is mostly dictated by renal function and glomerular filtration rate (GFR)

[c]Lithium carbonate is the most commonly prescribed form of lithium [43]. Lithium citrate does not appear to have a different toxicity profile from lithium carbonate [43]. Slow-release formulations of lithium should be avoided since they appear to increase risk for renal disease [59]

A major issue in lithium dosing is consideration of possible drug–drug interactions. Angiotensin converting enzyme (ACE) inhibitors, loop diuretics [15], NSAIDs [82, 83], cyclo-oxygenase 2 (COX2) inhibitors [84], and diuretics (including thiazide diuretics) [85], all have been associated with an up to 50 % increase in serum lithium levels, although the percent increase is highly variable among individuals. Therefore, it is advisable, whenever initiating these medications or adjusting their dose, to check serum lithium levels 5–7 days after a dose change. Because of the potential for mood relapse with lithium dose reduction [139] and the unpredictability of the extent to which a drug interaction will affect lithium levels, it is often best to keep the lithium dose constant when starting a medication with a potential drug–drug interaction (e.g., NSAIDs) in a chronic lithium user, check the lithium level 5–7 days afterward, and if necessary titrate the lithium dose to whichever lithium level the patient was previously stabilized on.

Close monitoring of renal function and lithium levels is a key to preventing AKI and CKD. Ideally this should be every 3 months in geriatric patients [102]. Using once-daily dosing and avoiding prolonged-release formulations has also been found to be helpful [67]. Both twice-daily dosing and prolonged-release formulations have been associated with increased renal disease risk. It has been hypothesized that single-dose/short-acting formulations give longer periods per day where the kidney is relatively unexposed to lithium, during which the kidney recovers [59]. Geriatric lithium levels and renal function do not appear to be markedly affected by environmental temperature in temperate climates where mean daily temperatures are seldom >20 °C [140, 141], although environmental temperatures (e.g., 40 °C) have been associated with lithium toxicity in tropical and desert climates [142].

7.5 Summary

In summary, most medical comorbidity in old age bipolar disorder is unrelated to lithium use. In addition, cautious dosing and frequent monitoring of lithium can prevent most lithium-related comorbidity. A key point is that the main alternatives—antiepileptics and atypical antipsychotics—have significant tolerability concerns of their own [7]. Given the superior effectiveness of lithium in a significant subset of patients with older age bipolar disorder [9], it continues to deserve to be a top choice for treatment of bipolar disorder in older age.

Clinical Pearls

- Lithium is associated with a number of renal, endocrine, neurological, and other effects in patients with older age bipolar disorder.
- Most medical comorbidities observed in older age bipolar disorder are unrelated to lithium and/or would also be observed with other bipolar pharmacotherapies.
- Most of the medical adverse effects attributable to lithium are avoidable through safe lithium dosing, prescribing, and appropriate laboratory monitoring.
- Other approaches to prevent lithium-associated medical effects in older age bipolar disorder include: vigilance about drug–drug interactions, lowering cardiovascular risk burden (which underlies many medical comorbidities observed in older lithium users), and collaborating closely with primary care practitioners and medical specialists.
- Given the superior effectiveness of lithium in a many patients, it continues to be the gold-standard treatment for older age bipolar disorders despite its potential for adverse medical effects.

References

1. Yatham LN, Kennedy SH, Parikh SV, Schaffer A, Beaulieu S, Alda M, et al. Canadian Network for Mood and Anxiety Treatments (CANMAT) and International Society for Bipolar Disorders (ISBD) collaborative update of CANMAT guidelines for the management of patients with bipolar disorder: update 2013. Bipolar Disord. 2013;15(1):1–44.
2. Grof P, Duffy A, Cavazzoni P, Grof E, Garnham J, MacDougall M, et al. Is response to prophylactic lithium a familial trait? J Clin Psychiatry. 2002;63(10):942–7.
3. Chen CH, Lee CS, Lee MT, Ouyang WC, Chen CC, Chong MY, et al. Variant GADL1 and response to lithium therapy in bipolar I disorder. N Engl J Med. 2014;370(2):119–28.
4. Geddes JR, Goodwin GM, Rendell J, Azorin JM, Cipriani A, Ostacher MJ, et al. Lithium plus valproate combination therapy versus monotherapy for relapse prevention in bipolar I disorder (BALANCE): a randomised open-label trial. The Lancet. 2010;375(9712):385–95.

5. Kessing LV, Hellmund G, Geddes JR, Goodwin GM, Andersen PK. Valproate v. lithium in the treatment of bipolar disorder in clinical practice: observational nationwide register-based cohort study. Br J Psychiatry. 2011;199(1):57–63.
6. Cipriani A, Hawton K, Stockton S, Geddes JR. Lithium in the prevention of suicide in mood disorders: updated systematic review and meta-analysis. BMJ. 2013;346:f3646.
7. Sajatovic M, Strejilevich SA, Gildengers AG, Dols A, Al Jurdi RK, Forester BP, et al. A report on older-age bipolar disorder from the International Society for Bipolar Disorders Task Force. Bipolar Disord. 2015;17(7):689–704.
8. Young RC, Schulberg HC, Gildengers AG, Sajatovic M, Mulsant BH, Gyulai L, et al. Conceptual and methodological issues in designing a randomized, controlled treatment trial for geriatric bipolar disorder: GERI-BD. Bipolar Disord. 2010;12(1):56–67.
9. Al Jurdi RK, Marangell LB, Petersen NJ, Martinez M, Gyulai L, Sajatovic M. Prescription patterns of psychotropic medications in elderly compared with younger participants who achieved a "recovered" status in the systematic treatment enhancement program for bipolar disorder. Am J Geriatr Psychiatry. 2008;16(11):922–33.
10. Shulman KI, Rochon P, Sykora K, Anderson G, Mamdani M, Bronskill S, et al. Changing prescription patterns for lithium and valproic acid in old age: shifting practice without evidence. BMJ. 2003;326(7396):960–1.
11. Rej S, Yu C, Shulman K, Herrmann N, Fischer HD, Fung K, et al. Medical comorbidity, acute medical care use in late-life bipolar disorder: a comparison of lithium, valproate, and other pharmacotherapies. Gen Hosp Psychiatry. 2015;37(6):528–32.
12. Oostervink F, Nolen WA, Kok RM, Board EA. Two years' outcome of acute mania in bipolar disorder: different effects of age and age of onset. Int J Geriatr Psychiatry. 2015;30(2):201–9.
13. Hwang YJ, Dixon SN, Reiss JP, Wald R, Parikh CR, Gandhi S, et al. Atypical antipsychotic drugs and the risk for acute kidney injury and other adverse outcomes in older adults: a population-based cohort study. Ann Intern Med. 2014;161(4):242–8.
14. Jin H, Shih PA, Golshan S, Mudaliar S, Henry R, Glorioso DK, et al. Comparison of longer-term safety and effectiveness of 4 atypical antipsychotics in patients over age 40: a trial using equipoise-stratified randomization. J Clin Psychiatry. 2013;74(1):10–8.
15. Juurlink DN, Mamdani MM, Kopp A, Rochon PA, Shulman KI, Redelmeier DA. Drug-induced lithium toxicity in the elderly: a population-based study. J Am Geriatr Soc. 2004;52(5):794–8.
16. Strejilevich SA, Urtueta-Baamonde M, Teitelbaum J, Martino DJ, Marengo E, Igoa A, et al. Clinical concepts associated with lithium underutilization in the treatment of bipolar disorder. Vertex. 2011;22(Suppl):3–20.
17. Ephraim E, Prettyman R. Attitudes of old age psychiatrists in England and Wales to the use of mood stabilizer drugs. Int Psychogeriatr. 2009;21(3):576–80.
18. Baldessarini RJ, Leahy L, Arcona S, Gause D, Zhang W, Hennen J. Patterns of psychotropic drug prescription for U.S. patients with diagnoses of bipolar disorders. Psychiatr Serv. 2007;58(1):85–91.
19. Rej S, Segal M, Low NC, Mucsi I, Holcroft C, Shulman K, et al. The McGill Geriatric Lithium-Induced Diabetes Insipidus Clinical Study (McGLIDICS). Can J Psychiatry. 2014;59(6):327–34.
20. Lala SV, Sajatovic M. Medical and psychiatric comorbidities among elderly individuals with bipolar disorder: a literature review. J Geriatr Psychiatry Neurol. 2012;25(1):20–5.
21. Ali MK, McKeever Bullard K, Imperatore G, Barker L, Gregg EW. Characteristics associated with poor glycemic control among adults with self-reported diagnosed diabetes—National Health and Nutrition Examination Survey, United States, 2007–2010. MMWR Morb Mortal Wkly Rep. 2012;61(Suppl):32–7.
22. Coresh J, Selvin E, Stevens LA, Manzi J, Kusek JW, Eggers P, et al. Prevalence of chronic kidney disease in the United States. JAMA. 2007;298(17):2038–47.

23. Lehmann SW, Lee J. Lithium-associated hypercalcemia and hyperparathyroidism in the elderly: what do we know? J Affect Disord. 2013;146(2):151–7.
24. van Melick EJ, Wilting I, Ziere G, Kok RM, Egberts TC. The influence of lithium on calcium homeostasis in older patients in daily clinical practice. Int J Geriatr Psychiatry. 2014;29(6):594–601.
25. Rej S, Begley A, Gildengers A, Dew MA, Reynolds CF 3rd, Butters MA. Psychosocial risk factors for cognitive decline in late-life depression: findings from the MTLD-III study. Can Geriatr J. 2015;18(2):43–50.
26. Paul R, Minay J, Cardwell C, Fogarty D, Kelly C. Meta-analysis of the effects of lithium usage on serum creatinine levels. J Psychopharmacol. 2010;24(10):1425–31.
27. Guo JJ, Keck PE, Li H, Patel NC. Treatment costs related to bipolar disorder and comorbid conditions among Medicaid patients with bipolar disorder. Psychiatr Serv. 2007;58(8):1073–8.
28. Dols A, Rhebergen D, Beekman A, Kupka R, Sajatovic M, Stek ML. Psychiatric and medical comorbidities: results from a bipolar elderly cohort study. Am J Geriatr Psychiatry. 2014;22(11):1066–74.
29. Konz HW, Meesters PD, Paans NP, van Grootheest DS, Comijs HC, Stek ML, et al. Screening for metabolic syndrome in older patients with severe mental illness. Am J Geriatr Psychiatry. 2014;22(11):1116–20.
30. Kessing LV, Vradi E, McIntyre RS, Andersen PK. Causes of decreased life expectancy over the life span in bipolar disorder. J Affect Disord. 2015;180:142–7.
31. Westman J, Hallgren J, Wahlbeck K, Erlinge D, Alfredsson L, Osby U. Cardiovascular mortality in bipolar disorder: a population-based cohort study in Sweden. BMJ Open. 2013;3(4):e002373.
32. Forty L, Ulanova A, Jones L, Jones I, Gordon-Smith K, Fraser C, et al. Comorbid medical illness in bipolar disorder. Br J Psychiatry. 2014;205(6):465–72.
33. Fenn HH, Bauer MS, Altshuler L, Evans DR, Williford WO, Kilbourne AM, et al. Medical comorbidity and health-related quality of life in bipolar disorder across the adult age span. J Affect Disord. 2005;86(1):47–60.
34. Sajatovic M, Friedman SH, Sabharwal J, Bingham CR. Clinical characteristics and length of hospital stay among older adults with bipolar disorder, schizophrenia or schizoaffective disorder, depression, and dementia. J Geriatr Psychiatry Neurol. 2004;17(1):3–8.
35. Sajatovic M, Popli A, Semple W. Ten-year use of hospital-based services by geriatric veterans with schizophrenia and bipolar disorder. Psychiatr Serv. 1996;47(9):961–5.
36. Regenold WT, Thapar RK, Marano C, Gavirneni S, Kondapavuluru PV. Increased prevalence of type 2 diabetes mellitus among psychiatric inpatients with bipolar I affective and schizoaffective disorders independent of psychotropic drug use. J Affect Disord. 2002;70(1):19–26.
37. Sajatovic M, Bingham CR, Campbell EA, Fletcher DF. Bipolar disorder in older adult inpatients. J Nerv Ment Dis. 2005;193(6):417–9.
38. Lehmann SW, Rabins PV. Factors related to hospitalization in elderly manic patients with early and late-onset bipolar disorder. Int J Geriatr Psychiatry. 2006;21(11):1060–4.
39. Gildengers AG, Whyte EM, Drayer RA, Soreca I, Fagiolini A, Kilbourne AM, et al. Medical burden in late-life bipolar and major depressive disorders. Am J Geriatr Psychiatry. 2008;16(3):194–200.
40. Abitbol R, Rej S, Segal M, Looper KJ. Diabetes mellitus onset in geriatric patients: does long-term atypical antipsychotic exposure increase risk? Psychogeriatrics. 2015;15(1):43–50.
41. Sylvestre JD, Yu C, Dawson B, Copps B, Segal M, Looper KJ, et al. Older adults with severe mental illness frequently require acute medical hospitalizations: an increased need for consultation-liaison services in future years? J Psychosom Res. 2015;79(1):87–8.

42. Kilbourne AM, Goodrich DE, Lai Z, Post EP, Schumacher K, Nord KM, et al. Randomized controlled trial to assess reduction of cardiovascular disease risk in patients with bipolar disorder: the self-management addressing heart risk trial (SMAHRT). J Clin Psychiatry. 2013;74(7):e655–62.
43. Rej S, Herrmann N, Shulman K. The effects of lithium on renal function in older adults—a systematic review. J Geriatr Psychiatry Neurol. 2012;25(1):51–61.
44. McKnight RF, Adida M, Budge K, Stockton S, Goodwin GM, Geddes JR. Lithium toxicity profile: a systematic review and meta-analysis. The Lancet. 2012;379(9817):721–8.
45. van Melick EJ, Meinders AE, Hoffman TO, Egberts TC. Renal effects of long-term lithium therapy in the elderly: a cross-sectional study. Int J Geriatr Psychiatry. 2008;23(7):685–92.
46. Bendz H, Aurell M, Balldin J, Mathe AA, Sjodin I. Kidney damage in long-term lithium patients: a cross-sectional study of patients with 15 years or more on lithium. Nephrol Dial Transplant. 1994;9(9):1250–4.
47. Wallin L, Alling C, Aurell M. Impairment of renal function in patients on long-term lithium treatment. Clin Nephrol. 1982;18(1):23–8.
48. Tyrer SP, Schacht RG, McCarthy MJ, Menard KN, Leong S, Shopsin B. The effect of lithium on renal haemodynamic function. Psychol Med. 1983;13(1):61–9.
49. Wilting I, Heerdink ER, Mersch PP, den Boer JA, Egberts AC, Nolen WA. Association between lithium serum level, mood state, and patient-reported adverse drug reactions during long-term lithium treatment: a naturalistic follow-up study. Bipolar Disord. 2009;11(4):434–40.
50. Grof P, Hux M, Dressler B, O'Sullivan K. Kidney function and response to lithium treatment. Prog Neuropsychopharmacol Biol Psychiatry. 1982;6(4–6):491–4.
51. Lassen E, Vestergaard P, Thomsen K. Renal function of patients in long-term treatment with lithium citrate alone or in combination with neuroleptics and antidepressant drugs. Arch Gen Psychiatry. 1986;43(5):481–2.
52. Rej S, Margolese HC, Low NC. Diabetes insipidus secondary to combination atypical antipsychotic and lithium use in a bipolar disorder patient: a case report. Primary Care Companion CNS Disord. 2011;13(4):pii: PCC.11l01138. doi:10.4088/PCC.11l01138.
53. Waller DG, Edwards JG, Polak A. Neuroleptics, lithium and renal function. Br J Psychiatry. 1985;146:510–4.
54. Vestergaard P, Amdisen A, Hansen HE, Schou M. Lithium treatment and kidney function. A survey of 237 patients in long-term treatment. Acta Psychiatr Scand. 1979;60(5):504–20.
55. Bucht G, Wahlin A. Renal concentrating capacity in long-term lithium treatment and after withdrawal of lithium. Acta Med Scand. 1980;207(4):309–14.
56. Nora RM, Hariprasad MK, Beke AZ. Urinary osmolality in lithium and non-lithium treated psychiatric patients. J Clin Psychiatry. 1981;42(6):254.
57. Miller AL, Bowden CL, Plewes J. Lithium and impairment of renal concentrating ability. J Affect Disord. 1985;9(2):115–9.
58. Lokkegaard H, Andersen NF, Henriksen E, Bartels PD, Brahm M, Baastrup PC, et al. Renal function in 153 manic-depressive patients treated with lithium for more than five years. Acta Psychiatr Scand. 1985;71(4):347–55.
59. Schou M, Amdisen A, Thomsen K, Vestergaard P, Hetmar O, Mellerup ET, et al. Lithium treatment regimen and renal water handling: the significance of dosage pattern and tablet type examined through comparison of results from two clinics with different treatment regimens. Psychopharmacology. 1982;77(4):387–90.
60. Plenge P, Mellerup ET, Bolwig TG, Brun C, Hetmar O, Ladefoged J, et al. Lithium treatment: does the kidney prefer one daily dose instead of two? Acta Psychiatr Scand. 1982;66(2):121–8.
61. Waller DG, Edwards JG, Naik R, Polak A. Renal function during lithium treatment. Q J Med. 1984;53(211):369–79.

62. Presne C, Fakhouri F, Noel LH, Stengel B, Even C, Kreis H, et al. Lithium-induced nephropathy: rate of progression and prognostic factors. Kidney Int. 2003;64(2):585–92.
63. Jorgensen F, Larsen S, Spanager B, Clausen E, Tango M, Brinch E, et al. Kidney function and quantitative histological changes in patients on long-term lithium therapy. Acta Psychiatr Scand. 1984;70(5):455–62.
64. Smith RE, Helms PM. Adverse effects of lithium therapy in the acutely ill elderly patient. J Clin Psychiatry. 1982;43(3):94–9.
65. Kinahan JC, NiChorcorain A, Cunningham S, Freyne A, Cooney C, Barry S, et al. Diagnostic accuracy of tests for polyuria in lithium-treated patients. J Clin Psychopharmacol. 2015;35(4):434–41.
66. Sajadi S, Yu C, Sylvestre J-D, Segal M, Looper K, Rej S. Does lower urine specific gravity predict decline in renal function and hypernatremia in older adults exposed to psychotropic medications? Clin Kidney J. 2016;9(2):268–72.
67. Rej S, Elie D, Mucsi I, Looper KJ, Segal M. Chronic kidney disease in lithium-treated older adults: a review of epidemiology, mechanisms, and implications for the treatment of late-life mood disorders. Drugs Aging. 2015;32(1):31–42.
68. Rej S, Senouci SI, Looper K, Segal M. Using hypernatraemic events to predict reduced renal function in elderly lithium patients: a brief report. Psychogeriatrics. 2013;13(1):25–8.
69. Rej S, Shulman K, Herrmann N, Harel Z, Fischer HD, Fung K, et al. Prevalence and correlates of renal disease in older lithium users: a population-based study. Am J Geriatr Psychiatry. 2014;22(11):1075–82.
70. Rej S, Looper K, Segal M. Do antidepressants lower the prevalence of lithium-associated hypernatremia in the elderly? A retrospective study. Can Geriatr J. 2013;16(2):38–42.
71. Batlle DC, von Riotte AB, Gaviria M, Grupp M. Amelioration of polyuria by amiloride in patients receiving long-term lithium therapy. N Engl J Med. 1985;312(7):408–14.
72. Bedford JJ, Weggery S, Ellis G, McDonald FJ, Joyce PR, Leader JP, et al. Lithium-induced nephrogenic diabetes insipidus: renal effects of amiloride. Clin J Am Soc Nephrol. 2008;3 (5):1324–31.
73. Boton R, Gaviria M, Batlle DC. Prevalence, pathogenesis, and treatment of renal dysfunction associated with chronic lithium therapy. Am J Kidney Dis. 1987;10(5):329–45.
74. Bendz H, Schon S, Attman PO, Aurell M. Renal failure occurs in chronic lithium treatment but is uncommon. Kidney Int. 2010;77(3):219–24.
75. Elie D, Segal M, Low NC, Mucsi I, Holcroft C, Shulman K, et al. Statins in the prevention of lithium-associated diabetes insipidus: preliminary findings. Kidney Int. 2015;87(4):862.
76. Dennison U, Clarkson M, O'Mullane J, Cassidy EM. The incidence and clinical correlates of lithium toxicity: a retrospective review. Ir J Med Sci. 2011;180(3):661–5.
77. Bellomo R, Ronco C, Kellum JA, Mehta RL, Palevsky P. Acute Dialysis Quality Initiative w. Acute renal failure—definition, outcome measures, animal models, fluid therapy and information technology needs: the Second International Consensus Conference of the Acute Dialysis Quality Initiative (ADQI) Group. Crit Care. 2004;8(4):R204–12.
78. Waring WS. Management of lithium toxicity. Toxicol Rev. 2006;25(4):221–30.
79. Oakley PW, Whyte IM, Carter GL. Lithium toxicity: an iatrogenic problem in susceptible individuals. Aust N Z J Psychiatry. 2001;35(6):833–40.
80. Roose SP, Nurnberger JI, Dunner DL, Blood DK, Fieve RR. Cardiac sinus node dysfunction during lithium treatment. Am J Psychiatry. 1979;136(6):804–6.
81. Chen KP, Shen WW, Lu ML. Implication of serum concentration monitoring in patients with lithium intoxication. Psychiatry Clin Neurosci. 2004;58(1):25–9.
82. Kristoff CA, Hayes PE, Barr WH, Small RE, Townsend RJ, Ettigi PG. Effect of ibuprofen on lithium plasma and red blood cell concentrations. Clin Pharmacy. 1986;5(1):51–5.
83. Reimann IW, Diener U, Frolich JC. Indomethacin but not aspirin increases plasma lithium ion levels. Arch Gen Psychiatry. 1983;40(3):283–6.

84. Phelan KM, Mosholder AD, Lu S. Lithium interaction with the cyclooxygenase 2 inhibitors rofecoxib and celecoxib and other nonsteroidal anti-inflammatory drugs. J Clin Psychiatry. 2003;64(11):1328–34.
85. Himmelhoch JM, Forrest J, Neil JF, Detre TP. Thiazide-lithium synergy in refractory mood swings. Am J Psychiatry. 1977;134(2):149–52.
86. Kirkham E, Skinner J, Anderson T, Bazire S, Twigg MJ, Desborough JA. One lithium level >1.0 mmol/L causes an acute decline in eGFR: findings from a retrospective analysis of a monitoring database. BMJ Open. 2014;4(11):e006020.
87. Laliberte V, Yu C, Rej S. Acute renal and neurotoxicity in older lithium users: how can we manage and prevent these events in patients with late-life mood disorders? J Psychiatry Neurosci. 2015;40(4):E29–30.
88. Crowe E, Halpin D, Stevens P. Early identification and management of chronic kidney disease: summary of NICE guidance. BMJ. 2008;337:a1530.
89. Chin HJ, Ahn SY, Ryu J, Kim S, Na KY, Kim KW, et al. Renal function and decline in functional capacity in older adults. Age Ageing. 2014;43(6):833–8.
90. Murray CJ, Atkinson C, Bhalla K, Birbeck G, Burstein R, Chou D, et al. The state of US health, 1990–2010: burden of diseases, injuries, and risk factors. JAMA. 2013;310(6):591–608.
91. Clos S, Rauchhaus P, Severn A, Donnan P. Long term effect of lithium maintenance therapy on estimated glomerular filtration rate (eGFR) in patients with affective disorders. Lancet Psychiatry. 2015;2(12):1075–83.
92. Kessing LV, Gerds TA, Feldt-Rasmussen B, Andersen PK, Licht RW. Use of lithium and anticonvulsants and the rate of chronic kidney disease: a nationwide population-based study. JAMA Psychiatry. 2015;72(12):1182–91.
93. Shine B, McKnight RF, Leaver L, Geddes JR. Long-term effects of lithium on renal, thyroid, and parathyroid function: a retrospective analysis of laboratory data. The Lancet. 2015;386 (9992):461–8.
94. Rej S, Beaulieu S, Segal M, Low NC, Mucsi I, Holcroft C, et al. Lithium dosing and serum concentrations across the age spectrum: from early adulthood to the tenth decade of life. Drugs Aging. 2014;31(12):911–6.
95. Singh LK, Nizamie SH, Akhtar S, Praharaj SK. Improving tolerability of lithium with a once-daily dosing schedule. Am J Ther. 2011;18(4):288–91.
96. Rej S, Abitbol R, Looper K, Segal M. Chronic renal failure in lithium-using geriatric patients: effects of lithium continuation versus discontinuation—a 60-month retrospective study. Int J Geriatr Psychiatry. 2013;28(5):450–3.
97. Rej S, Li BW, Looper K, Segal M. Renal function in geriatric psychiatry patients compared to non-psychiatric older adults: effects of lithium use and other factors. Aging Ment Health. 2014;18(7):847–53.
98. Albert U, De Cori D, Aguglia A, Barbaro F, Lanfranco F, Bogetto F, et al. Lithium-associated hyperparathyroidism and hypercalcaemia: a case-control cross-sectional study. J Affect Disord. 2013;151(2):786–90.
99. Pallan S, Khan A. Primary hyperparathyroidism: update on presentation, diagnosis, and management in primary care. Can Fam Phys. 2011;57(2):184–9.
100. Lally J, Lee B, McDonald C. Prevalence of hypercalcaemia in patients on maintenance lithium therapy monitored in primary care. Ir Med J. 2013;106(1):15–7.
101. Baird GS. Ionized calcium. Clin Chim Acta. 2011;412(9–10):696–701.
102. Ng F, Mammen OK, Wilting I, Sachs GS, Ferrier IN, Cassidy F, et al. The international society for bipolar disorders (ISBD) consensus guidelines for the safety monitoring of bipolar disorder treatments. Bipolar Disord. 2009;11(6):559–95.
103. Shulman KI, Sykora K, Gill SS, Mamdani M, Anderson G, Marras C, et al. New thyroxine treatment in older adults beginning lithium therapy: implications for clinical practice. Am J Geriatr Psychiatry. 2005;13(4):299–304.

104. Head L, Dening T. Lithium in the over-65s: who is taking it and who is monitoring it? A survey of older adults on lithium in the Cambridge Mental Health Services catchment area. Int J Geriatr Psychiatry. 1998;13(3):164–71.
105. Kraszewska A, Chlopocka-Wozniak M, Abramowicz M, Sowinski J, Rybakowski JK. A cross-sectional study of thyroid function in 66 patients with bipolar disorder receiving lithium for 10–44 years. Bipolar Disord. 2015;17(4):375–80.
106. Kraszewska A, Abramowicz M, Chlopocka-Wozniak M, Sowinski J, Rybakowski J. The effect of lithium on thyroid function in patients with bipolar disorder. Psychiatr Pol. 2014;48 (3):417–28.
107. Faggiano A, Del Prete M, Marciello F, Marotta V, Ramundo V, Colao A. Thyroid diseases in elderly. Minerva Endocrinol. 2011;36(3):211–31.
108. Berk M, Kapczinski F, Andreazza AC, Dean OM, Giorlando F, Maes M, et al. Pathways underlying neuroprogression in bipolar disorder: focus on inflammation, oxidative stress and neurotrophic factors. Neurosci Biobehav Rev. 2011;35(3):804–17.
109. Dols A, Sienaert P, van Gerven H, Schouws S, Stevens A, Kupka R, et al. The prevalence and management of side effects of lithium and anticonvulsants as mood stabilizers in bipolar disorder from a clinical perspective: a review. Int Clin Psychopharmacol. 2013;28(6):287–96.
110. Gold AB, Herrmann N, Lanctot KL. Lithium and its neuroprotective and neurotrophic effects: potential treatment for post-ischemic stroke sequelae. Curr Drug Targets. 2011;12 (2):243–55.
111. Svendal G, Fasmer OB, Engeland A, Berk M, Lund A. Co-prescription of medication for bipolar disorder and diabetes mellitus: a nationwide population-based study with focus on gender differences. BMC Med. 2012;10:148.
112. Schou M, Amdisen A, Trap-Jensen J. Lithium poisoning. Am J Psychiatry. 1968;125 (4):520–7.
113. Forester BP, Streeter CC, Berlow YA, Tian H, Wardrop M, Finn CT, et al. Brain lithium levels and effects on cognition and mood in geriatric bipolar disorder: a lithium-7 magnetic resonance spectroscopy study. Am J Geriatr Psychiatry. 2009;17(1):13–23.
114. Shulman KI, Sykora K, Gill S, Mamdani M, Bronskill S, Wodchis WP, et al. Incidence of delirium in older adults newly prescribed lithium or valproate: a population-based cohort study. J Clin Psychiatry. 2005;66(4):424–7.
115. Bohlega SA, Al-Foghom NB. Drug-induced Parkinson's disease. A clinical review. Neurosciences. 2013;18(3):215–21.
116. Shen HC, Li JY, Lo YK. Lithium intoxication-induced acute parkinsonism complicated with hyperparathyroidism and nephrogenic diabetes insipidus: report of a case. Acta Neurol Taiwan. 2007;16(4):231–3.
117. Marras C, Herrmann N, Fischer HD, Fung K, Gruneir A, Rochon P, et al. Lithium use in older adults is associated with increased prescribing of Parkinson's medications. Am J Geriatr Psychiatry. 2016;24(4):301–9.
118. Kessing LV, Sondergard L, Forman JL, Andersen PK. Lithium treatment and risk of dementia. Arch Gen Psychiatry. 2008;65(11):1331–5.
119. Forlenza OV, Diniz BS, Radanovic M, Santos FS, Talib LL, Gattaz WF. Disease-modifying properties of long-term lithium treatment for amnestic mild cognitive impairment: randomised controlled trial. Br J Psychiatry. 2011;198(5):351–6.
120. Mauer S, Vergne D, Ghaemi SN. Standard and trace-dose lithium: a systematic review of dementia prevention and other behavioral benefits. Aust N Z J Psychiatry. 2014;48(9):809–18.
121. Scheuing L, Chiu CT, Liao HM, Linares GR, Chuang DM. Preclinical and clinical investigations of mood stabilizers for Huntington's disease: what have we learned? Int J Biol Sci. 2014;10(9):1024–38.

122. Lan CC, Liu CC, Lin CH, Lan TY, McInnis MG, Chan CH, et al. A reduced risk of stroke with lithium exposure in bipolar disorder: a population-based retrospective cohort study. Bipolar Disord. 2015;17(7):705–14.
123. Bosche B, Schafer M, Graf R, Hartel FV, Schafer U, Noll T. Lithium prevents early cytosolic calcium increase and secondary injurious calcium overload in glycolytically inhibited endothelial cells. Biochem Biophys Res Commun. 2013;434(2):268–72.
124. Dreno B, Chosidow O, Revuz J, Moyse D, Study Investigator G. Lithium gluconate 8 % vs ketoconazole 2% in the treatment of seborrhoeic dermatitis: a multicentre, randomized study. Br J Dermatol. 2003;148(6):1230–6.
125. Gupta AK, Knowles SR, Gupta MA, Jaunkalns R, Shear NH. Lithium therapy associated with hidradenitis suppurativa: case report and a review of the dermatologic side effects of lithium. J Am Acad Dermatol. 1995;32(2 Pt 2):382–6.
126. Trepiccione F, Christensen BM. Lithium-induced nephrogenic diabetes insipidus: new clinical and experimental findings. J Nephrol. 2010;23(Suppl 16):S43–8.
127. Rej S, Segal M, Low NC, Mucsi I, Holcroft C, Shulman K, et al. In this correspondence, preliminary data in 100 lithium users found that urine osmolality correlated with chronic kidney disease, diabetes mellitus, and hypothyroidism. We hypothesize that GSK-3beta inhibition is a potential mechanism for lithium-associated medical illness. Med Hypotheses. 2015;84(6):602.
128. Sim JH, Himmel NJ, Redd SK, Pulous FE, Rogers RT, Black LN, et al. Absence of PKC-alpha attenuates lithium-induced nephrogenic diabetes insipidus. PLoS ONE. 2014;9 (7):e101753.
129. Kishore BK, Ecelbarger CM. Lithium: a versatile tool for understanding renal physiology. Am J Physiol Renal Physiol. 2013;304(9):F1139–49.
130. Sanches TR, Volpini RA, Massola Shimizu MH, Braganca AC, Oshiro-Monreal F, Seguro AC, et al. Sildenafil reduces polyuria in rats with lithium-induced NDI. Am J Physiol Renal Physiol. 2012;302(1):F216–25.
131. Gao C, Holscher C, Liu Y, Li L. GSK3: a key target for the development of novel treatments for type 2 diabetes mellitus and Alzheimer disease. Rev Neurosci. 2012;23(1):1–11.
132. Trepiccione F, Pisitkun T, Hoffert JD, Poulsen SB, Capasso G, Nielsen S, et al. Early targets of lithium in rat kidney inner medullary collecting duct include p38 and ERK1/2. Kidney Int. 2014;86(4):757–67.
133. Shulman KI, Mackenzie S, Hardy B. The clinical use of lithium carbonate in old age: a review. Prog Neuropsychopharmacol Biol Psychiatry. 1987;11(2–3):159–64.
134. Severus E, Taylor MJ, Sauer C, Pfennig A, Ritter P, Bauer M, et al. Lithium for prevention of mood episodes in bipolar disorders: systematic review and meta-analysis. Int J Bipolar Disord. 2014;2:15.
135. Aprahamian I, Santos FS, Dos Santos B, Talib L, Diniz BS, Radanovic M, et al. Long-term, low-dose lithium treatment does not impair renal function in the elderly: a 2-year randomized, placebo-controlled trial followed by single-blind extension. J Clin Psychiatry. 2014;75(7):e672–8.
136. Rej S, Looper K, Segal M. The effect of serum lithium levels on renal function in geriatric outpatients: a retrospective longitudinal study. Drugs Aging. 2013;30(6):409–15.
137. Machado-Vieira R, Otaduy MC, Zanetti MV, De Sousa RT, Dias VV, Leite CC, et al. A selective association between central and peripheral lithium levels in remitters in bipolar depression: a 3T-Li magnetic resonance spectroscopy study. Acta Psychiatr Scand. 2016;133 (3):214–20.
138. Sproule BA, Hardy BG, Shulman KI. Differential pharmacokinetics of lithium in elderly patients. Drugs Aging. 2000;16(3):165–77.
139. Fahy S, Lawlor BA. Discontinuation of lithium augmentation in an elderly cohort. Int J Geriatr Psychiatry. 2001;16(10):1004–9.

140. Rej S, AlAqeel B, Segal M, Low NC, Mucsi I, Holcroft C, et al. Is environmental temperature related to renal symptoms, serum lithium levels, and other laboratory test results in current lithium users? Hum Psychopharmacol. 2014;29(4):392–6.
141. Wilting I, Fase S, Martens EP, Heerdink ER, Nolen WA, Egberts AC. The impact of environmental temperature on lithium serum levels. Bipolar Disord. 2007;9(6):603–8.
142. Medhi B, Prakash O, Jose VM, Pradhan B, Chakrabarty S, Pandhi P. Seasonal variation in plasma levels of lithium in the Indian population: is there a need to modify the dose? Singap Med J. 2008;49(9):724–7.

Neuromodulation Therapies and Ketamine in Older Age Bipolar Disorder

8

Adriana P. Hermida and Oliver M. Glass

Clinical Vignette 8.1

Dr. C is a 65-year-old male physician with late onset depressive disorder who presented with a sad mood, low energy, poor motivation, anhedonia, a poor appetite, passive suicidal ideations, and an inability to do his job. His primary care physician prescribed sertraline 50 mg per day but it resulted in intolerable diarrhea. He was then tried on a low dose of escitalopram, which he could not tolerate due to the emergence of agitation. He was referred for TMS. He received TMS treatments five times per week at 120 % of motor threshold with 3000 pulses/session. The treatment sessions lasted five weeks. His mood improved and he was able to return to work. He did, however, have residual symptoms such as difficulty falling asleep and poor concentration. Several weeks later, Dr. C developed a manic episode, which presented as lack of sleep, elevated mood, and delusional thoughts. He believed God had given him special powers to save all the patients in the intensive care unit. He worked twenty-four hours a day and requested residents to round with him at midnight. He became extremely agitated and was sent to the emergency department, where he was found to be a potential danger to patients. After a psychiatric evaluation, he was admitted to the inpatient behavioral health unit. Lithium was initiated and titrated to the therapeutic range, but his response was poor. After failing several mood stabilizers and antipsychotics, a combination of valproic

A.P. Hermida (✉)
Department of Psychiatry and Behavioral Sciences,
Emory University School of Medicine, 12 Executive Park Drive NE,
Atlanta, GA 30329, USA
e-mail: ahermid@emory.edu

O.M. Glass
Department of Psychiatry and Behavioral Medicine, East Carolina University,
905 Johns Hopkins Dr, Greenville, NC 27834, USA
e-mail: glassol@ecu.edu

S.W. Lehmann and B.P. Forester (eds.), *Bipolar Disorder in Older Age Patients*,
DOI 10.1007/978-3-319-48912-4_8

acid and aripiprazole was able to partially control his symptoms. Dr. C, however, remained agitated, psychotic, refused to eat, and believed that people were trying to poison him. He was referred for ECT and received 8 right unilateral (RUL) treatments with excellent improvement in mood and psychosis. There was no residual cognitive impairment. He was able to return to work in 2 weeks, and did not receive maintenance ECT. One year later, Dr. C relapsed with a severe depressive episode, which included daily suicidal ideations. He failed several medication trials and was restarted on ECT, where he failed to respond to 8 bilateral treatments. Due to the lack of response to ECT and the severity of his depressive episode, he was referred and approved for a subcallosal cingulate deep brain stimulation (DBS) trial, where he experienced a significant improvement in mood. He was able to return to work 6 months later.

Learning Points

- During TMS treatment, patients can drive and generally continue their daily activities.
- ECT is effective in treating unipolar and bipolar depression.
- DBS trials typically enroll patients who have failed ECT.

8.1 Introduction

Neuromodulation therapies are important alternatives for the management of treatment-resistant mood disorders in older adults. Some of these therapies are relatively modern strategies such as the recently FDA-approved transcranial magnetic stimulation (TMS), vagal nerve stimulation (VNS), and deep brain stimulation (DBS), which is still being researched. Electroconvulsive therapy (ECT) has been available since its discovery by the Italian scientists Bini and Cerletti in 1938 and has been widely used in the USA since the 1940s. The discovery of electrical shocks for the induction of seizures preceded the use of lithium in medicine for mood stabilization (1949) and also the synthesis of the first antipsychotic drug, chlorpromazine (1951). The use of ECT has varied widely since then with a recent significant shift toward the use of ultra-brief-pulse width, right unilateral treatment, and its increased practice in outpatient settings.

The safety, efficacy, and specific clinical indications for the newer therapies have not been systematically studied in older adults. Despite the fact that ECT has been widely used in geriatric patients, there are limited evidence-based data about its use in this population.

Older individuals are particularly vulnerable to polypharmacy given increased medical comorbidities with advancing age. Polypharmacy can be particularly dangerous as older adults exhibit pharmacokinetic changes such us decreased renal blood flow, decreased hepatic drug clearance, changes in protein binding, decreased lean body mass and total body water, all of which significantly affect the volume of distribution. These changes can cause adverse side effects and toxicity. Neuromodulation techniques are not pharmacotherapies and, therefore, have the potential of limiting polypharmacy in older adults with psychiatric disorders. While the vast majority of neuromodulation therapy research focuses on unipolar depression, there is an increasing amount of research examining the safety and efficacy of ECT in individuals with bipolar depression.

Bipolar disorder is often underdiagnosed or misdiagnosed [1]. Therefore, some patients who are incorporated into neuromodulation studies on depression may have bipolar depression rather than unipolar depression. Furthermore, older adults with bipolar disorder (OABD) may have a better response rate to antidepressants, but whether they are less likely to switch into manic or mixed episodes when compared to younger patients is still to be determined [2]. Unfortunately, there is limited research that solely evaluates neuromodulation on OABD.

8.2 Electroconvulsive Therapy (ECT)

ECT is a neuromodulation therapy that induces seizures by the transmission of electrical impulses into the brain with the intention of providing symptom improvement for a wide range of mental illnesses. The impulse is commonly provided by an electrical energy device, which transmits an electrical current toward leads attached to the patient's scalp. Modern ECT devices produce trains of rectangular, constant-current pulses with alternating polarity; the waveform is characterized by *amplitude* (the current strength during the pulse), *pulse width* (PW, the duration of each pulse), pulse-pair repetition *frequency* (the number of pairs of a positive and a negative pulse per second), and stimulus train *duration*. The current amplitude is reported in amperes (A) or in milliamperes. ECT devices provide either individual dials or software menu settings for independent adjustment of stimulus parameters or a single dial that increments the total charge of the stimulus by a percentage of maximal charge by automatically setting the various stimulus parameters following a preprogrammed schedule [3]. This electrical impulse generates electroencephalogram (EEG) evidence for seizure activity. Patients are given anesthesia, along with a muscle relaxant such as succinylcholine or rocuronium to inhibit tonic-clonic movement and to minimize post-ECT symptoms such as muscle soreness. Often beta-blockers and anticholinergic agents are administered to compensate for the para-sympathetic and sympathetic release that occurs during ECT.

ECT is considered a highly effective acute treatment in older age patients with mood disorders; however, data on the safety and efficacy of maintenance ECT in this population is promising but sparse [4]. It has been reported that elderly patients may have a higher immediate response rate than younger patients [5, 6], where one study saw a response rate of 73 % for patients aged 60–74 compared to 54 % in adult patients [6]. According to recent data, one-third of patients who undergo ECT are aged 65 years or older and 15.6 % of older age patients with affective disorders receive ECT [7]. There might be several reasons for why patients aged 65 years or older receive ECT: greater medical comorbidities, which makes them more vulnerable to side effects and drug–drug interactions related to pharmacotherapy, higher rates of medication intolerance, and frailty, which can lead to a faster ECT referral. Additionally, late onset psychotic depression predicts a better response to ECT, making this a potentially favorable treatment modality [8]. There are reports indicating that the more severe the presentation, the better the response to ECT. This can be explained by the possibility that this subset of individuals often present with a more organic presentation such as psychotic depression and less often with a confounding comorbidity such as an underlying personality disorder [8]. Older adults with depression complicated by psychosis and catatonia respond very well to ECT. ECT is considered a safe and well-tolerated procedure even when administered to frail older adults with medical comorbidity [9].

OABD remains a severe illness often associated with comorbid disorders such as substance abuse, alcohol use disorders, dysthymia, generalized anxiety disorder, panic disorder [10], and delirium. All of these comorbidities must be considered when considering ECT use in OABD.

The treatment of bipolar depression with ECT brings a set of challenges, most notably the concomitant use of anticonvulsants as mood stabilizers. The earlier practice of stopping all psychotropic medications before and during a course of ECT is no longer a common practice [8]. However, there is controversy in the field and difference in opinion regarding the combination of antiepileptic drugs (AEDs) and ECT [11]. The American Psychiatry Association guidelines advise stopping AEDs during ECT if AEDs are prescribed for a psychiatric indication [12], whereas the Royal College of Psychiatrists guidelines state that AEDs can be continued during a course of ECT when they are used as mood stabilizers [13, 14]. Thus, guidelines have been contradictory.

In a survey examining different ECT practices, Thirthalli and colleagues noted widely varying preferences regarding concomitant treatment with ECT and anticonvulsants. One-third of the clinicians (33 %) preferred to continue the antiepileptic drug at full dose; about half (51 %) stated that they would reduce the anticonvulsant dose to half and about 16 % preferred to stop anticonvulsants completely during ECT [15].

Virupaksha et al. [11] published a retrospective chart review of individuals with bipolar disorder undergoing ECT. Seventy-nine patients had concomitant use of AEDs while 122 were not treated with AEDs. All patients had bilateral ECTs [bifrontal ECTs: n = 82 (40.8 %) or bitemporal ECTs: n = 119(59.2 %)]. Both groups achieved comparable symptomatic improvement at the end of the ECT course; however, AED patients required a significantly higher number of ECT sessions to achieve improvement. Rubner et al. [16] reported on 189 patients, 87 (46.0 %) patients received combination therapy. Of these 87 patients, only nine (10.3 %) reported difficulty inducing an adequate seizure. When AEDs are going to be continued, a change of anesthetic agent or an altered anesthetic dose is recommended. Additionally, the AED dose should be reduced or withheld the night before and the morning of ECT. Mukherjee et al. [17] recommends lowering the Lithium serum level to less than 0.4 mmol/l on the day of ECT and found that the combination of AEDs and ECT seems to be safe.

Another challenge of using ECT for the treatment of bipolar depression is the risk of a switch to mania or modifying the illness to one that is rapid cycling, which could become more difficult to treat. Similar to findings with regard to antidepressant treatment of individuals with bipolar disorder, there is also a higher risk of manic switches with ECT in bipolar depression [18, 19]. Following expert recommendations in the field of the treatment of bipolar depression, providers should have caution when using antidepressants alone [20]. Since bipolar disorder requires the use of mood stabilizers, it can make sense to continue anticonvulsant medications during ECT for mood stabilization purposes. If there is concern of the anticonvulsant interfering with seizure activity, the dose could be lowered or held the night before the ECT session. Additionally, benzodiazepines should be reduced to the minimum tolerated dose and always be reversed with a benzodiazepine reversal agent to assist with normalizing the seizure threshold during the ECT session. Seizure titration is the preferred method to determine stimulus dosing during the acute course of ECT to ensure adequate electrical charge during the treatment.

There is insufficient evidence to determine which electrode placement is most efficacious in treating bipolar disorder. Some experts recommend the use of bilateral treatments. However, no evidence-based data support this particular approach. The suggestion of using bilateral electrode placement for bipolar disorder is supported by the concept that bipolar illness needs a more aggressive type of treatment since it is thought to be a more difficult to treat condition compared to unipolar depression. In a recent report by Medda et al. [21], 130 patients, with an average age of 52, were compared. The patients in the study had diagnoses of unipolar major depression (UP), bipolar I (BP I), and bipolar II (BP II). The individuals with UP responded most effectively to ECT. On the contrary, BP I was less responsive and showed more residual symptomatology. The study's data showed that BP I patients reported more manic and psychotic features than UP and BP II on final evaluation.

Bitemporal (BT) lead placement, which is also known as bilateral (BL), despite popular belief, has not been proven to be more efficacious than RUL in improving psychiatric symptoms [22]. A major concern of BT lead placement is its significant cognitive side effects such as acute confusion, retrograde, and anterograde amnesia. Even though the cognitive side effects are thought to be mostly temporary, they are nonetheless discomforting to the patient and may last up to six months. Initially, to minimize cognitive impairment post-ECT, the choice of using RUL lead placement is often made. RUL is highly effective in treating a wide variety of psychiatric patients, but those who do not respond adequately to RUL treatment may require a trial of another lead placement.

The exact mechanism of action of ECT is still not clear, but ECT has been shown to have neurotrophic effects in adult patients with major depressive disorder [23, 24]. Increases in gray matter volume in medial temporal lobes, inferior temporal cortices, and the right anterior cingulate have been correlated to clinical improvement measured by the Hamilton Rating Scale for Depression (HRSD) [23].

In pharmacotherapy-resistant depression, ECT increases hippocampus and amygdala volumes [24]. Common assumptions that the elderly are more susceptible to cognitive impairment following ECT compared to younger adults has not been supported by published research [25]. It has been suggested that smaller hippocampal volumes may predict a more robust clinical response [26]. RUL brief-pulse ECT has been shown to improve mood in bipolar depression and has not been shown to adversely affect general neurocognitive function [27]. RUL and BT brief-pulse ECT have been shown to improve global cognitive functioning (MMSE), anterograde memory, and verbal learning in OABD patients [25].

Side effects from ECT include headache, nausea, muscle soreness, post-ictal agitation, and delirium. Some elderly patients after ECT may experience increased speech latency secondary to a hypoactive delirium [28]. A sensitive assessment for delirium post-ECT includes serial 7s or naming the months of the year backwards. The length of the ECT seizure has been correlated with a heightened chance for developing delirium [29].

ECT is an effective neuromodulation therapy which can treat unipolar and bipolar depression in adult and OABD patients [21]. Data on the treatment of OABD patients with mania is lacking.

8.3 Transcranial Magnetic Stimulation

Transcranial magnetic stimulation (TMS) is a noninvasive treatment that uses a computerized, electromechanical medical device to produce and deliver magnetic stimulation using brief duration, rapidly alternating, or pulsed, magnetic fields to induce electrical currents directed at spatially discrete regions of the cerebral cortex [30]. Within the brain, the magnetic field is converted into an electrical current modifying neuronal activity in the dorsolateral prefrontal cortex (DLPFC). Functional imaging studies have shown that in major depressive disorders, the left prefrontal cortex is less active than the right. Thus, repeated subconvulsive stimulations of this area elicit activity in circuits involving regulatory pathways that interact with the limbic system [31]. Currently, repetitive TMS (rTMS) devices are capable of delivering pulses with frequencies of up to 20 cycles per second. Most commonly, the stimulation parameter is performed at a 10 Hz frequency over the left DLPFC, with sessions five times per week at 120 % of motor threshold for 3000 pulses/session for four to six weeks [32].

TMS has shown potential benefit in treating bipolar depression. According to one retrospective study that sampled adult patients with bipolar depression, the severity of the depression, failures of two or more antidepressants or mood stabilizers, older age, number of prior depressive episodes predicted the need for more than 15 sessions to achieve remission [33]. In this same study, patients had an average of 3.5 depressive episodes.

TMS has been reported to cause mood changes that are specific to the side of the brain stimulated [34]. A study by Grisaru et al. [35] reported on the effect of right versus left prefrontal TMS on mania. Sixteen patients were enrolled with an average age of 36 years (20–52). Patients were randomized to right or left TMS stimulation. The study's results suggested that TMS stimulation of the right prefrontal cortex had a better therapeutic effect in mania. A later study by the same group in which right TMS was compared to sham right TMS in 19 patients of mean age 41.6 years (19–65) did not support the therapeutic effect of right TMS in the treatment of mania [36]. Saba et al. [37] reported on eight manic patients who received five treatments of 15-s, 10-Hz rTMS stimulation at 80 % of the motor threshold over the right DLPFC. The patients demonstrated significant improvement in manic symptoms measured by the Mania Assessment Scale (MAS) and Clinical Global Impression (CGI) scale. Additionally, Michael and Erfurth [38] reported on eight manic patients who successfully received right prefrontal rTMS as an augmentation to partially effective mood stabilization pharmacotherapy. The patients achieved sustained reduction of manic symptoms during the 4 weeks of treatment. Loo et al. [39] performed a review on the safety of rTMS for treating unipolar and bipolar depression in the general population and concluded that it is associated with a low risk of induced hypomania and accidental seizures.

Deep transcranial magnetic stimulation (dTMS) is a new type of TMS which uses a H1 coil and has the capacity to stimulate deeper than conventional TMS (eight shape coil). Conventional TMS can penetrate 2 cm into the brain while deep TMS (H-coil) penetrates approximately 5 cm into the brain. Potentially, deep TMS, as opposed to conventional TMS, can stimulate fibers connecting the subgenual cingulate gyrus to the prefrontal cortex, thereby inducing a more robust antidepressant effect.

According to one study [40], dTMS has shown the ability to decrease depressive symptoms in adult patients with unipolar and bipolar disorder. The initial sessions were daily, and lasted four weeks. At the completion of the 4-week interval, weekly or biweekly maintenance dTMS was effective in maintaining euthymia at the 12-month follow-up in unipolar and bipolar depressed patients [38].

Similar to concerns regarding ECT-induced mania, TMS may potentially be associated with treatment-emergent mania [41, 42]. Although TMS requires the inconvenience of daily sessions, frequent treatment also allows for close monitoring of patients to detect emergent mania and other possible TMS associated adverse effects. Common side effects related to TMS include tension type headache in 10–20 % of subjects, painful scalp sensations in about 39 % of patients, facial twitching in 1 in 3 patients and a very low risk of inducing seizure 0.003 % per treatment exposure and <0.1 % per acute treatment course. In contrast to ECT, no major cognitive effects have been reported in patients who receive rTMS. Potential benefits of TMS over ECT include the administration of the treatment without anesthesia and the convenience of outpatient treatment that does not restrict patients from driving.

Currently, TMS is not approved for mania in the USA and the available literature is limited in the older population.

8.4 Deep Brain Stimulation (DBS)

DBS is a neurosurgical neuromodulation therapy in which strategic areas of the brain are electrically stimulated. The mechanism of action of DBS is more complex than just functional inhibition caused by high-frequency local stimulation. There is evidence of both excitatory and inhibitory effects on brain regions adjacent to and remote from the site of stimulation [43]. DBS has been experimentally used for the treatment of depression by targeting different sites such as the ventral capsule/ventral striatum [44], cingulate gyrus [45], medial forebrain bundle [46], and nucleus accumbens [47]. The most common region of device implantation is in the subcallosal cingulate area [48].

DBS has FDA approval for the treatment of Parkinson's disease, dystonia, essential tremor, and obsessive-compulsive disorder (the latter approved through a humanitarian device exemption). The procedure requires the impulse to be sent through implanted electrodes usually, 24 h a day. The implantation of the electrodes in the intended location requires placement under local anesthesia with minor sedation [49]. The electrodes are connected to cables that travel subcutaneously to the impulse generator. The implantation of the impulse generator requires general anesthesia, and the battery is replaced every 3–5 years [49]. After installation of the DBS system, parameters can be modified through a transcutaneous programming device.

Chronic stimulation with DBS on the subcallosal cingulate has been shown to be a safe and effective for treatment-resistant depression in patients with bipolar disorder [48]. The efficacy of DBS treatment in patients with bipolar depression and MDD has been shown to be similar [48]. DBS-induced mania has been described when the device is implanted in the subthalamic nucleus during Parkinson's disease treatment [50]; however, symptoms of mania have not been demonstrated during stimulation of the subcallosal cingulate. Whether DBS of the subcallosal cingulate may trigger or prevent hypomanic or manic episodes in geriatric bipolar depressed patients is still to be determined. The patients participating in DBS trials for mood disorders are typically not older adults. However, DBS for the treatment of movement disorders has been performed safely on older patients. DBS in the subcallosal cingulate white matter and nucleus accumbens has been reported to be safe in terms of cognitive side effects [51]. DBS is the most invasive of the neuromodulation therapies as it requires neurosurgery. The treatment is promising for those patients who fail ECT, but it is still considered investigational and "off label" for mood disorders with limitation of its applicability in the geriatric population.

8.5 Magnetic Seizure Therapy (MST)

MST combines elements of ECT with TMS, effectively reducing depressive symptoms in unipolar and bipolar depressed patients, with fewer side effects than ECT [52]. MST, which is still an experimental modulation therapy, specifically applies high intensity rTMS to induce a seizure [53]. MST does not involve impedance of the skull, which allows for a more focal seizure restricted to the superficial cortex. Seizures are elicited under general anesthesia by a magnetic field. In a study involving 10 subjects, aged 18–65, with MDD or bipolar depression, six were responders, and three achieved remission status. MST has been shown to produce fewer cognitive side effects compared to RUL brief-pulse ECT, as demonstrated by faster orientation, attention, and retrograde memory recovery from treatments [52, 54]. According to available data, reorientation time after MST may take as little as 2 min [52], showing potential as a treatment for bipolar depressed elderly patients prone to post-ECT memory impairment. No study has currently examined the effect of MST solely on bipolar depressed patients, and no data are available regarding whether a switch to mania may occur with MST. Due to the limited amount of data, MST as a treatment for bipolar depression in the geriatric population is promising at best.

8.6 Trancranial Direct Current Stimulation (tDCS)

tDCS works by delivering a weak electrical current through two electrodes attached to the scalp, powered by a portable battery stimulator [55]. The mechanism of action of tDCS is not fully understood, but it is known to specifically modulate spontaneous neuronal network activity rather than depolarization of the neuronal membrane [56]. In young healthy individuals, improvement of working memory performance [57] and visuomotor coordination [58] has been observed after tDCS. Although studies in the geriatric population are lacking, tDCS is nonetheless promising in an older adult population given the cognitive improvements seen in younger patients. tDCS holds the advantage of being generally inexpensive and may potentially be administered in a home or non-specialized clinical environment in the near future [55]. Adverse effects associated with tDCS include a burning sensation, headache, tingling, itching, and discomfort [59]. A study by Brunoni et al. [60] examined the effects of tDCS on 31 depressed patients, 14 of whom had bipolar disorder. Five sessions of tDCS were performed over the left DLPFC, each lasting 20 min. After the fifth session, a reduction of depressive symptoms was noted in unipolar and bipolar depressed patients, with beneficial effects lasting one month [60]. Whether a switch to mania can occur in bipolar depressed patients undergoing tDCS is still unknown.

8.7 Focal Electrically Administered Seizure Therapy (FEAST)

In an attempt to further optimize ECT-style treatments, FEAST initiates focal seizures in the prefrontal cortex with subsequent generalization. FEAST may result in fewer cognitive side effects compared to ECT while also retaining similar antidepressant efficacy. Individuals who receive right unilateral FEAST develop early-ictal increases in regional cerebral blood flow [61]. Post-ictally, the same individuals experience reduced perfusion in bilateral frontal and occipital cortices and increased perfusion in the left motor cortex and precuneus [61]. In an open label trial, examination of both unipolar and bipolar depressed patients aged 53 ± 2, resulted in a significant antidepressant effect when patients were treated with FEAST [62]. A 46.1 ± 35.5 % improvement on HRSD when compared to baseline was seen [62]. After treatment with FEAST, reorientation has been demonstrated to be as quick as about 5 min [62].

8.8 Ketamine Infusion

Ketamine is a dissociative anesthetic drug that acts as an *N*-methyl-D-aspartic acid receptor (NMDAR) antagonist [63]. Available intravenously, intramuscularly, and intranasally, ketamine has demonstrated transient antidepressant effects [64]. Specifically, ketamine has been shown to be effective in MDD and bipolar depression in recent studies [64]. Studies have not specifically analyzed whether ketamine is effective for mixed bipolar episodes due to exclusion from studies to date. When ketamine is provided as an anesthetic agent for ECT, it can prolong the seizure and provide possible independent antidepressant effects [64, 65]. In bipolar depressed patients aged 18–65, significant improvement in depression lasting up to three days when compared to placebo [66, 67] has been demonstrated. Additionally, ketamine treatment has demonstrated rapid antisuicidal effects (within 1 h) in bipolar depressed patients after just a single infusion [67]. There are no current available data describing a switch to mania or hypomania with the use of ketamine. In a study evaluating older adults (mean age of 83 ± 3), ketamine was found to increase sympathetic stimulation and mild depression of respiratory rate. The same study concluded that ketamine is nonetheless a safe anesthetic agent [68].

8.9 Discussion

In patients who are depressed and experiencing psychotic symptoms, ECT has been shown to be superior to TMS. The onset of clinical benefit from ECT is more rapid in comparison with traditional antidepressant pharmacotherapy. However, this benefit comes at the expense of exposure to generalized anesthesia. While the neuromodulating therapies listed in this chapter are promising, ECT has the strongest data to support its use in patients with bipolar depression, with cognitive side effects posing the greatest risk for discontinuation. While there have been advances in our understanding of neuromodulation therapies, there is an ongoing improvement in ECT practice. Among the approaches of modern ECT to mitigate cognitive side effects are alterations of electrical stimulus dosing, electrode placement, pulse amplitude, shape, and width. When comparing ECT to MST, the median ECT stimulation strength in the brain is 3–11 times higher than that for MST [69]. As a result, there have been discussions with regard to lowering ECT current amplitudes as a means of reducing cognitive side effects [69]. FEAST has a potential advantage over ECT in its capacity for spatial targeting and its low dosing capability [62]. Ketamine infusion leads to rapid antidepressant and antisuicidal effects in patients with bipolar depression. When ketamine is used as an anesthetic agent in ECT, it has the potential of improving seizure quality and potentiating ECT's antidepressant effect. However, double-blind randomized clinical trials have failed to demonstrate sustained antidepressant effects of ketamine when used as an anesthetic agent in ECT [70].

Neuromodulation therapies are exciting avenues of research for psychiatric illnesses. The limited data in geriatric bipolar disorder may be related to the fact that investigators and/or device companies are wary of the potential adverse effects of these therapies in older adult population. Additionally, treatment-emergent mania and the challenges of conducting informed consent may also be barriers impacting the inclusion of older adults with bipolar disorder in neuromodulation therapy studies.

8.10 Summary and Conclusions

See Table 8.1 for a summary comparison of neuromodulation therapies.

Future neuromodulation studies should include older adults with major depression and bipolar disorder. This will help to better understand the potential efficacy and safety of these treatments in older, medically complex populations with treatment-resistant depression.

Clinical Pearls

ECT

- In ECT, right unilateral lead placement may minimize cognitive side effects compared to bifrontal, left anterior right temporal, or bitemporal lead placements
- Older adults generally have higher medical comorbidity due to medical complexity and are, therefore, at higher risk for polypharmacy. Treatment of bipolar disorder (depression, mania, mixed episodes) with ECT may

Table 8.1 Comparison of neuromodulation therapies

Modulation therapy	General anesthesia	Cognitive side effects	Indicated when failure to respond to one antidepressant in current episode	Treatment-resistant depression	Switch to mania	Seizurogenic
ECT	Yes	Yes	–	+	Cases reported	Yes
TMS	No	No	+	±	Cases reported	No
DBS	Yes	Possible	–	+	Cases reported	No
MST	Yes	Minimal	–	+	Unavailable literature	Yes
FEAST	Yes	Minimal	–	+	Unavailable literature	Yes
tDCS	No	No	+	±	Unavailable literature	Possible

allow for a reduction in polypharmacy to achieve remission, thus lowering the risk of drug–drug interactions.

- Older adults with depression complicated by catatonic and psychotic features generally have better response rates to ECT than those without psychosis or catatonia.
- Older age is generally a positive predictor of ECT response.
- ECT has demonstrated efficacy in treating unipolar and bipolar depression.
- Acute mania, acute depression, and mixed episodes in bipolar illness can be effectively treated with ECT.

TMS

- TMS requires daily sessions for at least four weeks to demonstrate antidepressant effects.
- While studies are limited, available data show that rTMS improves depressive symptoms in adult-aged bipolar patients. More data are needed to support its use in older adults with bipolar disorder.

DBS

- Due to the invasiveness, cost, and complexity of DBS, more studies are needed before this experimental therapy becomes a clinical option outside of very specific trials.
- In Parkinson's disease, DBS has reportedly shown the potential of inducing mania when targeting the subthalamic nucleus.

- As seen in this chapter's clinical vignette, DBS is a therapy that is reserved for patients who have failed less invasive neuromodulation treatments.

MST

- MST combines elements of ECT and TMS, producing fewer cognitive side effects compared to RUL ECT.
- MST allows for a focal seizure restricted to the superficial cortex.
- Available literature indicates that MST is a promising option in treating bipolar depression.

tDCS

- tDCS is generally inexpensive and has the potential of being administered in non-specialized clinical environments.
- tDCS has demonstrated efficacy in treating bipolar depressed patients in small studies.

FEAST

- FEAST initiates focal seizures in the prefrontal cortex with subsequent generalization and may be a neuromodulation therapy that produces fewer cognitive side effects compared to ECT.
- FEAST has shown significant antidepressant effects in both unipolar and bipolar depressed patients with no current data on treatment-emergent mania.

Ketamine Infusion

- Ketamine is an NMDA receptor antagonist, with significant transient antidepressant effects when administered intranasal or intravenously.
- Ketamine can prolong seizure time in ECT when used as an anesthetic agent, with potential independent antidepressant effects and theoretically less cognitive adverse effects. Large double-blind randomized clinical trials are needed to investigate these findings further.
- Ketamine has been found to possess rapid antisuicidal effects within 60 min in patients with bipolar depression.

References

1. Hoyle S, Elliott L, Comer L. Available screening tools for adults suffering from bipolar affective disorder in primary care: an integrative literature review. J Am Assoc Nurse Pract. 2015;27(5):280–9.
2. Forester BP, Ajilore O, Spino C, Lehmann SW. Clinical characteristics of patients with late life bipolar disorder in the community: data from the NNDC registry. Am J Geriatr Psychiatry. 2015;23(9):977–84.
3. Peterchev AV, Rosa MA, Deng ZD, Prudic J, Lisanby SH. Electroconvulsive therapy stimulus parameters: rethinking dosage. J ECT. 2010;26(3):159–74.
4. van Schaik AM, Comijs HC, Sonnenberg CM, Beekman AT, Sienaert P, Stek ML. Efficacy and safety of continuation and maintenance electroconvulsive therapy in depressed elderly patients: a systematic review. Am J Geriatr Psychiatry. 2012;20(1):5–17.
5. Tew JD Jr, Mulsant BH, Haskett RF, Prudic J, Thase ME, Crowe RR, et al. Acute efficacy of ECT in the treatment of major depression in the old-old. Am J Psychiatry. 1999;156 (12):1865–70.
6. O'Connor MK, Knapp R, Husain M, Rummans TA, Petrides G, Smith G, et al. The influence of age on the response of major depression to electroconvulsive therapy: a CORE Report. Am J Geriatr Psychiatry Fall. 2001;9(4):382–90.
7. Kerner N, Prudic J. Current electroconvulsive therapy practice and research in the geriatric population. Neuropsychiatry (London). 2014;4(1):33–54.
8. Greenberg RM, Kellner CH. Electroconvulsive therapy: a selected review. Am J Geriatr Psychiatry. 2005;13(4):268–81.
9. Damm J, Eser D, Schule C, Obermeier M, Moller HJ, Rupprecht R, et al. Influence of age on effectiveness and tolerability of electroconvulsive therapy. J ECT. 2010;26(4):282–8.
10. Goldstein BI, Herrmann N, Shulman KI. Comorbidity in bipolar disorder among the elderly: results from an epidemiological community sample. Am J Psychiatry. 2006;163(2):319–21.
11. Virupaksha HS, Shashidhara B, Thirthalli J, Kumar CN, Gangadhar BN. Comparison of electroconvulsive therapy (ECT) with or without anti-epileptic drugs in bipolar disorder. J Affect Disord. 2010;127(1–3):66–70.
12. American Psychiatric Association Group. The practice of electroconvulsive therapy: recommendations for treatment, training, and privileging. A Task Force Report of the American Psychiatric Association. 2nd ed. Washington, DC: APA; 2001.
13. Scott A. College guidelines on electroconvulsive therapy: an update for prescribers. 2005;11:150–6.
14. Royal College of Psychiatrists. The ECT Handbook. 2005. (The Third Report of the Royal College of Psychiatrists' Special Committee on ECT (Council Report CR128)).
15. Thirthalli J, Rakesh G, Gangadhar BN. Antiepileptic drugs-ECT combination: need for systematic studies. World J Biol Psychiatry. 2010;11(7):919–20.
16. Rubner P, Koppi S, Conca A. Frequency of and rationales for the combined use of electroconvulsive therapy and antiepileptic drugs in Austria and the literature. World J Biol Psychiatry. 2009;10(4 Pt 3):836–45.
17. Mukherjee S. Combined ECT and lithium therapy. Convuls Ther. 1993;9(4):274–84.
18. Lee J, Arcand L, Narang P, Lippmann S. ECT-induced Mania. Innov Clin Neurosci. 2014;11 (11–12):27–9.
19. Li DJ, Li HJ, Lin CH. Electroconvulsive therapy-induced manic episode for a patient with bipolar depression: a case report. J ECT. 2015;31(2):e30–1.
20. Ghaemi SN. Antidepressants in bipolar depression: the clinical debate. Aust NZ J Psychiatry. 2012;46(4):298–301.
21. Medda P, Perugi G, Zanello S, Ciuffa M, Cassano GB. Response to ECT in bipolar I, bipolar II and unipolar depression. J Affect Disord. 2009;118(1–3):55–9.

22. Semkovska M, Landau S, Dunne R, Kolshus E, Kavanagh A, Jelovac A, et al. Bitemporal versus high-dose unilateral twice-weekly electroconvulsive therapy for depression (EFFECT-Dep): a pragmatic, randomized non-inferiority trial. Am J Psychiatry. 2016;173(4):408–17.
23. Ota M, Noda T, Sato N, Okazaki M, Ishikawa M, Hattori K, et al. Effect of electroconvulsive therapy on gray matter volume in major depressive disorder. J Affect Disord. 2015;1 (186):186–91.
24. Tendolkar I, van Beek M, van Oostrom I, Mulder M, Janzing J, Voshaar RO, et al. Electroconvulsive therapy increases hippocampal and amygdala volume in therapy refractory depression: a longitudinal pilot study. Psychiatry Res. 2013;214(3):197–203.
25. Verwijk E, Comijs HC, Kok RM, Spaans HP, Tielkes CE, Scherder EJ, et al. Short- and long-term neurocognitive functioning after electroconvulsive therapy in depressed elderly: a prospective naturalistic study. Int Psychogeriatr. 2014;26(2):315–24.
26. Joshi SH, Espinoza RT, Pirnia T, Shi J, Wang Y, Ayers B, et al. Structural plasticity of the hippocampus and amygdala induced by electroconvulsive therapy in major depression. Biol Psychiatry. 2016;79(4):282–92.
27. Kessler U, Schoeyen HK, Andreassen OA, Eide GE, Malt UF, Oedegaard KJ, et al. The effect of electroconvulsive therapy on neurocognitive function in treatment-resistant bipolar disorder depression. J Clin Psychiatry. 2014;75(11):e1306–13.
28. Reti IM, Krishnan A, Podlisky A, Sharp A, Walker M, Neufeld KJ, et al. Predictors of electroconvulsive therapy postictal delirium. Psychosomatics. 2014;55(3):272–9.
29. Hassamal S, Pandurangi A, Venkatachalam V, Levenson J. Delayed onset and prolonged ECT-related delirium. Case Rep Psychiatry. 2013;2013:840425.
30. Perera T, George MS, Grammer G, Janicak PG, Pascual-Leone A, Wirecki TS. The clinical TMS society consensus review and treatment recommendations for TMS therapy for major depressive disorder. Brain Stimul. 2016;9(3):336–46.
31. George MS. Transcranial magnetic stimulation for the treatment of depression. Expert Rev Neurother. 2010;10(11):1761–72.
32. Riva-Posse P, Hermida AP, McDonald WM. The role of electroconvulsive and neuromodulation therapies in the treatment of geriatric depression. Psychiatr Clin North Am. 2013;36 (4):607–30.
33. Cohen RB, Brunoni AR, Boggio PS, Fregni F. Clinical predictors associated with duration of repetitive transcranial magnetic stimulation treatment for remission in bipolar depression: a naturalistic study. J Nerv Ment Dis. 2010;198(9):679–81.
34. Grisaru N, Yaroslavsky Y, Belmaker RH. Is TMS an antibipolar treatment? In: George MS, Belmaker RH, editors. Transcranial magnetic stimulation in neuropsychiatry. 1st ed. DC: American Psychiatric Press; 2000. p. 201–7.
35. Grisaru N, Chudakov B, Yaroslavsky Y, Belmaker RH. Transcranial magnetic stimulation in mania: a controlled study. Am J Psychiatry. 1998;155(11):1608–10.
36. Kaptsan A, Yaroslavsky Y, Applebaum J, Belmaker RH, Grisaru N. Right prefrontal TMS versus sham treatment of mania: a controlled study. Bipolar Disord. 2003;5(1):36–9.
37. Saba G, Rocamora JF, Kalalou K, Benadhira R, Plaze M, Lipski H, et al. Repetitive transcranial magnetic stimulation as an add-on therapy in the treatment of mania: a case series of eight patients. Psychiatry Res. 2004;128(2):199–202.
38. Michael N, Erfurth A. Treatment of bipolar mania with right prefrontal rapid transcranial magnetic stimulation. J Affect Disord. 2004;78(3):253–7.
39. Loo CK, McFarquhar TF, Mitchell PB. A review of the safety of repetitive transcranial magnetic stimulation as a clinical treatment for depression. Int J Neuropsychopharmacol. 2008;11(1):131–47.
40. Rapinesi C, Bersani FS, Kotzalidis GD, Imperatori C, Del Casale A, Di Pietro S, et al. Maintenance deep transcranial magnetic stimulation sessions are associated with reduced depressive relapses in patients with unipolar or bipolar depression. Front Neurol. 2015;9(6):16.

41. Xia G, Gajwani P, Muzina DJ, Kemp DE, Gao K, Ganocy SJ, et al. Treatment-emergent mania in unipolar and bipolar depression: focus on repetitive transcranial magnetic stimulation. Int J Neuropsychopharmacol. 2008;11(1):119–30.
42. Dolberg OT, Schreiber S, Grunhaus L. Transcranial magnetic stimulation-induced switch into mania: a report of two cases. Biol Psychiatry. 2001;49(5):468–70.
43. Vitek JL. Mechanisms of deep brain stimulation: excitation or inhibition. Mov Disord. 2002;17(Suppl 3):S69–72.
44. Malone DA Jr, Dougherty DD, Rezai AR, Carpenter LL, Friehs GM, Eskandar EN, et al. Deep brain stimulation of the ventral capsule/ventral striatum for treatment-resistant depression. Biol Psychiatry. 2009;65(4):267–75.
45. Mayberg HS, Lozano AM, Voon V, McNeely HE, Seminowicz D, Hamani C, et al. Deep brain stimulation for treatment-resistant depression. Neuron. 2005;45(5):651–60.
46. Schlaepfer TE, Bewernick BH, Kayser S, Madler B, Coenen VA. Rapid effects of deep brain stimulation for treatment-resistant major depression. Biol Psychiatry. 2013;73(12):1204–12.
47. Schlaepfer TE, Cohen MX, Frick C, Kosel M, Brodesser D, Axmacher N, et al. Deep brain stimulation to reward circuitry alleviates anhedonia in refractory major depression. Neuropsychopharmacology. 2008;33(2):368–77.
48. Holtzheimer PE, Kelley ME, Gross RE, Filkowski MM, Garlow SJ, Barrocas A, et al. Subcallosal cingulate deep brain stimulation for treatment-resistant unipolar and bipolar depression. Arch Gen Psychiatry. 2012;69(2):150–8.
49. Coenen VA, Amtage F, Volkmann J, Schlapfer TE. Deep brain stimulation in neurological and psychiatric disorders. Dtsch Arztebl Int. 2015;112(31–32):519–26.
50. Ugurlu TT, Acar G, Karadag F, Acar F. Manic episode following deep brain stimulation of the subthalamic nucleus for Parkinson's disease: a case report. Turk Neurosurg. 2014;24(1):94–7.
51. Moreines JL, McClintock SM, Holtzheimer PE. Neuropsychologic effects of neuromodulation techniques for treatment-resistant depression: a review. Brain Stimul. 2011;4(1):17–27.
52. Cretaz E, Brunoni AR, Lafer B. Magnetic seizure therapy for unipolar and bipolar depression: a systematic review. Neural Plast. 2015;2015:521398.
53. Alexopoulos GS, Kelly RE Jr. Research advances in geriatric depression. World Psychiatry. 2009;8(3):140–9.
54. Galvez V, Ho KA, Alonzo A, Martin D, George D, Loo CK. Neuromodulation therapies for geriatric depression. Curr Psychiatry Rep. 2015;17(7):59.
55. Elder GJ, Taylor JP. Transcranial magnetic stimulation and transcranial direct current stimulation: treatments for cognitive and neuropsychiatric symptoms in the neurodegenerative dementias? Alzheimers Res Ther. 2014;6(9):74.
56. Nitsche MA, Cohen LG, Wassermann EM, Priori A, Lang N, Antal A, et al. Transcranial direct current stimulation: state of the art 2008. Brain Stimul. 2008;1(3):206–23.
57. Zaehle T, Sandmann P, Thorne JD, Jancke L, Herrmann CS. Transcranial direct current stimulation of the prefrontal cortex modulates working memory performance: combined behavioural and electrophysiological evidence. BMC Neurosci 2011;12:2-2202-12-2.
58. Antal A, Nitsche MA, Kruse W, Kincses TZ, Hoffmann KP, Paulus W. Direct current stimulation over V5 enhances visuomotor coordination by improving motion perception in humans. J Cogn Neurosci. 2004;16(4):521–7.
59. Tortella G, Casati R, Aparicio LV, Mantovani A, Senco N, D'Urso G, et al. Transcranial direct current stimulation in psychiatric disorders. World J Psychiatry. 2015;5(1):88–102.
60. Brunoni AR, Ferrucci R, Bortolomasi M, Vergari M, Tadini L, Boggio PS, et al. Transcranial direct current stimulation (tDCS) in unipolar vs. bipolar depressive disorder. Prog Neuropsychopharmacol Biol Psychiatry. 2011;35(1):96–101.
61. Chahine G, Short B, Spicer K, Schmidt M, Burns C, Atoui M, et al. Regional cerebral blood flow changes associated with focal electrically administered seizure therapy (FEAST). Brain Stimul. 2014;7(3):483–5.

62. Nahas Z, Short B, Burns C, Archer M, Schmidt M, Prudic J, et al. A feasibility study of a new method for electrically producing seizures in man: focal electrically administered seizure therapy [FEAST]. Brain Stimul. 2013;6(3):403–8.
63. Newport DJ, Carpenter LL, McDonald WM, Potash JB, Tohen M, Nemeroff CB, et al. Ketamine and other NMDA antagonists: early clinical trials and possible mechanisms in depression. Am J Psychiatry. 2015;172(10):950–66.
64. Fond G, Loundou A, Rabu C, Macgregor A, Lancon C, Brittner M, et al. Ketamine administration in depressive disorders: a systematic review and meta-analysis. Psychopharmacology. 2014;231(18):3663–76.
65. Salehi B, Mohammadbeigi A, Kamali AR, Taheri-Nejad MR, Moshiri I. Impact comparison of ketamine and sodium thiopental on anesthesia during electroconvulsive therapy in major depression patients with drug-resistant; a double-blind randomized clinical trial. Ann Card Anaesth. 2015;18(4):486–90.
66. Diazgranados N, Ibrahim L, Brutsche NE, Newberg A, Kronstein P, Khalife S, et al. A randomized add-on trial of an N-methyl-D-aspartate antagonist in treatment-resistant bipolar depression. Arch Gen Psychiatry. 2010;67(8):793–802.
67. Zarate CA Jr, Brutsche NE, Ibrahim L, Franco-Chaves J, Diazgranados N, Cravchik A, et al. Replication of ketamine's antidepressant efficacy in bipolar depression: a randomized controlled add-on trial. Biol Psychiatry. 2012;71(11):939–46.
68. Stefansson T, Wickstrom I, Haljamae H. Hemodynamic and metabolic effects of ketamine anesthesia in the geriatric patient. Acta Anaesthesiol Scand. 1982;26(4):371–7.
69. Won Hee L, Lisanby SH, Laine AF, Peterchev AV. Stimulation strength and focality of electroconvulsive therapy and magnetic seizure therapy in a realistic head model. Conf Proc IEEE Eng Med Biol Soc. 2014;2014:410–3.
70. Loo CK, Katalinic N, Garfield JB, Sainsbury K, Hadzi-Pavlovic D, Mac-Pherson R. Neuropsychological and mood effects of ketamine in electroconvulsive therapy: a randomised controlled trial. J Affect Disord. 2012;142(1–3):233–40.

Psychotherapy and Psychosocial Interventions, Family Psychoeducation, and Support for Older Age Bipolar Disorder

9

Dimitris N. Kiosses, Lindsey C. Wright and Robert C. Young

9.1 Introduction

Psychological interventions are critical in the treatment of bipolar disorders (BDs) as an adjunct to pharmacotherapy and other somatic treatments. These interventions are particularly important in older adults, who face psychosocial challenges, cognitive difficulties, high rates of medical comorbidity, disability, and increased rates of suicide [1, 2]. In this chapter, we review outpatient psychological treatments for older adults with bipolar disorders (OABDs). We broadly define as psychological any intervention, program, or model that includes psychological approaches, e.g., psychotherapeutic, psychosocial, skills training, psychoeducational, and family support interventions. We discuss potentially relevant clinical issues, such as disability, cognitive impairment, emotion regulation, and suicidality. Finally, a clinical vignette and a list of clinical "pearls" highlight important therapeutic targets for this population.

D.N. Kiosses (✉) · R.C. Young
Westchester Division, Department of Psychiatry, New York Presbyterian Hospital-Weill Cornell Medicine, 21 Bloomingdale Road, White Plains NY 10605, USA
e-mail: dkiosses@med.cornell.edu

R.C. Young
e-mail: ryoung@med.cornell.edu

L.C. Wright
323 West 96th Street, Apt 906, New York, NY 10032, USA
e-mail: lcw2128@cumc.columbia.edu

S.W. Lehmann and B.P. Forester (eds.), *Bipolar Disorder in Older Age Patients*,
DOI 10.1007/978-3-319-48912-4_9

9.2 Literature Search

We selected studies in older adults with bipolar patients through searches of PUBMED (1968–2015), PsychINFO (1968–2015), and Cochrane database. The searches used combinations of the following keywords: psychosoc*, psychother*, psychoedu*, family support, bipolar, mood disorders, old*, and elder* (the * denotes any combination of the word). We also explored previous reviews and meta-analyses in this population [1–5]. As a comparison, we selected articles, reviews, and meta-analyses on psychological interventions for BD in young and middle-aged adults [6–13].

The searches generated 257 articles. Forty-four of these articles were literature reviews (including systematic reviews and meta-analyses) and twelve reported results from clinical trials. Two of the latter twelve articles discussed a day hospital treatment for older adults with unipolar or bipolar depression [14] and an inpatient dual-diagnosis program for patients with alcohol dependence and unipolar or bipolar affective disorder [15]. One trial focused on an educational intervention for families living with a bipolar patient [16]. Three were clinical trials involving young to middle-aged patients (average age <55 years): smoking cessation for people with severe mental illness [17] (mean age = 47.2 years); a pharmacist-psychiatrist collaborative medication therapy management clinic for patients with severe mental illness [18] (mean age = 49 years; 7 %, $N = 5$, BD); and a psychoeducational program for euthymic patients with BD [19] (mean age = 52).

The main focus of this chapter is a review of the remaining six (out of the twelve) clinical trials' articles that concentrate on older adults with bipolar disorders (OABDs) (i.e., the study participants or a designated group of participants had an average age of 60 years or older). These six articles reported results of four distinct clinical trials (three RCTs) that include the following four outpatient interventions: a manualized psychosocial skills and psychoeducation training program [Helping Older People Experience Success (HOPES)] [20, 21]; an intensive clinical and psychosocial management program [Enhanced Clinical Intervention (ECI)] [22]; a medication adherence intervention [Medication Adherence Skills Training for Bipolar Disorder (MAST-BD)] [23]; and a bipolar disorder medical care model [Bipolar Medical Care Model (BCM)] [24, 25]. Table 9.1 summarizes the studies and the interventions in these six manuscripts.

In summary, the four distinct clinical trials shared the following characteristics: (1) The whole sample or a subgroup of the sample had a diagnosis of BD I, II, or NOS; (2) the average age of the whole sample (or a designated subsample of older adults) was 60 years or older; and (3) each trial tested an outpatient psychological intervention. In the following section, we present a detailed description of each intervention and summarize the study findings.

Table 9.1 Description of studies of psychological interventions for older adults with bipolar disorder

Articles	Groups	RCT	Total *N*	Mean age	Sample description	Recruitment	Attrition
Bartels et al. [20], Mueser et al. [21] (same sample)	HOPES versus TAU	Yes	183	60.2	20 % BD, 28 % schizophrenia, 28 % schizoaffective, 24 % MDD	Community Mental Health Centers	Social skills: attendance across sites 75 % year 1, 70 % year 2; Preventive health care: attendance 66 % across sites
Fagiolini et al. [22]	SCBD versus SCBD + ECI	Yes	463	40.2 (39 participants were ≥65 years of age)	BD I (n = 313), BD II (n = 87), NOS (n = 53), or schizoaffective disorder bipolar type (n = 10)	University Specialty Clinics for BD; Behavioral Health Clinic	Whole sample: 32 % discontinued over 2 years
Kilbourne et al. [24, 25] (same sample)	BCM versus TAU	Yes	58	55.3 (30 % were ≥60 years of age)	BD I (77 %), BD II (5 %), or BD NOS (18 %), and cardiovascular disease risk factors	VA Mental Health Facility	Self-management: 85 % of participants completed all session; Care management: 73 % completed at least 6 contacts
Depp et al. [23]	MAST-BD	No	21	60 (range: 53–73 years)	BD I (62 %), BD II (38 %)	Different sources (e.g., VA, geropsychiatry service)	76 % of participants completed the intervention; 86 % of sessions were attended by completers

(continued)

Table 9.1 (continued)

Articles	Groups	Outcomes	Summary of results
Articles	Groups	Outcomes	Summary of results
Bartels et al. [20], Mueser et al. [21] (same sample)	HOPES versus TAU	Functioning, symptoms, self-efficacy, and service use	HOPES had greater improvement than TAU in performance measures of social skill, psychosocial and community functioning, negative symptoms, self-efficacy, and service use
Fagiolini et al. [22]	SCBD versus SCBD + ECI	Clinical status and quality of life	No significant differences in improvement in Clinical Global Index (CGI) and the Global Assessment of Functioning (GAF), but ECI participants had significantly greater improvement in quality of life. No significant differences in treatment outcomes were found between patients of different ages, except for a greater GAF improvement in late-life versus adult participants
Kilbourne et al. [24, 25] (same sample)	BCM versus TAU	Physical and mental health-related quality of life, functioning and bipolar symptoms, self-management efficacy	BCM participants had greater improvement in physical health-related quality of life, no difference in mental health-related quality of life, functioning, symptoms, and self-management efficacy
Depp et al. [23]	MAST-BD	Feasibility and acceptability, adherence to psychiatric medications, medication management ability, attitudes toward medication, symptoms, and health-related quality of life	Evidence of feasibility (76 % completed the intervention and 86 % of sessions were attended), acceptability (participants reported high treatment satisfaction) and improvement in medication adherence, medication management ability, depressive symptoms, and quality of life

BCM Bipolar Medical Care Model, *ECI* Enhanced Clinical Intervention, *HOPES* Helping Older People Experience Success, *MAST-BD* Medication Adherence Skills Training for Bipolar Disorder, *SCBD* Specialized Care for Bipolar Disorder, *TAU* Treatment as Usual

9.3 Helping Older People Experience Success (HOPES)

HOPES is a manualized psychosocial skills and psychoeducation training program developed for older adults with severe mental illness, including bipolar disorder, schizophrenia, schizoaffective disorder, and major depression, living in the community. The aim of the intervention is to improve overall psychosocial function, while reducing long-term medical burden [20, 21, 26]. The HOPES program includes one year of intensive skills training and health management, followed by a 1-year maintenance period. Both the first intensive year and second maintenance years include weekly skills classes, bimonthly community practice trips, and one-on-one meetings with a nurse, monthly in the first year, with decreased frequency in the second year (Table 9.1).

9.3.1 Intensive Psychosocial Skills Training

HOPES interventions are grounded in the principles of social skills training through the use of modeling and role-playing techniques, provision of positive and corrective feedback, and completion of homework assignments. The curriculum includes seven modules: communicating effectively, making and keeping friends, making the most of leisure time, healthy living, using medications effectively, and making the most of a healthcare visit [21]. Each module includes 6–8 component skills with one specific skill taught each week by a master's prepared rehabilitation specialist. Participants practice the skills in community group outings. Another form of community practice involved the participant identifying an "indigenous supporter" (family member, friend, clinician, spouse) who could help facilitate opportunities to practice the targeted skills in a safe and natural space.

9.3.2 Healthcare Management

HOPES care management is delivered by registered professional nurses who evaluate each participant's medical history and current healthcare needs. The nurses and participants set health-related goals and focus on preventative and primary healthcare benchmarks. The skills training clinicians and registered nurses meet weekly to coordinate each component of HOPES.

9.3.3 Comment

As indicated in Table 9.1, one RCT study demonstrated that HOPES participants had greater improvement than treatment as usual (TAU) in measures of performance skills, psychosocial and community functioning, symptoms, and self-efficacy[1] at 1, 2, and 3 years [20, 21].

The multicomponent HOPES intervention is appropriate for older adults with severe mental illness, including BD, who face a combination of psychosocial and medical issues and have persistent impairment in multiple areas of functioning (e.g., work and self-care). The benefits of the program were unrelated to psychiatric diagnosis, i.e., psychotic disorders (schizophrenia–schizoaffective) versus mood disorders (MDD and BD). Nevertheless, because of the small percentage of older adults with BD in the sample, evaluation and potential adaptation of the HOPES program specifically for older adults with BD are needed. Furthermore, because study participants had persistent impairment in functioning, validation of the HOPES program in older adults with higher level of functioning is recommended.

9.4 Enhanced Clinical Intervention (ECI)

Enhanced clinical intervention (ECI) is a manualized intensive clinical and psychosocial management program provided by a nurse or masters-level clinician and consists of four educational components (including education about BD, pharmacotherapy, sleep, and social rhythm hygiene), five management components (including review of symptoms, medication side effects, discussion of early warning signs, and 24-h on-call service), and a support component [22]. ECI clinicians meet with patients for 20–30 min before a scheduled appointment with the psychiatrist. Patients receive ECI weekly for 12 weeks, every other week for the following 8 weeks and monthly for the duration of treatment (mean = 20 months; range: 18–34 months). If patients had a recurrence of mood episode, they would return to weekly visits.

9.4.1 Comment

One study, an RCT, compared Specialized Care for Bipolar Disorder (SCBD) versus SCBD with ECI [22] in patients with a wide age range including adolescents ($N = 75$, 12–18 years of age), young and middle-aged adults ($N = 349$, 19–64 years of age), and older adults ($N = 39$, 65 years of age and older). SCBD is a manualized system of clinical disease management for bipolar patients, which includes assessment of psychiatric symptoms and standardized algorithm-driven pharmacotherapy [22]. Because SCBD does not include a psychosocial component,

[1]According to Albert Bandura, perceived self-efficacy is “the belief in one’s capabilities to organize and execute the courses of action required to manage prospective situations.” Bandura A. Self-efficacy: Toward a Unifying Theory of Behavioral Change. Psychological Review 1977;84 (2): 191–215.

the Enhanced Clinical Intervention (ECI) was added to SCBD. As indicated in Table 9.1, the groups showed comparable improvement on the Clinical Global Index (CGI), the Global Assessment of Functioning (GAF), and Quality of Life Enjoyment and Satisfaction Questionnaire over 18 months of treatment [22]. However, participants in the SCBD + ECI group had greater improvement in the quality-of-life measures. Even though there were no separate analyses in the group of older adults, there were no significant differences in treatment outcomes among age groups [22].

Future investigations may concentrate on the application of ECI in older adults with BD and identification of the most useful and efficacious components in improving symptoms and quality of life in this population.

9.5 Bipolar Medical Care Model

The Bipolar Medical Care Model (BCM) [24, 25] is an adaptation of the Bipolar Disorder Collaborative Chronic Care Model [27, 28] and aims to improve medical outcomes and reduce cardiovascular risk in patients with BD [25; mean age = 55.3, range = 30–73]. The model proposes that effective strategies to reduce symptoms are necessary to improve adherence to medical treatment, promote health behavior change, and achieve optimal health outcomes [25]. It includes three main components: self-management education, care management, and guideline implementation (Table 9.1).

9.5.1 Self-Management Component

This component is based on the Life Goals Program, a group psychoeducational program for BD [29]. The program is enhanced with additional material on the cardiovascular disease risk, on diet and exercise, and on engagement of general medical providers. The self-management component is delivered by a care manager in four two-hour group sessions [25] and complementary phone sessions.

9.5.2 Care Management Component

In this component, a nurse care manager served as a liaison between patients and providers, addressed patients' health concerns, referred urgent issues to appropriate medical and mental health providers, reinforced self-management, and followed patient's progress over time [25]. This component was delivered by regular phone calls for up to 6 months.

9.5.3 Guideline Implementation Component

Continuing medical education sessions addressed cardiovascular disease risk factors following the American Diabetes Association and American Heart Association guidelines, for all primary care and mental health providers.

9.5.4 Comment

In an RCT, BCM was associated with significantly greater improvement in physical health-related quality of life compared to TAU, but there were no significant differences between the two groups in other outcomes including symptoms and functioning (Table 9.1). Evaluation of specific components of BCM and effects in older patients is needed.

9.6 Medication Adherence Skills Training for Bipolar Disorder (MAST-BD)

Medication Adherence Skills Training for Bipolar Disorder is a 12-week manualized group intervention that combines educational (weeks 1–3), motivational (weeks 4–6), medication management skills (weeks 7–9), and symptom management training (weeks 10–12). Each part is comprised of three, 90-min sessions. The content of each session is derived from psychosocial interventions typically used for younger adults with BD and included elements of cognitive behavioral therapy and structured group therapy [30, 31]. The medication adherence component was derived from the Functional Adaptation Skills Training program, which is an intervention targeted for older adults with psychotic disorders [32] (Table 9.1).

9.6.1 Comment

Non-adherence to pharmacotherapy is associated with increased risk for relapse, recurrence, hospitalization, and high healthcare costs [12, 23, 33]. MAST-BD is a promising and needed intervention that focuses on this critical issue of medication adherence in older adults with BD. In a pilot study [23], MAST-BD provided the evidence of feasibility, acceptability, and improvement in medication adherence, medication management ability, depressive symptoms, and quality of life (Table 9.1). Future investigations may evaluate its effects in a randomized controlled trial.

9.7 Limitations

The studies and these interventions have the following limitations:

1. Only 3 out of the 4 studies are RCTs (Table 9.1). Further, the interventions that were tested in an RCT were long-term interventions (from 6 months to 2 years), which makes it difficult to apply for acute treatment.
2. Only the MAST-BD intervention (which was not tested in an RCT) is designed for and tested exclusively in older adults with BD. HOPES is designed for older adults with severe mental illness, including patients with schizophrenia, schizoaffective, major depression, and BD. ECI and BCM were tested in the studies of mixed-aged samples (ECI study: 8.4 % of the sample, i.e., 39 participants, were older adults aged 65 or older; BCM study: 30 %, i.e., 18 participants, were 60 years or older).
3. All interventions had multiple components, which highlights the clinical complexities of treating BD. Future investigations may investigate the beneficial effects of individual components in older patients with BD.

9.8 Other Interventions for Young and Middle-Aged Adults

Because of the sparse literature on RCTs in older bipolar patients, we include other promising interventions that have been tested in RCTs in mixed samples of both young and middle-aged adults (cognitive behavioral therapy, interpersonal and social rhythm therapy, family-focused therapy, and psychoeducation). In the section below, we briefly describe each intervention and summarize our conclusion.

9.8.1 Cognitive Behavioral Therapy, Interpersonal and Social Rhythm Therapy, and Family-Focused Therapy

In young to middle-aged adults, these three interventions have been studied separately [34–42], but also as part of the Systematic Treatment Enhancement Program for BD (STEP-BD) [43, 44].

Cognitive behavioral therapy has been adapted for BD and includes (1) psychoeducation on the course of BD, medication adherence, and stress management; (2) scheduling of life events; (3) cognitive restructuring; (4) problem-solving training; (5) plans for early detection and intervention; and (6) selected interventions for comorbidity [43, 45, 46].

Interpersonal and social rhythm therapy [11] consists of psychoeducation, social rhythm therapy, and interpersonal psychotherapy. Psychoeducation focuses on pharmacotherapy, medication side effects, and early episode warning signs and detection of prodromal symptoms [11]. Social rhythm therapy identifies strategies to prevent the disruption of social routines and sleep/wake cycles [47]. Interpersonal psychotherapy focuses on reducing interpersonal difficulties because of grief, role transitions, role disputes, and interpersonal deficits. An additional area of "grief for the lost healthy self" was added to interpersonal and social rhythm therapy [11].

Family-focused therapy includes psychoeducational sessions focusing on symptoms, course of illness, treatment, and self-management of BD [48]. In the intermediate phase, after psychoeducation, patients and family members participated in exercises to enhance communication skills. In the final phase, families focused on solving problems related to the illness.

9.8.1.1 Conclusion

Results from the STEP-BD study and other RCTs on the individual effects of each intervention (CBT, interpersonal and social rhythm therapy, family-focused therapy) [9, 34–42] are encouraging for young and middle-aged adults, but future investigations are needed to examine these therapies in older adults with BD, especially in those who are 75 years of age or older.

9.8.2 Psychoeducation

Psychoeducation has been a significant component of the interventions for older bipolar patients, as we described above, but to our knowledge, there are no clinical trials of stand-alone psychoeducation in older adults with BD [12, 34]. Psychoeducation has been widely utilized in a group or individual format as a stand-alone intervention or as an adjunct to other psychosocial interventions for young to middle-aged adults with BD and their families [12, 34, 42, 49–51]. It helps patients and their families develop skills to identify early signs and symptoms, monitor the patients' sleep patterns and symptoms, and avoid relapse [12, 42, 49–51].

9.8.2.1 Conclusion

Again, studies of stand-alone psychoeducational programs have concentrated mainly on young and middle-aged adults, and future investigations focusing on older adults with BD are needed.

9.9 Clinical Issues Related to Bipolar Disorder in Older Adults

Emotion regulation, suicidality, social and family support, disability, cognitive impairment, and caregiver tension and burden are critical issues in older adults that need to be systematically assessed and addressed. These issues are important for

OABD, especially in those who are 75 years or older, a population that has not been adequately investigated. The following section highlights these clinical challenges.

9.9.1 Emotion Regulation

Because of emotional lability in BD, assessment and regulation of negative and positive emotions in patients with BD are critical. Emotion regulation strategies have been effective in improving depression and reducing disability in older adults with unipolar or bipolar major depression and varying degrees of cognitive functioning, including older patients with major depression and significant cognitive impairment, or middle-aged and older adults after successful electroconvulsive therapy (ECT) [52, 53]. Emotion regulation techniques that follow the process model of emotion regulation [54] may be effective in the management of emotions associated with a depression, hypomanic, or manic state. These techniques include situation selection (i.e., selecting situations that promote adaptive positive emotions and reduce negative emotions), situation modification (i.e., modifying situations to promote adaptive positive emotions and reduce negative emotions), attentional deployment (i.e., shifting attention to promote adaptive positive emotions and reduce negative emotions), cognitive change (i.e., changing the appraisal of a situation to modify the emotional response, similar to "cognitive restructuring" that is used in cognitive behavioral therapy) or response modulation (i.e., utilizing direct efforts to alter one's emotional responses).

9.9.2 Suicidality

According to the latest statistics from the Centers for Disease Control and Prevention [55], suicide rates in older adults are alarmingly high and older white men (aged 85 and older) have the highest rate of suicide (54/100,000) [55]. Even though the suicide risk appears to be higher in young adults than in older adults with BD [56, 57], studies on suicide risk in older adults with BD are sparse [58, 59]. In a study of 1354 older adults who died by suicide, BD had a stronger association with suicide (OR 9.20; 95 % CI 4.38–19.33) than depression (OR 6.44; 95 % CI 5.45–7.61) or anxiety disorders (OR 4.65; 95 % CI 4.07–5.32) [60]. Despite the need for interventions to prevent suicide in older adults with mood disorders, no interventions for older patients with BDs have been designed or tested. Clinicians must assess suicidal ideation, past suicide attempts, as well as risk and protective factors for suicide in older adults with BD [58, 61].

9.9.3 Social and Family Support

Decreased social support is critical in older adults with severe mental illness [62], including BDs, and is associated with increased isolation and decreased pleasure [63, 64]. Belonging to a large family network and having increased instrumental support are associated with a shorter bipolar episode [64]. Social support and family support become increasingly important as disability and cognitive impairment increase [65]. Therefore, clinicians must evaluate the social and family support of an older adult with BD and seek to increase social support and reduce interpersonal tension in the family.

9.9.4 Disability

Disability is prevalent in older adults and is associated with increased depression, medical morbidity and mortality, and reduced quality of life of patients and caregivers [66, 67]. Careful assessment of disability domains, the impact of disability on an individual's emotions and quality of life, and its contribution to increased family stress is critical.

9.9.5 Cognitive Impairment

Cognitive impairment, especially deficits in executive functioning, memory, psychomotor speed, and sustained attention, is associated with BD in adults of all ages [13, 68–75]. Cognitive deficits may contribute to reduced quality of life, increased disability, and, in some cases, poor treatment outcomes [13, 76, 77]. Clinicians should assess the specific cognitive deficits and their impact on daily functioning and interference with adherence to pharmacotherapy or psychosocial treatments. A formal neuropsychological assessment may be necessary to fully evaluate these cognitive deficits.

9.9.6 Family/Caregiver Participation

BD has a significant impact on both the individual with BD and the family. Furthermore, family stress may contribute to worsening of bipolar symptoms. It is important to engage family members and/or caregivers as part of the treatment for older adults who are faced with increased medical illnesses, disability, and cognitive impairment. However, most family interventions for BD focus on young and middle-aged patients [78]. Caregiver participation may exacerbate potential caregiver burden. Clinicians need to evaluate a caregiver's availability and motivation to help, disability, and cognitive impairment. Caregivers of older adults with major depression and cognitive impairment have shown high treatment satisfaction and found their participation in treatment to be productive [52].

Clinical Vignette 9.1

Mr. Y, a recently retired 68-year-old, was hospitalized for a manic episode. His episode was characterized by alcohol abuse and extramarital affairs, reduced sleep, and increased energy that led to significant interpersonal tension with his wife and adult son. During his hospitalization, he cycled into a depressive syndrome with features that included guilt, hopelessness, and suicidal ideation. Mr. Y responded to ECT. He was discharged with a continuation management program (psychiatrist and therapist). The therapist and the psychiatrist had continuous communication during the treatment.

Mr. Y and his treatment team focused on the following clinical areas identified in our chapter: assessment of cognitive deficits, medication adherence, emotion regulation, apathy and lack of initiation, psychoeducation, and reduction of interpersonal tension. The following sections discuss the 12-week acute treatment following discharge and biweekly or monthly booster sessions for the next 6 months.

Assessment of Cognitive Deficits

Mr. Y had short-term memory difficulties due to ECT, and the psychotherapist used compensatory strategies and tools, including reminders, a notebook to summarize treatment and highlight the homework, and a weekly schedule to reduce apathy and increase engagement in activities. As expected, after 4 weeks, Mr. Y's short-term memory had significantly improved, based on subjective reports by patient and his family

Suicidal Ideation

Mr. Y had re-emergent passive suicidal ideation, without any intent or plan, after his discharge. His suicidal thoughts were fueled by his hopelessness and guilt related to his manic behavior. Mr. Y ruminated about his extramarital affairs and about how much he hurt his family. The therapist explored with Mr. Y the effect that his behavior had on his family, confronting the all-or-none thinking that there "was no way out" and regulating negative emotions during stressful situations that triggered his suicidal ideation.

Medication Adherence

The therapist educated Mr. Y about the side effects of medication (lithium and antidepressant medication) and discussed the pros and cons of medication adherence and relapse prevention. Mr. Y demonstrated insight and identified the pros of medication adherence and relapse prevention (i.e., reduce symptoms, promote recovery, improve his functioning, and prevent another episode) and was encouraged to discuss the potential side effects of medication with his psychiatrist.

Emotion Regulation

Mr. Y identified problems, concerns, and triggers of negative emotions, such as guilt, feelings of worthlessness, hopelessness, and anxiety. For each problem, Mr. Y developed emotion regulation strategies to reduce these negative emotions. These strategies, based on Gross' process model of emotion regulation [54], included situation selection (selecting the situations the patient is exposed to), situation modification (modifying potentially emotion-eliciting situations), distraction (shifting patient's attention within a situation), cognitive reappraisal (changing patient's perspective about a situation, which is mostly utilized in cognitive behavioral therapy), and response modulation (utilizing direct efforts to alter patient's emotional responses, e.g., stress management tools). Distraction (e.g., concentrating on a pleasurable or rewarding activity when feeling sad) and situation selection (e.g., avoiding upsetting conversations or situations) were effective emotion regulation strategies in the beginning of treatment, when the patient's short-term memory was impaired. Cognitive reappraisal (e.g., changing patient's perspective on medication adherence) was used later in the treatment when the cognitive functioning was significantly improved.

Interpersonal Tension with Wife and Adult Son

Tension between the patient and his family was high due to patient's prior manic symptoms and risky behavior. His wife wanted to separate and did not want to participate in treatment, while the son said that he did not trust his father any longer. The interpersonal tension contributed significantly to patient's depression. The therapist used practical, hands-on strategies to de-escalate the tension, e.g., prepared to stop the discussion if tension increased. The patient was able to temporarily move in with his son, while the wife was convinced to begin couples treatment to explore whether the marriage can be saved. Weekly sessions with the patient and either the son or the wife helped educate the family as well as promote the rebuilding of trust between the patient and his family.

Psychoeducation and Recognition of Early Symptoms

Mr. Y and the therapist discussed extensively the early signs and symptoms of his episodes. Mr. Y's wife and son also participated in the discussion. The therapist created a list of early signs and symptoms and how they can be recognized and reduced. Mr. Y incorporated his family's help in identifying at-risk situations and developed a step-by-step plan on how to deal with these signs and symptoms.

Learning Points

- Psychological intervention for bipolar disorder in older adults needs to include a multidimensional approach consisting of medication adherence,

emotion regulation, psychoeducation, evaluation and treatment of suicidal ideation, and reduction of interpersonal conflicts.
- Evaluation of cognitive deficits and strengths is important for the treatment of older adults with bipolar disorder.
- Maintenance evaluation and early recognition of symptoms are critical for relapse prevention.

9.10 Summary

- Psychological approaches are critical in the treatment of OABD, in conjunction with pharmacotherapy and other somatic treatments.
- Clinical issues that are important for older adults and need to be systematically assessed and addressed include emotion regulation, suicidality, family and social support, disability, cognitive impairment, and caregiver participation.
- There is a paucity of peer-reviewed literature of randomized controlled clinical trials of psychological approaches including psychotherapies, skills training, psychosocial, family-focused, and psychoeducation interventions used for the management of OABD.
- Three interventions have demonstrated efficacy in randomized controlled trials in a subgroup of OABD: Helping Older People Experience Success (HOPES), Enhanced Clinical Intervention (ECI), and Bipolar Medical Care Model (BCM).
- Medication Adherence Skills Training for Bipolar Disorder (MAST-BD), a promising intervention for medication adherence for OABD, needs to be further investigated in an RCT.
- Most psychotherapy intervention studies focus on young and middle-aged older adults. Further investigation of such interventions in adults 75 years or older with BD is needed.

Clinical Pearls

- Cognitive Impairment: The clinician must evaluate a patient's cognitive performance and explore how cognitive impairment impacts daily functioning and treatment. Screening tools such as the Mini Mental State Exam (MMSE) [79] or the Montreal Cognitive Assessment (MOCA) [80] are helpful, but a formal neuropsychological evaluation is recommended to fully assess cognitive deficits.

- Questions to consider: What domains of cognitive performance are impaired and how severe are these deficits? What are the patient's cognitive strengths and limitations? How do cognitive limitations affect daily functioning, medication adherence, and insight? How do cognitive deficits affect the administration of a psychosocial intervention? What compensatory strategies (e.g., reminders, notebooks, and signs) that may help improve functional capacity?

- Disability and Functioning: The clinician shall assess the patient's areas of physical and behavioral disability and impairment in functioning.

  - Questions to consider: What is the patient's overall psychosocial and occupational functioning? What domains of functioning have been affected (e.g., interpersonal, activities of daily living)? Is the patient currently involved in adaptive pleasurable and rewarding activities?

- Maladaptive Negative or Positive Emotions: The clinician must explore negative emotions and their triggers and develop practical emotion regulation techniques to reduce negative emotions and their impact on a patient's life. The clinician will also identify adaptive and maladaptive positive emotions and help the patient promote adaptive and regulate maladaptive positive emotions.

  - Questions to consider: What are the negative emotions that the patient experiences? What situations trigger these negative emotions? How do these negative emotions affect the patient's thinking and actions? What strategies can be used to reduce these negative emotions? Are there any positive emotions, e.g., pleasure and hyperthymia that contribute to risky behavior? How does the patient feel about the impact of these emotions on daily functioning and quality of life?

- Suicide Risk: The clinician must thoroughly assess suicide risk (e.g., substance abuse, disability, pain, and family history of suicide) and protective factors (e.g., religion and family support) and explore any previous suicide attempts. Access to firearms and other lethal means must be evaluated.

  - Questions: Does the individual have a history of suicidal ideation or attempts? What precipitated any prior suicide attempts? What symptoms (manic, hypomanic, depression) were associated with suicidal ideation or past suicide attempts? Are there any protective factors, including religiosity?

- Social Support: The clinician must evaluate family and social support and the effect of BD on his or her relationships.
  - Questions: Has the patient been isolated from his or her social circle or the family? What were the effects of manic, hypomanic, or depression symptoms on the patient's family and social network?
- Caregiver/Family Member/Significant Other Participation: The clinician will explore whether a caregiver is available and willing to participate in treatment. Reduction of interpersonal tension between the patient and family members or significant others is critical. The clinician must assess caregiver's cognitive and functional abilities.
  - Questions: What was the effect of a patient's behavior on the relationship with his or her family? Is the caregiver/family member/significant other willing and available to participate in treatment? Are the family and the patient educated about the symptoms and course of illness, medications and their potential side effects, and importance of adherence to medication treatment?

References

1. Sajatovic M, Chen P. Geriatric bipolar disorder. Psychiatr Clin N Am. 2011;34(2):319–33.
2. Sajatovic M. Treatment of bipolar disorder in older adults. Int J Geriatr Psychiatry. 2002;17(9):865–73.
3. Dines P, Hu W, Sajatovic M. Depression in later-life: an overview of assessment and management. Psychiatr Danub. 2014;26(Suppl 1):78–84.
4. Reiser R, Truong D, Nguyen T, Wachsmuth W, Marquett R, Feit A, et al. Cognitive behavioral therapy for older adults with bipolar disorder. In: Gallagher-Thompson D, Steffen A, Thompson LW, editors. Handbook of behavioral and cognitive therapies with older adults. New York: Springer Science + Business Media; 2008. p. 249–63.
5. Gebretsadik M, Jayaprabhu S, Grossberg GT. Mood disorders in the elderly. Med Clin N Am. 2006;90(5):789–805.
6. Gitlin M, Frye MA. Maintenance therapies in bipolar disorders. Bipolar Disord. 2012;14(Suppl 2):51–65.
7. Goldberg JF. Bipolar disorder with comorbid substance abuse: diagnosis, prognosis, and treatment. J Psychiatr Pract. 2001;7(2):109–22.
8. Miklowitz DJ. A review of evidence-based psychosocial interventions for bipolar disorder. J Clin Psychiatry. 2006;67(Suppl 11):28–33 (Review).
9. Castle DJ, Berk L, Lauder S, Berk M, Murray G. Psychosocial interventions for bipolar disorder. Acta Neuropsychiatr. 2009;21:275–84.
10. Swartz HA, Swanson J. Psychotherapy for bipolar disorder in adults: a review of the evidence. Focus (Am Psychiatr Publ). 2014 Summer;12(3):251–266.

11. Swartz HA, Levenson JC, Frank E. Psychotherapy for bipolar II disorder: the role of interpersonal and social rhythm therapy. Prof Psychol Res Pr. 2012;43(2):145–53.
12. Depp CA, Moore DJ, Patterson TL, Lebowitz BD, Jeste DV. Psychosocial interventions and medication adherence in bipolar disorder. Dialogues Clin Neurosci. 2008;10(2):239–50.
13. Popovic D, Yildiz A, Murphy P, Colom F. Unexplored areas of psychotherapy in bipolar disorder. Harv Rev Psychiatry. 2014;22(6):373–8.
14. Canuto A, Meiler-Mititelu C, Herrmann FR, Delaloye C, Giannakopoulos P, Weber K. Longitudinal assessment of psychotherapeutic day hospital treatment for elderly patients with depression. Int J Geriatr Psychiatry. 2008;23(9):949–56.
15. Farren CK, Mc Elroy S. Treatment response of bipolar and unipolar alcoholics to an inpatient dual diagnosis program. J Affect Disord. 2008;106(3):265–72.
16. Jönsson PD, Wijk H, Danielson E, Skärsäter I. Outcomes of an educational intervention for the family of a person with bipolar disorder: a 2-year follow-up study. J Psychiatr Ment Health Nurs. 2011;18(4):333–41.
17. Gilbody S, Peckham E, Man MS, Mitchell N, Li J, Becque T, et al. Bespoke smoking cessation for people with severe mental ill health (SCIMITAR): a pilot randomised controlled trial. Lancet Psychiatry. 2015;2(5):395–402.
18. Tallian KB, Hirsch JD, Kuo GM, Chang CA, Gilmer T, Messinger M, et al. Development of a pharmacist-psychiatrist collaborative medication therapy management clinic. J Am Pharm Assoc (2003). 2012;52(6):e252–8.
19. Even C, Richard H, Thuile J, Friedman S, Rouillon F. Characteristics of voluntary participants versus nonparticipants in a psychoeducation program for euthymic patients with bipolar disorder. J Nerv Ment Dis. 2007;195(3):262–5.
20. Bartels SJ, Pratt SI, Mueser KT, Forester BP, Wolfe R, Cather C, et al. Long-term outcomes of a randomized trial of integrated skills training and preventive healthcare for older adults with serious mental illness. Am J Geriatr Psychiatry. 2014;22(11):1251–61.
21. Mueser KT, Pratt SI, Bartels SJ, Swain K, Forester B, Cather C, et al. Randomized trial of social rehabilitation and integrated health care for older people with severe mental illness. J Consult Clin Psychol. 2010;78(4):561–73.
22. Fagiolini A, Frank E, Axelson DA, Birmaher B, Cheng Y, Curet DE, et al. Enhancing outcomes in patients with bipolar disorder: results from the Bipolar Disorder Center for Pennsylvanians Study. Bipolar Disord. 2009;11(4):382–90.
23. Depp CA, Lebowitz BD, Patterson TL, Lacro JP, Jeste DV. Medication adherence skills training for middle-aged and elderly adults with bipolar disorder: development and pilot study. Bipolar Disord. 2007;9(6):636–45.
24. Kilbourne AM, Post EP, Nossek A, Sonel E, Drill LJ, Cooley S, et al. Service delivery in older patients with bipolar disorder: a review and development of a medical care model. Bipolar Disord. 2008;10(6):672–83.
25. Kilbourne AM, Post EP, Nossek A, Drill L, Cooley S, Bauer MS. Improving medical and psychiatric outcomes among individuals with bipolar disorder: a randomized controlled trial. Psychiatr Serv. 2008;59(7):760–8.
26. Pratt SI, Bartels SJ, Mueser KT, Forester B. Helping older people experience success: an integrated model of psychosocial rehabilitation and health care management for older adults with serious mental illness. Am J Psychiatr Rehabil. 2008;11:41–60.
27. Bauer MS, McBride L, Williford WO, Glick H, Kinosian B, Altshuler L, et al. Cooperative Studies Program 430 Study Team. Collaborative care for bipolar disorder: part I. Intervention and implementation in a randomized effectiveness trial. Psychiatr Serv. 2006;57(7):927–36.
28. Simon GE, Ludman EJ, Bauer MS, Unützer J, Operskalski B. Long-term effectiveness and cost of a systematic care program for bipolar disorder. Arch Gen Psychiatry. 2006;63(5):500–8.
29. Bauer MS, McBride L. Structured group psychotherapy for bipolar disorder: the life goals program. 2nd ed. New York: Springer Publishing Company; 2003.
30. Basco M, Rush AJ. Cognitive-behavioral therapy for bipolar disorder. New York: Guilford Press; 1996. p. 35.

31. Bauer M, McBride C. Structured group therapy for bipolar disorder: the life goals program. New York: Springer; 2003.
32. Patterson TL, McKibbin C, Taylor M, Goldman S, Davila-Fraga W, Bucardo J, et al. Functional adaptation skills training (FAST): a pilot psychosocial intervention study in middle-aged and older patients with chronic psychotic disorders. Am J Geriatr Psychiatry. 2003;11:17–23.
33. Sajatovic M, Chen P, Dines P, Shirley ER. Psychoeducational approaches to medication adherence in patients with bipolar disorder. Dis Manage Health Outcomes. 2007;15(3):181–92.
34. Hollon SD, Ponniah K. A review of empirically supported psychological therapies for mood disorders in adults. Depress Anxiety. 2010;27(10):891–932.
35. Miklowitz DJ, George EL, Richards JA, Simoneau TL, Suddath RL. A randomized study of family-focused psychoeducation and pharmacotherapy in the outpatient management of bipolar disorder. Arch Gen Psychiatry. 2003;60(9):904–12.
36. Rae MM, Tompson M, Miklowitz DJ, Goldstein MJ, Hwang S, Mintz J. Family focused treatment vs. individual treatment for bipolar disorder. Results of a randomized clinical trial. J Consult Clin Psychol. 2003;71:482–92.
37. Frank E, Kupfer DJ, Thase ME, Mallinger AG, Swartz HA, Fagiolini AM, et al. Two-year outcomes for interpersonal and social rhythm therapy in individuals with bipolar I disorder. Arch Gen Psychiatry. 2005;62(9):996–1004.
38. Lam DH, Watkins ER, Hayward P, Bright J, Wright K, Kerr N, et al. A randomized controlled study of cognitive therapy for relapse prevention for bipolar affective disorder: outcome of the first year. Arch Gen Psychiatry. 2003;60(2):145–52.
39. Lam DH, Hayward P, Watkins ER, Wright K, Sham P. Relapse prevention in patients with bipolar disorder: cognitive therapy outcome after 2 years. Am J Psychiatry. 2005;162(2):324–9.
40. Scott J, Paykel E, Morriss R, Bentall R, Kinderman P, Johnson T, et al. Cognitive-behavioural therapy for severe and recurrent bipolar disorders: randomised controlled trial. Br J Psychiatry. 2006;188:313–20.
41. Colom F, Vieta E, Sánchez-Moreno J, Palomino-Otiniano R, Reinares M, Goikolea JM, et al. Group psychoeducation for stabilised bipolar disorders: 5-year outcome of a randomised clinical trial. Br J Psychiatry. 2009;194(3):260–5.
42. Colom F, Vieta E, Martinez-Aran A, Reinares M, Goikolea JM, Benabarre A, et al. A randomized trial on the efficacy of group psychoeducation in the prophylaxis of recurrences in bipolar patients whose disease is in remission. Arch Gen Psychiatry. 2003;60(4):402–7.
43. Miklowitz DJ, Otto MW, Frank E, Reilly-Harrington NA, Wisniewski SR, Kogan JN, et al. Psychosocial treatments for bipolar depression: a 1-year randomized trial from the Systematic Treatment Enhancement Program. Arch Gen Psychiatry. 2007;64(4):419–26.
44. Sachs GS, Thase ME, Otto MW, Bauer M, Miklowitz D, Wisniewski SR, et al. Rationale, design, and methods of the systematic treatment enhancement program for bipolar disorder (STEP-BD). Biol Psychiatry. 2003;53:1028–42.
45. Newman C, Leahy R, Beck AT, Reilly-Harrington N, Gyulai L. Bipolar disorder: a cognitive therapy approach. New York: American Psychological Association; 2002.
46. Lam D, Jones S, Hayward P, Bright J. Cognitive therapy for bipolar disorder. New York: Wiley; 1999.
47. Gruber J, Miklowitz DJ, Harvey AG, Frank E, Kupfer D, Thase ME, et al. Sleep matters: sleep functioning and course of illness in bipolar disorder. J Affect Disord. 2011;134(1–3):416–20.
48. Miklowitz DJ, Goldstein MJ. Bipolar disorder: a family-focused treatment approach. New York: Guilford Press; 1997.
49. Simon GE, Ludman EJ, Bauer MS, Unützer J, Operskalski B. Long-term effectiveness and cost of a systematic care program for bipolar disorder. Arch Gen Psychiatry. 2006;63(5):500–8.
50. Bauer MS. The collaborative practice model for bipolar disorder: design and implementation in a multi-site randomized controlled trial. Bipolar Disord. 2001;3(5):233–44.

51. Reinares M, Colom F, Sánchez-Moreno J, Torrent C, Martínez-Arán A, Comes M, et al. Impact of caregiver group psychoeducation on the course and outcome of bipolar patients in remission: a randomized controlled trial. Bipolar Disord. 2008;10(4):511–9.
52. Kiosses DN, Ravdin LD, Gross JJ, Raue P, Kotbi N, Alexopoulos GS. Problem adaptation therapy for older adults with major depression and cognitive impairment: a randomized clinical trial. JAMA Psychiatry. 2015;72(1):22–30.
53. Kiosses DN, Alexopoulos GS. REBUILD: A post-ECT psychosocial intervention to reduce residual depression symptoms and disability. Bethesda: American Association for Geriatric Psychiatry; 2014.
54. Gross JJ. Emotion regulation: conceptual and empirical foundations. In: Gross JJ, editor. Handbook of emotion regulation. 2nd ed. New York: Guilford; 2014. p. 3–20.
55. Centers for Disease Control and Prevention, National Center for Injury Prevention and Control. Web-based Injury Statistics Query and Reporting System (WISQARS). http://www.cdc.gov/injury/wisqars/fatal_injury_reports.html. Accessed 24 Apr 2016
56. Tsai SY, Kuo CJ, Chen CC, Lee HC. Risk factors for completed suicide in bipolar disorder. J Clin Psychiatry. 2002;63:469–76.
57. Shulman K, Tohen M, Satlin A, Mallya G, Kalunian D. Mania compared to depression in old age. Am J Psychiatry. 1992;149:341–5.
58. Aizenberg D, Olmer A, Barak Y. Suicide attempts amongst elderly bipolar patients. J Affect Disord. 2006;91(1):91–4.
59. Sajatovic M, Strejilevich SA, Gildengers AG, Dols A, Al Jurdi RK, Forester BP, et al. A report on older-age bipolar disorder from the International Society for Bipolar Disorders Task Force. Bipolar Disord. 2015;17(7):689–704.
60. Juurlink DN, Herrmann N, Szalai JP, Kopp A, Redelmeier DA. Medical illness and the risk of suicide in the elderly. Arch Intern Med. 2004;164(11):1179–84.
61. Dervic K, Carballo JJ, Baca-Garcia E, Galfalvy HC, Mann JJ, Brent DA, et al. Moral or religious objections to suicide may protect against suicidal behavior in bipolar disorder. J Clin Psychiatry. 2011;72(10):1390–6.
62. Speer DC. Differences in social resources and treatment history among diagnostic groups of older adults. Hosp Community Psychiatry. 1992;43(3):270–4.
63. Kilbourne AM. Bipolar disorder in late life: future directions in efficacy and effectiveness research. Curr Psychiatry Rep. 2005;7(1):10–7.
64. Beyer JL, Greenberg RL, Marino P, Bruce ML, Al Jurdi RK, Sajatovic M, et al. Social support in late life mania: GERI-BD. Int J Geriatr Psychiatry. 2014;29(10):1028–32.
65. Kiosses DN, Rosenberg PB, McGovern A, Fonzetti P, Zaydens H, Alexopoulos GS. Depression and suicidal ideation during two psychosocial treatments in older adults with major depression and dementia. J Alzheimers Dis. 2015;48(2):453–62.
66. Gildengers A, Tatsuoka C, Bialko C, Cassidy KA, Dines P, Emanuel J, et al. Correlates of disability in depressed older adults with bipolar disorder. Cut Edge Psychiatry Pract. 2013;2013(1):332–8.
67. Depp CA, Mausbach BT, Eyler LT, Palmer BW, Cain AE, Lebowitz BD, et al. Performance-based and subjective measures of functioning in middle-aged and older adults with bipolar disorder. J Nerv Ment Dis. 2009;197(7):471–5.
68. Tsai SY, Kuo CJ, Chung KH, Huang YL, Lee HC, Chen CC. Cognitive dysfunction and medical morbidity in elderly outpatients with bipolar disorder. Am J Geriatr Psychiatry. 2009;17(12):1004–11.
69. Tsai SY, Lee HC, Chen CC, Huang YL. Cognitive impairment in later life in patients with early-onset bipolar disorder. Bipolar Disord. 2007;9(8):868–75.
70. Aprahamian I, Ladeira RB, Diniz BS, Forlenza OV, Nunes PV. Cognitive impairment in euthymic older adults with bipolar disorder: a controlled study using cognitive screening tests. Am J Geriatr Psychiatry. 2014;22(4):389–97.

71. Rej S, Butters MA, Aizenstein HJ, Begley A, Tsay J, Reynolds CF 3rd, et al. Neuroimaging and neurocognitive abnormalities associated with bipolar disorder in old age. Int J Geriatr Psychiatry. 2014;29(4):421–7.
72. Aprahamian I, Nunes PV, Forlenza OV. Cognitive impairment and dementia in late-life bipolar disorder. Curr Opin Psychiatry. 2013;26(1):120–3.
73. Young RC, Murphy CF, Heo M, Schulberg HC, Alexopoulos GS. Cognitive impairment in bipolar disorder in old age: literature review and findings in manic patients. J Affect Disord. 2006;92(1):125–31.
74. Canuto A, Giannakopoulos P, Moy G, Rubio MM, Ebbing K, Meiler-Mititelu C, et al. Neurocognitive deficits and personality traits among euthymic patients with mood disorders in late life. J Neurol Sci. 2010;299(1–2):24–9.
75. Schouws SN, Stek ML, Comijs HC, Beekman AT. Risk factors for cognitive impairment in elderly bipolar patients. J Affect Disord. 2010;125(1–3):330–5.
76. Gildengers A, Tatsuoka C, Bialko C, Cassidy KA, Al Jurdi RK, Gyulai L, et al. Correlates of treatment response in depressed older adults with bipolar disorder. J Geriatr Psychiatry Neurol. 2012;25(1):37–42.
77. Martino DJ, Marengo E, Igoa A, Scápola M, Ais ED, Perinot L, et al. Neurocognitive and symptomatic predictors of functional outcome in bipolar disorders: a prospective 1 year follow-up study. J Affect Disord. 2009;116(1–2):37–42.
78. Reinares M, Bonnín CM, Hidalgo-Mazzei D, Sánchez-Moreno J, Colom F, Vieta E. The role of family interventions in bipolar disorder: a systematic review. Clin Psychol Rev. 2015;3 (43):47–57.
79. Folstein MF, Folstein SE, McHugh PR. "Mini-mental state." A practical method for grading the cognitive state of patients for the clinician. J Psychiatr Res. 1975;12(3):189–98.
80. Nasreddine ZS, Phillips NA, Bédirian V, Charbonneau S, Whitehead V, Collin I, Cummings JL, Chertkow H. The Montreal Cognitive Assessment, MoCA: a brief screening tool for mild cognitive impairment. J Am Geriatr Soc. 2005;53(4):695–9.

Complementary and Integrative Therapies for Older Age Bipolar Disorder

10

Maria Cristina Poscablo-Stein and Adriana P. Hermida

10.1 Introduction

There is growing awareness and use of complementary and alternative medicine in the USA to treat a variety of physical and mental disorders as well as optimize overall wellness. Complementary and alternative medicine (CAM) is defined as a group of diverse medical and healthcare systems, practices, and products that are not presently considered to be part of conventional medicine [1]. Within CAM, therapies can be categorized into various domains, including mind–body interventions such as meditation and yoga, body-based methods such as chiropractic and massage therapy, and biologics such as herbs and dietary supplements (i.e., nutraceuticals), as well as whole medical systems (e.g., traditional Chinese medicine and Ayurveda). In December 2008, the National Center for Complementary and Integrative Health (NCCIH), formerly the National Center for Complementary and Alternative Medicine (NCCAM), surveyed Americans on their use of CAM as part of the 2007 National Health Interview Survey [2]. They reported that 38 % of US adults used some form of CAM in the last year with the highest use (44 %) in adults between 50 and 59. Non-vitamin, non-mineral natural products were the most popular CAM modality reported. There were significant increases in the use of several therapies including yoga, meditation, and fish oil supplementation between 2002 and 2007 [2].

M.C. Poscablo-Stein · A.P. Hermida (✉)
Department of Psychiatry and Behavioral Sciences, Emory University School of Medicine, 12 Executive Park Drive NE, Suite 331, Atlanta, GA 30329, USA
e-mail: ahermid@emory.edu

M.C. Poscablo-Stein
e-mail: cristina.poscablo-stein@emory.edu

S.W. Lehmann and B.P. Forester (eds.), *Bipolar Disorder in Older Age Patients*,
DOI 10.1007/978-3-319-48912-4_10

The prevalence of CAM use in US adults older than 65 is reported to be between 41 and 87 % with similar reports internationally [3–8]. Estimates from the National Health Interview Survey in 2002 showed that approximately 82 % of older adults with self-reported depression or anxiety used some form of CAM compared with about 61 % reported by those without such conditions, though only about one-fifth were using CAM for their mental health disorder [9]. It has been reported that older adults with mood disorders commonly use herbal and nutritional supplements, with higher use in bipolar disorder (44 %) versus major depression (16 %) [10]. Although little is known about patterns of CAM use in patients with bipolar disorder, there is some evidence that increased utilization of CAM may be related to decreased perception of effectiveness of medications on bipolar symptoms as well as interpersonal and occupational functioning [11].

Studies examining CAM therapies for the treatment of bipolar disorder in the geriatric population are lacking. However, there have been a number of recent reviews of randomized controlled trials (RCTs) examining CAM therapies in depression and anxiety [12, 13]. More recently, several reviews of CAM therapies in adult bipolar disorder have been published [14–16] and much of this chapter draws from this evidence base.

Although medications are the mainstay of treatment in geriatric bipolar disorder, they are associated with long-term adverse cardio-metabolic and other side effects. Moreover, their use can be limited by comorbid medical conditions and interactions with medications commonly prescribed in the elderly. Adherence to medications is often problematic, in part because of intolerable physical side effects [17, 18]. These factors highlight the need for safer and better tolerated adjunctive treatments for bipolar disorder patients, particularly in older age.

This chapter aims to review several complementary and alternative treatments for bipolar disorder. Due to the paucity of peer-reviewed publications of clinical trials examining CAM therapies in geriatric bipolar disorder, the majority of information presented here comes from the literature on adult bipolar disorder and unipolar depression. Table 10.1 summarizes selected CAM therapies that show the most promise as adjunctive treatments for bipolar disorder.

10.2 Nutraceuticals

Nutraceuticals are dietary supplements of naturally occurring substances such as vitamins and minerals. They can be obtained and used without a prescription as they are considered natural health products such as herbal remedies. Nutraceuticals are derived from food sources and are believed to have additional health benefits beyond their basic nutritional value.

Patients with bipolar disorder may be at risk for mood shifts when they are deficient in certain micronutrients [19, 20]. Indeed, screening for vitamin deficiencies such as folic acid, vitamin B12, and vitamin D is part of the standard psychiatric evaluation and treatment of mood disorders. However, much less is

Table 10.1 Complementary and integrative medicine interventions for bipolar disorder

Intervention	Mechanism of action	Effectiveness in bipolar disorder	Adverse effects/notable interactions
Omega-3 fatty acids	Regulation of neurotransmission, involved in cell survival and protection against neuro-inflammation	Mixed evidence for mild–moderate effect in bipolar depression; no effect on mania	Gastrointestinal symptoms, fishy aftertaste, caution with warfarin and NSAID's as may affect bleeding time
SAM-e	Methyl donor required for synthesis of neurotransmitters	Negative study in treatment refractory bipolar depression; more research needed	Induction of mania, gastrointestinal symptoms, headache
Folic acid and B12	Cofactors in neurotransmitter synthesis	Limited data in bipolar disorder	Induction of mania, interaction with SSRI's
Inositol	Glucose isomer, precursor in phosphatidylinositol bisphosphate second messenger system activated by neurotransmitters	One positive RCT in bipolar depression one study showing positive trend but underpowered so statistically nonsignificant	Induction of mania, headache
St. John's Wort	Decrease reuptake of monoamine neurotransmitters, monoamine oxidase inhibition	No studies in bipolar disorder; extensively studied in unipolar depression with positive effects	Serotonin syndrome, induction of mania, potent CYP3A4 inducer, mild CYP2C9/1A2 inducer
N-acetylcysteine (NAC)	Precursor of glutathione, the main antioxidant in tissues	Few studies show benefit in reducing depression in patients already on mood stabilizers, no effect on mania	Well tolerated, gastrointestinal discomfort
Coenzyme Q10	Cofactor in electron transport chain and generation of ATP, membrane stabilizer, antioxidant	One small open-label trial in bipolar depression with improvement in depressive symptoms	Well tolerated, gastrointestinal symptoms
Meditation	Reduce emotional reactivity, reduce stress, promote well-being	Some studies showing reduced depression and anxiety, improved attention in bipolar depression	Physical discomfort, dissociative experience
Exercise	Positive effect on neurogenesis, reduce inflammation and oxidative stress, and improve cardiovascular function	Several small uncontrolled studies showing benefit for depression; more studies in unipolar depression	Physical injury, induction of mania
Bright light therapy	Circadian rhythm regulation via suprachiasmatic nucleus and melatonin production, monoaminergic modulation	Mixed results in bipolar depression; effective in seasonal affective disorder	Headache, eye irritation, induction of mania, photosensitivity with psychotropics

known about the relationship between mood and nutritional deficiencies, in part due to inadequate biomarkers for many micronutrients and variation in the individual dietary needs of each patient [20]. There are no studies examining the role of various micronutrients in older age bipolar disorder, but several micronutrients have been studied in adult bipolar disorder and are reviewed here.

10.2.1 Omega-3 Fatty Acids

Clinical Vignette 10.1 Mr. R is a 71-year-old male with bipolar disorder, previous stroke, and mild cognitive impairment. He has been taking valproate for mood stabilization for many years. Mr. R has had several depressive episodes and has taken a number of antidepressants including fluoxetine, escitalopram, and most recently sertraline with good results. He was also prescribed quetiapine in the past but stopped due to elevated triglycerides. While Mr. R reported overall satisfaction with his current regimen to his psychiatrist at his last visit, he also reported occasional anhedonia and amotivation, and delayed ejaculation. This is not a new problem, and he reports that he has “just gotten used to it.” Mr. R read about the health benefits of fish oil and omega-3 fatty acids and wonders if it might help with his depression. His psychiatrist tells him the evidence for omega-3 fatty acids in bipolar disorder is not clear, but he would consider recommending supplementation if the patient was interested. Two weeks later, Mr. R returned for follow-up. At this visit, his psychiatrist recommended 1 g of purified eicosapentaenoic acid (EPA) daily and reduced his sertraline dose by 25 %. He counseled Mr. R on possible effects on bleeding in light of his aspirin use. Mr. R came for follow-up every 4–6 weeks for the next 6 months. Although Mr. R noted no worsening depression despite decreasing his sertraline dose, he cannot tell whether it is made any noticeable improvement in his mood. However, he is happy to report reduced sexual side effects and no adverse effects from the supplement. As a result, Mr. R decides to continue with this regimen indefinitely.

Learning Points

- Medication side effects can limit conventional treatment options for bipolar disorder.
- Adjunctive nutritional supplementation may be helpful, especially when potential benefits outweigh low risks.
- Frequent follow-up should occur with any medication or supplement change to monitor for worsening or improving of clinical condition.

Fish oil is the most widely used non-vitamin, non-mineral supplement used by the adults in the USA. The percentage of adults reporting use rose from 4.8 % in 2007 to 7.8 % in 2012 according to data collected as part of the National Health Interview Survey [21]. Omega-3 fatty acids are essential polyunsaturated fatty acids that must be obtained from the diet. The three main omega-3 fatty acids are alpha-linolenic acid (ALA), found in dark leafy vegetables, flax seeds, and nuts, eicosapentaenoic acid (EPA) and docosahexaenoic acid (DHA), found primarily in cold-water fish such as salmon and tuna. In contrast, omega-6 fatty acids are found in foods such as vegetable oils, margarine, and animal fat and are common in Western diets. Indeed, it has been proposed that the imbalance in ratio favoring omega-6 to omega-3 fatty acids in modern diets has contributed to the rise in chronic inflammatory diseases such as heart disease, obesity, diabetes, and mental health disorders including depression, bipolar disorder, and schizophrenia [22]. Thus, there is growing interest in omega-3 fatty acid supplementation and the potential to prevent a wide range of pathologic processes and health conditions related to aging such as cognitive decline, osteoarthritis, and cardiovascular disease [23–25].

Omega-3 fatty acid supplementation has also been studied as potential monotherapy and adjunctive treatment for mood disorders. A number of mechanisms have been proposed to explain omega 3-fatty acid psychotropic effects. These include regulation of neurotransmission, cell survival, and neuro-inflammation [26]. Omega-3 fatty acids are also thought to inhibit signal transduction pathways similar to the mechanism of valproate and lithium [24]. Epidemiologic studies have shown rates of fish consumption (which are high in omega-3 fatty acids) to be inversely correlated with rates of bipolar disorder and major depression [27, 28]. Erythrocyte membrane EPA and DHA contents have been used as biomarkers for omega-3 fatty acid status [29]. Epidemiologic studies have observed lowered EPA and/or DHA levels in adults with bipolar disorder [30, 31]. A recent study by McNamara and colleagues replicated these findings of erythrocyte cell membrane DHA deficits in first episode bipolar mania and mixed presentation patients compared to healthy controls [32]. Interestingly, patients were then treated with lithium and quetiapine, but no changes in fatty acid composition were noted despite symptomatic improvement, suggesting that changes in mood symptoms were not mediated by fatty acid status.

There have been numerous clinical trials examining the role of omega-3 fatty acids in major depressive disorder and have been reviewed by Lin et al., Williams et al., and Su et al., but few studies have looked at omega-3 supplementation in bipolar disorder [33–35]. Stoll and colleagues were the first to report on the beneficial role of omega-3 supplementation in bipolar patients [36]. In this double-blind placebo-controlled RCT ($N = 44$) comparing omega-3 supplementation to conventional pharmacologic treatment, subjects with a mean age of 41.4 treated with 9.6 g/day EPA/DHA had significant reduction in depressive symptoms and longer remission over 4 months compared to placebo (olive oil). There was no effect on mania. Another RCT of 75 patients (mean age 45–49) treated with 1 or 2 g EPA versus placebo adjunctively showed a small reduction in depressive symptoms at both doses as measured by the Hamilton Depression Rating Scale (HAM-D) but with no difference in manic symptoms [37]. Hirashima and coworkers reported on a small study of younger female patients with bipolar I disorder treated with EPA 5 g/DHA 3 g versus non-treatment [38]. They did not find a difference in manic and depressive symptoms among the groups but did find a decrease in T2 signaling on MRI, suggesting an increase in cell membrane fluidity. Subsequent studies of varying duration and dosages yielded similar results, with no improvement in manic symptoms [39, 40]. A recent meta-analysis of omega-3 fatty acids role in depression reported on a total of 7 RCTs in adults and children with bipolar disorder [41]. In this study, pooled analysis of 3 RCTs did support omega-3 fatty acids' effectiveness in bipolar depression.

Omega-3 fatty acids seem to be safe and well tolerated. A fishy aftertaste and gastrointestinal symptoms can occur with increasing dose. Omega-3 fatty acids could potentially affect bleeding time but there have been no cases of abnormal bleeding even when used in conjunction with anticoagulant medications [42]. In summary, omega 3-fatty acids may be modestly effective in bipolar depression but do not seem to be effective in bipolar mania. However, there are conflicting data regarding their efficacy given variations in doses and formulations. Future studies in larger samples are needed to determine optimum dosages.

10.2.2 S-adenosylmethionine (SAM-e)

S-adenosylmethionine (SAM-e) is a compound that is synthesized in the body from the amino acid methionine. It is available as a dietary supplement and has been studied for its antidepressant effects in unipolar depression [43]. SAM-e, via 1-carbon metabolism pathway, contributes methyl groups required for the synthesis of neurotransmitters, including serotonin and epinephrine as well as phosphatidylcholine, important in intracellular cell signaling [44]. In 2014, authors from McLean Hospital reported on a small double-blind, placebo-controlled RCT examining oral SAM-e adjunctive treatment for bipolar depression [45]. Patients aged 18 to 65 were included if they met criteria for bipolar I or II disorder based on DSM-IV TR criteria and had persistent moderate depression as defined by a score on the Montgomery-Asberg Depression Rating Scale (MADRS) ≥15 for the last three months. To reduce risk of inducing switch to the manic state, which had been reported previously with intravenous administration of SAM-e, a brief trial including 4 weeks of oral dose titration followed by 2 weeks of monitoring without medication was planned [46, 47]. Patients received SAM-e for 3 days of the week before the dose was increased. Maximum dosage was 1600 mg/day and was consistent with usual over-the-counter dosages. The authors reported no difference in depression response above the placebo response. However, the study was underpowered and was done in a treatment refractory population. Patients may require higher oral doses (compared to older studies which used intravenous administration). Further studies should be completed in larger, possibly less depressed samples to elucidate any benefit of SAM-e in bipolar depression.

10.2.3 Amino Acids

N-acetylcysteine (NAC) is an amino acid with anti-inflammatory and antioxidant properties. *N*-acetylcysteine is a bioavailable form of cysteine, which is the direct rate-limiting precursor for glutathione. Glutathione is the main antioxidant substrate for tissue, and perturbations in glutathione synthesis have been implicated in a number of psychiatric conditions including schizophrenia and bipolar disorder [48–50]. Berk and colleagues conducted a 24-week trial of NAC (1 g twice daily) versus placebo in 75 patients (mean age of 44.6 years) bipolar disorder already on medication [51]. The authors reported that NAC significantly reduced depressive symptoms as measured on the Montgomery-Asberg Depression Rating Scale and Bipolar Depression Rating Scale. There were no effects on mania although the baseline mania levels were low at baseline. Analysis of cognitive function in the same sample of patients revealed no change in cognitive status at 6 months [52]. A subsequent report in a similar population ($N = 149$, mean age 45.8 years) by the same group showed no benefit of maintenance treatment with NAC combined with treatment as usual as measured by change in mood symptoms, functionality, and quality of life [53]. NAC appears to be well tolerated with few adverse effects reported across numerous studies. Side effects include gastrointestinal discomfort headache, and rarely pruritus and rash [54].

Two small RCTs suggest that branched chain amino acids may be beneficial in attenuating symptoms of acute mania [55, 56]. The branched chain amino acids—leucine, isoleucine, and valine—compete with tyrosine and phenylalanine (catecholamine precursors) for entry into the brain. This, in turn, reduces the synthesis of norepinephrine and dopamine and subsequent dopaminergic neurotransmission [56]. In a study of 25 bipolar patients ranging in age from 19 to 62 on inpatient units with acute mania, patients were randomized to receive a 60-g branched chain amino acid mixture versus a placebo drink in addition to treatment as usual for seven days [56]. Those patients receiving the amino acid mixture had significantly reduced scores on YMRS after 6 h compared to placebo. However, intention to treat analysis after 2-week follow-up showed no difference between groups.

10.2.4 Inositol

Inositol is a glucose isomer, which is the precursor in the phosphatidyl-inositol second messenger system activated by many neurotransmitters in the brain. In 2000, there was a small pilot investigation of adjunctive inositol versus D-glucose placebo in 24 adults with bipolar depression over six weeks [57]. The mean age of participants was 43 years. Patients were on stable doses of lithium, valproate, or carbamazepine at study entry which were maintained unchanged throughout the study. The authors reported no statistically significant difference in depression between the group treated with 4 g inositol three times daily and the group treated with placebo. However, more patients in the inositol group (50 %) responded to treatment compared to placebo (30 %). Five of six inositol responders maintained their response after 24-week follow-up. A subsequent study of inositol 19 g daily added to therapeutic doses of lithium or valproate yielded similar results, though results in this study were statistically significant [58].

10.2.5 Folic Acid

Folic acid is a vitamin involved in DNA repair, methylation, and the synthesis of various neurotransmitters. An early study examined the role of folic acid supplementation in euthymic patients with unipolar depression, bipolar disorder, and schizoaffective disorder on lithium over 52 weeks [59]. Subset analysis of those patients with bipolar disorder ($N = 17$) did not show a significant difference in depressive symptoms as measured by the Beck Depression Inventory (BDI) over the course of the study when patients were treated with 200 μg of folic acid daily compared to placebo. However, the sample was small and depression levels were likely too low (BDI average score 1.6 at baseline) to detect any effect. Only one study to date has examined folic acid supplementation for acute mania [60]. In this more recent study in Iran, 88 adults with acute mania admitted to an inpatient psychiatric hospital were treated with sodium valproate plus 2 mg of folic acid or sodium valproate plus placebo for three weeks. The authors showed that while both groups showed improvement in manic symptoms over the study time, the group receiving adjunctive treatment with folic acid had greater and statistically significant improvement in Young Mania Rating Scale scores (mean 7.1 vs. 10.1, $p = 0.005$).

10.2.6 Coenzyme Q10

There is a growing body of evidence that alterations in energy metabolism and increased oxidative stress play roles in the neurobiology of bipolar disorder—in all phases of the illness as well as neuro-progression over time [61–63]. Mitochondrial dysfunction and the formation of reactive oxidative and nitrosative species (i.e., through increased inflammation) cause direct damage to membrane lipids, mitochondria, DNA, and functional proteins. As a result, several cellular processes are affected and may contribute to unipolar and bipolar depression. These include dysfunction in intracellular signaling, neurotransmission, neuroplasticity, cellular proliferation/growth, mitochondrial processes, and apoptosis [64].

Coenzyme Q10 (CoQ10) is present in the mitochondria of cells throughout the body and is a cofactor in the electron transport chain, within a series of redox reactions required for the synthesis of adenosine triphosphate (ATP). It is also a powerful antioxidant. CoQ10 has been studied in the treatment of various medical disorders involving mitochondrial impairment such as Parkinson's disease and fibromyalgia and has gained recent attention in unipolar and bipolar depression

[65]. Forester and coworkers reported an open-label trial of Coenzyme Q10 in older adults with a current episode of bipolar depression [66]. Patients were treated with 800 mg/day for four weeks, which was added to their existing medication regimen. There were 19 subjects included in the sample with a mean age of 63 years. The authors reported a significant reduction in MADRS score ($p = 0.001$) from baseline to week 4 of treatment. Exploratory analysis showed that CoQ10 may improve specific symptoms of lassitude, sadness, and poor concentration [66]. Randomized control trials are needed to further assess its effectiveness for bipolar depression.

10.3 St. John's Wort

St. John's Wort or *Hypericum perforatum* is a flowering plant found throughout the world that has been used for medicinal purposes for millennia. Though it has been most extensively studied in the treatment of depression, researchers have been interested in its application to a number of other psychiatric conditions [67]. Unfortunately, there have been no clinical trials to date specifically in bipolar disorder.

Evidence in the depression literature supports use of high-quality, standardized preparations of St. John's Wort in mild-to-moderate major depression and has been extensively reviewed. There have been dozens of randomized trials, and a recent meta-analysis demonstrated it to be better than placebo and comparable to conventional antidepressants [68]. Hyperforin and hypericin are the active components in St. John's Wort. It is typically dosed as 900 mg in divided doses two or three times daily, which is equivalent to approximately 1.0 mcg hypericin and 0.5–5 % hyperforin though some may need up to 1800 mg/day for more severe depression [67]. Its mechanisms of action are purported to be wide-based reuptake inhibition of serotonin, dopamine, and norepinephrine as well as MAO-inhibition. It may also have some modulatory effects on GABA and glutamate [69].

There are limited data on St. John's Wort in older adults. An RCT involving mostly female older adults demonstrated equivalent efficacy of St. John's Wort (800 mg) compared to fluoxetine (20 mg) with minimal adverse effects [70]. Importantly, cost-effective analysis showed potential economic benefit of St. John's Wort, with several hundred dollars saved per individual compared to sertraline and venlafaxine [71].

St. John's Wort is quite tolerable with mild dermatologic reactions and gastrointestinal symptoms as the most commonly reported side effects. In 2010, Kasper and colleagues assessed the tolerability of St. John's Wort across several randomized control trials compared to paroxetine and other selective serotonin reuptake inhibitors. The authors reported comparable adverse reaction rates for St. John's Wort to placebo and lower adverse reactions compared to paroxetine and other SSRIs [72]. Treatment with St. John's Wort carries the risk of inducing mania/hypomania, with multiple cases of St. John's Wort-induced mania reported in the literature [73, 74]. It is a potent CYP3A4 inducer and a mild inducer of CYP2C9 and CYP1A2 [75]. Psychotropic drugs are metabolized largely by these enzymes, and therefore, their induction can decrease psychotropic drug levels if taken simultaneously. Clinically significant drug interactions include effects on warfarin, cyclosporine, HIV protease inhibitors, theophylline, oral contraceptives, and digoxin. Specifically, St. John's Wort can reduce warfarin levels via CYP2C9 induction and decrease levels of cyclosporine, HIV protease inhibitors, and oral contraceptives via CYP3A4 induction. St. John's Wort can reduce the absorption and distribution of digoxin through induction of P-glycoprotein transport protein [76]. It is not recommended to use SSRIs concomitantly with St. John's Wort given risk of serotonin syndrome and decreasing psychotropic effectiveness due to liver enzyme induction [67].

In summary, there is some evidence to extrapolate from studies conducted in adults with major depression to support the use of St. John's Wort in older patients with bipolar disorder, particularly in those who cannot tolerate antidepressants. However, it is important to counsel patients that, while tolerable, St. John's Wort is not without adverse effects. Clinicians should carefully consider possible drug–drug interactions, which could potentially decrease the effectiveness of various medications in the elderly. Moreover, the lack of regulation/standardization by the Food and Drug Administration and potential for variable amounts of active plant product across formulations further increases the potential for adverse consequences from drug–herb interactions. Thus, it may be wise to avoid St. John's Wort when taking medications with significant drug interactions as described above. Further work is needed to more clearly identify potential use of St. John's Wort in older adults with bipolar depression, when used in conjunction with mood stabilizers.

10.4 Mindfulness Meditation

Clinical Vignette 10.2

Ms. L is a 68-year-old female with bipolar disorder who has been seeing her current psychiatrist regularly for the last 7 years. She is widowed and plans to retire from her job as a paralegal in the next two years. She has had several episodes of depression since age 28 and two distinct manic episodes in her lifetime. Her history is also relevant for severe depression 10 years ago when her husband died, for which she was hospitalized and was treated with ECT. She has been on a number of medications during her life and most recently maintained on lithium and venlafaxine. She reports despite "feeling good most of the time" she occasionally struggles with sadness, anhedonia, and feeling dissatisfied with her life from time to time. Ms. L reports ongoing difficulties with keeping focused at work and has been treated with small doses of stimulants in the past. While the medications helped, she sometimes struggled with the side effect of insomnia. Her cognitive complaints never progressed and only mildly impacted her work. Ms. L did not want to change her medications and asked her psychiatrist if he could recommend a non-pharmacological treatment to help with residual depressive symptoms and her cognition. Her psychiatrist was aware that the patient enjoyed yoga and meditation as hobbies, and recommended an 8-week course in mindfulness training as an adjunctive treatment. After attending a Mindfulness-Based Cognitive Therapy course (MBCT), Ms. L reported improvement in residual depressive symptoms, noting increased awareness of small daily pleasures that uplift her mood. She finds the meditation relaxing and it helps her insomnia.

Learning Points

- Bipolar patients often complain of residual symptoms or comorbid psychiatric conditions.
- Evidence-based behavioral therapies should be considered to address these problems as an alternative to additional psychopharmacologic approaches for stable patients.
- Clinicians should take patient's preferences into account when considering treatment modalities (i.e., are they open to a mindfulness approach, etc.).

Mindfulness meditation and mindfulness-based interventions have grown in popularity, and their clinical benefits have been studied in an array of psychiatric conditions, physical illnesses including pain, and general well-being [77–80]. While the concept of mindfulness originated from Eastern spiritual, and cultural contemplative traditions (e.g., Buddhism), it has also been described in psychological terms as paying attention on purpose to the present moment with nonjudgmental attitude to one's inner and outer experiences [81]. Both Mindfulness-Based Cognitive Therapy (MBCT) and Mindfulness-Based Stress Reduction (MBSR) were developed by clinical groups to address physical and mental health issues [82–85]. While MBSR has been studied in a number of psychiatric conditions over the years since its inception, there have been several recent studies examining the effectiveness of MBCT in adults with bipolar disorder, though none exclusively in the geriatric population [86–88]. The studies have enrolled mixed ages from 18 to 65 with average age around 40. MBCT combines mindfulness training with cognitive therapy and was initially developed to prevent relapse in major depressive disorder [89]. MBCT has been shown to be more effective in treating residual symptoms of depression and improving quality of life compared to maintenance antidepressant therapy in patients with fully or partially remitted major depressive disorder (MDD) [90]. An open-label, nonrandomized controlled trial comparing MBCT (cohort $N = 23$) versus sertraline (cohort $N = 20$) as a first-line treatment for acute major depressive disorder found significant reductions in HAM-D scores but no difference between groups, suggesting MBCT may be a viable alternative to medication for acute depression [91].

A small study of 12 adult patients with bipolar disorder with residual depressive symptoms used a modified version of the MBCT protocol to examine possible changes in mood, attention, and well-being [86]. Although the conditions were not controlled, the authors reported a decrease in depressive symptoms, fewer attention difficulties, an increase in mindfulness, and improvements in emotional regulation, positive effect, and psychological well-being. Subsequent analysis of the same study sample found patient reports of improved executive functioning, memory, and ability to initiate and complete tasks after 3 months of follow-up [92]. Perich and coworkers reported on a small RCT of MBCT + treatment as usual (TAU) versus treatment as usual in bipolar patients (N = 48 MBCT, N = 47 TAU) [88]. The authors reported no benefit of MBCT versus TAU in time to recurrence of mood symptoms or number of recurrences over 12-month follow-up but did demonstrate some improvement in anxiety. However, the study was limited by a short follow-up period relative to previous studies and a high dropout rate in both groups. There is an ongoing 3-prong randomized clinical trial comparing MBCT plus medication management versus an active psycho-education intervention plus medication management versus medication management alone in outpatient bipolar patients with subthreshold depressive symptoms. Results from this study have not yet been published [93].

Mindfulness-Based Cognitive Therapy may exert effects across a broad spectrum of neurocognitive symptoms in bipolar disorder. There is evidence in the literature demonstrating neurocognitive deficits in bipolar patients in various phases of the illness. In particular, patients with bipolar disorder have been found to have impairment in attention, working memory, processing speed, and verbal learning and these neurocognitive deficits contribute to functional impairment even in the euthymic state [94–97]. There is some evidence that MBCT may modulate cognitive processes in these patients. Howell and colleagues completed a pilot EEG study to examine attention control in bipolar patients [98]. Bipolar patients exhibited decreased attention readiness and activation of irrelevant information compared to healthy controls. After an 8-week MBCT course, the patients exhibited improvements in attention readiness and attenuated activation of non-relevant information processing.

Mindfulness training may help to modulate emotional reactivity and anxiety in individuals with bipolar disorder. In a study of 23 bipolar disorder patients and 10 healthy controls, patients reported high levels of anxiety and stress as well as low scores on working memory during neuropsychological testing pre-MBCT intervention [99]. After MBCT, the patients reported improvements in mindfulness, anxiety, emotional regulation, and working memory and verbal fluency. Additionally, fMRI analysis showed increased activation of the medial prefrontal cortex in these patients, which is a region associated with cognitive flexibility in bipolar disorder. Bipolar patients may also exhibit alterations in emotional processing.

Emotional processing as measured by event-related potentials and heart rate variability are exaggerated in patients with bipolar disorder compared to normal adults [100]. These measures of emotional processing were attenuated after an 8-week MBCT course [99].

10.5 Exercise and Yoga

Physical exercise has been evaluated for its potential impact on psychiatric disorders. Patients with bipolar disorder report less regular exercise than other adults [101]. In addition to physical health benefits, exercise may help to improve mood through several proposed mechanisms. Exercise is thought to affect a multiplicity of neurobiological systems involved in neurogenesis, neurotransmission, and neuro-inflammation [102]. The relationship between exercise and neurogenesis is best explained by brain-derived neurotrophic factor (BDNF) [103]. BDNF levels are increased in the brain during chronic antidepressant administration and BDNF is a biomarker of disease activity in psychiatric illnesses [104]. In fact, BDNF levels seem to be decreased in mania and depression and are recovered following resolution of acute mania [105]. Additionally, BDNF is remarkably responsive to exercise [106]. Other postulated benefits of exercise on mood include effects on endorphins, the hypothalamic pituitary adrenal (HPA) axis and cortisol production, and systemic inflammation [102]. Specifically, the release of endorphins during exercise enhances mood and feelings of well-being. Pro-inflammatory markers such as IL-6 and TNF-α have been shown to be elevated in both mania and bipolar depression, and exercise has been associated with smaller increases in inflammatory cytokine response to acute stress [107, 108]. Therefore, one may hypothesize that exercise might reduce symptoms of bipolar disorder via attenuated inflammatory responses but this warrants further investigation. Finally, exercise might play a role in reducing cortisol levels, which may be elevated in depression [102].

Although there have been numerous trials examining the utility of exercise in unipolar depression, the data in bipolar disorder are limited. A recent review of 31 studies of exercise and bipolar disorder showed that physical activity was associated with fewer depressive symptoms, better quality of life, and increased functioning [109]. However, the review was limited in that many of the studies were cross-sectional and none was randomized control trials. Ng and colleagues reported on a retrospective study of inpatients admitted to a private hospital for acute bipolar disorder [110]. They compared participants ($N = 24$) and nonparticipants ($N = 74$) in a voluntary exercise program, and although they reported no difference in overall functioning, the participants reported decreased depression, anxiety, and stress. Several other open trial studies of exercise interventions showed benefits on well-being, reducing weight, cholesterol, and glucose levels, as well as improving depressive symptoms [111, 112]. In 2010, Van Citters and colleagues reported on a pilot study of an individualized health promotion program for 76 individuals with severe mental illness. Nineteen (25 %) of the patients had bipolar disorder [113]. One-third of the study participants were older than age 50. During the 9-month study, which focused on physical activity and dietary behaviors, there was a significant increase in exercise, reduction in waist circumference, and satisfaction with fitness and mental functioning among the study subjects as a whole [113]. Concern has been raised that exercise may induce manic symptoms [114]. However, it is very possible that the relationship simply reflects core symptomatology of the phases of illness (i.e., increased energy and activation leading to more exercise in mania compared to depression). Nevertheless, the physical and mental health benefits of exercise are promising in light of high rates of comorbid cardiovascular disease and premature mortality and morbidity from obesity and diabetes in patients with bipolar disorder [115, 116].

Yoga is a physical, mental, and spiritual practice originating from India that has gained popularity in Western cultures and is considered a form of complementary alternative medicine. It has been studied as monotherapy and adjunctive treatment for depression and has been reviewed in mood and anxiety disorders [117] but studies are of variable quality. Its potential effects on mood may be related to reducing sympathetic activity while improving parasympathetic tone, regulating the HPA axis activity, and influencing monoamines [12]. These effects may have a positive effect on emotion regulation and stress reactivity [118, 119]. There are no randomized clinical trials examining yoga in bipolar disorder. However, a recent survey of 86 yoga practitioners with bipolar disorder found that patients commonly reported positive emotional effects (e.g., reduced anxiety), improved cognition (e.g., acceptance and focus), and physical benefits (e.g., weight loss and increased energy) [120].

10.6 Bright Light Therapy

Light therapy has been used in psychiatric practice for some time, most extensively for seasonal affective disorder. There has been growing interest in its application to bipolar disorder. Circadian rhythm dysfunction has been implicated in bipolar disorder in all phases of the illness including euthymia [121]. Compared to healthy controls, individuals with bipolar disorder showed advances in cycle phase, higher percentage of nocturnal sleep, and lower average daily activity [122]. The mechanisms by which light therapy regulates mood are not completely clear. However, several mechanisms have been suggested, including modulating effects on serotonin possibly via enhanced 5-HT transmission, melatonin regulation, and synchronization of the circadian rhythm [123, 124]. In a study of 49 adult patients (mean age 39) with bipolar depression and HAM-D scores >18, individuals were randomized to sleep deprivation and light therapy plus medication or to medication alone [125]. The authors demonstrated a robust and statistically significant decrease in depressive symptoms as early as 48 h and maintained over 7 weeks of follow-up in patients treated with sleep deprivation and light therapy plus medication. Tseng and coworkers conducted a meta-analysis of 9 studies which included 489 patients with bipolar depression treated with light therapy [126]. They reported that patients treated with light therapy, with and without total sleep deprivation, had a reduction in disease severity. Light therapy is purported to be safe with minor side effects of sleep onset difficulties, eye irritation, and blurred vision reported [126]. However, light therapy has been shown to induce mixed states in a case series of bipolar women [127]. Unfortunately, no studies have examined bright light therapy specifically in older age adults with bipolar disorder and so generalizability to this population is limited.

10.7 Summary

Management of bipolar disorder in the geriatric population poses unique challenges. Clinicians must weigh the benefits of standard pharmacologic treatments against multiple risks in the elderly, including adverse effects related to drug–drug interactions and worsening of comorbid medical illnesses such as diabetes and cardiovascular disease. Moreover, high rates of residual symptoms and functional impairment highlight the need for additional treatments to improve patients' quality of life and well-being. High-quality CAM studies are essentially nonexistent in older age bipolar disorder, and further research is needed to identify effective and safe interventions for this population. However, this should not preclude the judicious use of complementary therapies as adjunctive treatments to standard approaches that have shown promise in younger bipolar patients as well as those with other mood disorders. Although there is no available consensus or treatment algorithm for CAM modalities, we recommend the following the clinical pearls below based on available literature to date.

Clinical Pearls

- Clinicians should strive to develop an integrative treatment model that incorporates conventional treatments with select CAM therapies that have a strong evidence base. From the nutraceuticals, there is increasing evidence for omega-3 fatty acid supplementation in bipolar depression. Though St. John's Wort has been studied extensively in mood disorders, its use in older age bipolar disorder may be limited by its interactions with certain medications. Inositol may be promising for bipolar depression though larger studies are needed in the future.
- CAM therapies without supportive safety and effectiveness data should not be used, especially in cases of severe and acute depression and/or

mania. Therapies reviewed here with questionable effectiveness include folic acid and branched chain amino acids.

- CAM therapies such as mindfulness meditation may be most useful as adjunctive treatments when residual symptoms or other psychiatric symptoms (e.g., anxiety and insomnia) are present.
- CAM therapies can be considered as part of a comprehensive treatment plan that not only addresses the core symptoms of bipolar disorder, but also general physical and mental well-being.

References

1. National Center for Complementary and Integrative Health Bethesda 2008 [updated Mar 2015]. Available from: https://nccih.nih.gov/health/integrative-health-cvsa.
2. Barnes PM, Bloom B, Nahin RL. Complementary and alternative medicine use among adults and children: United States, 2007. Natl Health Stat Rep. 2008;12:1–23.
3. Schnabel K, Binting S, Witt CM, Teut M. Use of complementary and alternative medicine by older adults—a cross-sectional survey. BMC Geriatr. 2014;14:38.
4. Astin JA, Pelletier KR, Marie A, Haskell WL. Complementary and alternative medicine use among elderly persons: one-year analysis of a Blue Shield Medicare supplement. J Gerontol Ser A Biol Sci Med Sci. 2000;55(1):M4–9.
5. Cheung CK, Wyman JF, Halcon LL. Use of complementary and alternative therapies in community-dwelling older adults. J Altern Complement Med (New York, NY). 2007;13 (9):997–1006.
6. Cohen RJ, Ek K, Pan CX. Complementary and alternative medicine (CAM) use by older adults: a comparison of self-report and physician chart documentation. J Gerontol Ser A Biol Sci Med Sci. 2002;57(4):M223–7.
7. Najm W, Reinsch S, Hoehler F, Tobis J. Use of complementary and alternative medicine among the ethnic elderly. Altern Ther Health Med. 2003;9(3):50–7.
8. Williamson AT, Fletcher PC, Dawson KA. Complementary and alternative medicine. Use in an older population. J Gerontol Nurs. 2003;29(5):20–8.
9. Grzywacz JG, Suerken CK, Quandt SA, Bell RA, Lang W, Arcury TA. Older adults' use of complementary and alternative medicine for mental health: findings from the 2002 National Health Interview Survey. J Altern Complement Med (New York, NY). 2006;12(5):467–73.
10. Keaton D, Lamkin N, Cassidy KA, Meyer WJ, Ignacio RV, Aulakh L, et al. Utilization of herbal and nutritional compounds among older adults with bipolar disorder and with major depression. Int J Geriatr Psychiatry. 2009;24(10):1087–93.
11. Jarman CN, Perron BE, Kilbourne AM, Teh CF. Perceived treatment effectiveness, medication compliance, and complementary and alternative medicine use among veterans with bipolar disorder. J Altern Complement Med (New York, NY). 2010;16(3):251–5.
12. Ravindran AV, da Silva TL. Complementary and alternative therapies as add-on to pharmacotherapy for mood and anxiety disorders: a systematic review. J Affect Disord. 2013;150(3):707–19.
13. van der Watt G, Laugharne J, Janca A. Complementary and alternative medicine in the treatment of anxiety and depression. Curr Opin Psychiatry. 2008;21(1):37–42.

14. Andreescu C, Mulsant BH, Emanuel JE. Complementary and alternative medicine in the treatment of bipolar disorder–a review of the evidence. J Affect Disord. 2008;110(1–2):16–26.
15. Sarris J, Mischoulon D, Schweitzer I. Adjunctive nutraceuticals with standard pharmacotherapies in bipolar disorder: a systematic review of clinical trials. Bipolar Disord. 2011;13(5–6):454–65.
16. Sarris J, Lake J, Hoenders R. Bipolar disorder and complementary medicine: current evidence, safety issues, and clinical considerations. J Altern Complement Med (New York, NY). 2011;17(10):881–90.
17. Fleck DE, Keck PE Jr, Corey KB, Strakowski SM. Factors associated with medication adherence in African American and white patients with bipolar disorder. J Clin Psychiatry. 2005;66(5):646–52.
18. Miklowitz DJ, Johnson SL. The psychopathology and treatment of bipolar disorder. Annu Rev Clin Psychol. 2006;2:199–235.
19. Bourre JM. Effects of nutrients (in food) on the structure and function of the nervous system: update on dietary requirements for brain. Part 1: micronutrients. J Nutr Health Aging. 2006;10(5):377–85.
20. Kaplan BJ, Crawford SG, Field CJ, Simpson JS. Vitamins, minerals, and mood. Psychol Bull. 2007;133(5):747–60.
21. Clarke TC, Black LI, Stussman BJ, Barnes PM, Nahin RL. Trends in the use of complementary health approaches among adults: United States, 2002–2012. Natl Health Stat Rep. 2015;79:1–16.
22. Simopoulos AP. Importance of the ratio of omega-6/omega-3 essential fatty acids: evolutionary aspects. World Rev Nutr Diet. 2003;92:1–22.
23. Ubeda N, Achon M, Varela-Moreiras G. Omega 3 fatty acids in the elderly. Br J Nutr. 2012;107(Suppl 2):S137–51.
24. Kotwal S, Jun M, Sullivan D, Perkovic V, Neal B. Omega 3 Fatty acids and cardiovascular outcomes: systematic review and meta-analysis. Circ Cardiovasc Qual Outcomes. 2012;5(6):808–18.
25. Lopez HL. Nutritional interventions to prevent and treat osteoarthritis. Part I: focus on fatty acids and macronutrients. PM & R: J Inj Funct Rehabil. 2012;4(5 Suppl):S145–54.
26. Su KP, Matsuoka Y, Pae CU. Omega-3 polyunsaturated fatty acids in prevention of mood and anxiety disorders. Clin Psychopharmacol Neurosci: Off Sci J Kor College Neuropsychopharmacol. 2015;13(2):129–37.
27. Tanskanen A, Hibbeln JR, Tuomilehto J, Uutela A, Haukkala A, Viinamaki H, et al. Fish consumption and depressive symptoms in the general population in Finland. Psychiatric Ser (Washington, DC). 2001;52(4):529–31.
28. Noaghiul S, Hibbeln JR. Cross-national comparisons of seafood consumption and rates of bipolar disorders. Am J Psychiatry. 2003;160(12):2222–7.
29. Harris WS. The omega-3 index: clinical utility for therapeutic intervention. Curr Cardiol Rep. 2010;12(6):503–8.
30. McNamara RK, Jandacek R, Rider T, Tso P, Dwivedi Y, Pandey GN. Selective deficits in erythrocyte docosahexaenoic acid composition in adult patients with bipolar disorder and major depressive disorder. J Affect Disord. 2010;126(1–2):303–11.
31. Ranjekar PK, Hinge A, Hegde MV, Ghate M, Kale A, Sitasawad S, et al. Decreased antioxidant enzymes and membrane essential polyunsaturated fatty acids in schizophrenic and bipolar mood disorder patients. Psychiatry Res. 2003;121(2):109–22.
32. McNamara RK, Jandacek R, Tso P, Blom TJ, Welge JA, Strawn JR, et al. First-episode bipolar disorder is associated with erythrocyte membrane docosahexaenoic acid deficits: Dissociation from clinical response to lithium or quetiapine. Psychiatry Res. 2015;230(2):447–53.
33. Lin PY, Su KP. A meta-analytic review of double-blind, placebo-controlled trials of antidepressant efficacy of omega-3 fatty acids. J Clin Psychiatry. 2007;68(7):1056–61.

34. Williams AL, Katz D, Ali A, Girard C, Goodman J, Bell I. Do essential fatty acids have a role in the treatment of depression? J Affect Disord. 2006;93(1–3):117–23.
35. Su KP, Wang SM, Pae CU. Omega-3 polyunsaturated fatty acids for major depressive disorder. Expert Opin Investig Drugs. 2013;22(12):1519–34.
36. Stoll AL, Severus WE, Freeman MP, Rueter S, Zboyan HA, Diamond E, et al. Omega 3 fatty acids in bipolar disorder: a preliminary double-blind, placebo-controlled trial. Arch Gen Psychiatry. 1999;56(5):407–12.
37. Frangou S, Lewis M, McCrone P. Efficacy of ethyl-eicosapentaenoic acid in bipolar depression: randomised double-blind placebo-controlled study. Br J Psychiatry: J Ment Sci. 2006;188:46–50.
38. Hirashima F, Parow AM, Stoll AL, Demopulos CM, Damico KE, Rohan ML, et al. Omega-3 fatty acid treatment and T(2) whole brain relaxation times in bipolar disorder. Am J Psychiatry. 2004;161(10):1922–4.
39. Keck PE Jr, Mintz J, McElroy SL, Freeman MP, Suppes T, Frye MA, et al. Double-blind, randomized, placebo-controlled trials of ethyl-eicosapentanoate in the treatment of bipolar depression and rapid cycling bipolar disorder. Biol Psychiatry. 2006;60(9):1020–2.
40. Chiu CC, Huang SY, Chen CC, Su KP. Omega-3 fatty acids are more beneficial in the depressive phase than in the manic phase in patients with bipolar I disorder. J Clin Psychiatry. 2005;66(12):1613–4.
41. Sarris J, Mischoulon D, Schweitzer I. Omega-3 for bipolar disorder: meta-analyses of use in mania and bipolar depression. J Clin Psychiatry. 2012;73(1):81–6.
42. Eritsland J, Arnesen H, Gronseth K, Fjeld NB, Abdelnoor M. Effect of dietary supplementation with n-3 fatty acids on coronary artery bypass graft patency. Am J Cardiol. 1996;77(1):31–6.
43. Papakostas GI. Evidence for S-adenosyl-L-methionine (SAM-e) for the treatment of major depressive disorder. J Clin Psychiatry. 2009;70(Suppl 5):18–22.
44. Mischoulon D, Fava M. Role of S-adenosyl-L-methionine in the treatment of depression: a review of the evidence. Am J Clin Nutr. 2002;76(5):1158s–61s.
45. Murphy BL, Babb SM, Ravichandran C, Cohen BM. Oral SAMe in persistent treatment-refractory bipolar depression: a double-blind, randomized clinical trial. J Clin Psychopharmacol. 2014;34(3):413–6.
46. Carney MW, Chary TK, Bottiglieri T, Reynolds EH. The switch mechanism and the bipolar/unipolar dichotomy. Br J Psychiatry: J Ment Sci. 1989;154:48–51.
47. Lipinski JF, Cohen BM, Frankenburg F, Tohen M, Waternaux C, Altesman R, et al. Open trial of S-adenosylmethionine for treatment of depression. Am J Psychiatry. 1984;141 (3):448–50.
48. Steullet P, Cabungcal JH, Monin A, Dwir D, O'Donnell P, Cuenod M, et al. Redox dysregulation, neuroinflammation, and NMDA receptor hypofunction: a "central hub" in schizophrenia pathophysiology? Schizophr Res. 2016;176(1):41–51.
49. Tuncel OK, Sarisoy G, Bilgici B, Pazvantoglu O, Cetin E, Unverdi E, et al. Oxidative stress in bipolar and schizophrenia patients. Psychiatry Res. 2015;228(3):688–94.
50. Brown NC, Andreazza AC, Young LT. An updated meta-analysis of oxidative stress markers in bipolar disorder. Psychiatry Res. 2014;218(1–2):61–8.
51. Berk M, Copolov DL, Dean O, Lu K, Jeavons S, Schapkaitz I, et al. *N*-acetyl cysteine for depressive symptoms in bipolar disorder—a double-blind randomized placebo-controlled trial. Biol Psychiatry. 2008;64(6):468–75.
52. Dean OM, Bush AI, Copolov DL, Kohlmann K, Jeavons S, Schapkaitz I, et al. Effects of *N*-acetyl cysteine on cognitive function in bipolar disorder. Psychiatry Clin Neurosci. 2012;66(6):514–7.
53. Berk M, Dean OM, Cotton SM, Gama CS, Kapczinski F, Fernandes B, et al. Maintenance *N*-acetyl cysteine treatment for bipolar disorder: a double-blind randomized placebo controlled trial. BMC Med. 2012;10:91.

54. Deepmala, Slattery J, Kumar N, Delhey L, Berk M, Dean O, et al. Clinical trials of *N*-acetylcysteine in psychiatry and neurology: a systematic review. Neurosci Biobehav Rev. 2015;55:294–321.
55. McTavish SF, McPherson MH, Harmer CJ, Clark L, Sharp T, Goodwin GM, et al. Antidopaminergic effects of dietary tyrosine depletion in healthy subjects and patients with manic illness. Br J Psychiatry: J Ment Sci. 2001;179:356–60.
56. Scarna A, Gijsman HJ, McTavish SF, Harmer CJ, Cowen PJ, Goodwin GM. Effects of a branched-chain amino acid drink in mania. Br J Psychiatry: J Ment Sci. 2003;182:210–3.
57. Chengappa KN, Levine J, Gershon S, Mallinger AG, Hardan A, Vagnucci A, et al. Inositol as an add-on treatment for bipolar depression. Bipolar Disord. 2000;2(1):47–55.
58. Eden Evins A, Demopulos C, Yovel I, Culhane M, Ogutha J, Grandin LD, et al. Inositol augmentation of lithium or valproate for bipolar depression. Bipolar Disord. 2006;8(2):168–74.
59. Coppen A, Chaudhry S, Swade C. Folic acid enhances lithium prophylaxis. J Affect Disord. 1986;10(1):9–13.
60. Behzadi AH, Omrani Z, Chalian M, Asadi S, Ghadiri M. Folic acid efficacy as an alternative drug added to sodium valproate in the treatment of acute phase of mania in bipolar disorder: a double-blind randomized controlled trial. Acta Psychiatr Scand. 2009;120(6):441–5.
61. Clay HB, Sillivan S, Konradi C. Mitochondrial dysfunction and pathology in bipolar disorder and schizophrenia. Int J Dev Neurosci: Off J Int Soc Dev Neurosci. 2011;29(3):311–24.
62. Stork C, Renshaw PF. Mitochondrial dysfunction in bipolar disorder: evidence from magnetic resonance spectroscopy research. Mol Psychiatry. 2005;10(10):900–19.
63. Berk M, Kapczinski F, Andreazza AC, Dean OM, Giorlando F, Maes M, et al. Pathways underlying neuroprogression in bipolar disorder: focus on inflammation, oxidative stress and neurotrophic factors. Neurosci Biobehav Rev. 2011;35(3):804–17.
64. Moylan S, Berk M, Dean OM, Samuni Y, Williams LJ, O'Neil A, et al. Oxidative & nitrosative stress in depression: Why so much stress? Neurosci Biobehav Rev. 2014;45:46–62.
65. Morris G, Anderson G, Berk M, Maes M. Coenzyme Q10 depletion in medical and neuropsychiatric disorders: potential repercussions and therapeutic implications. Mol Neurobiol. 2013;48(3):883–903.
66. Forester BP, Harper DG, Georgakas J, Ravichandran C, Madurai N, Cohen BM. Antidepressant effects of open label treatment with coenzyme Q10 in geriatric bipolar depression. J Clin Psychopharmacol. 2015;35(3):338–40.
67. Sarris J St. John's wort for the treatment of psychiatric disorders. Psychiatric Clin N Am. 2013;36(1):65–72.
68. Linde K, Mulrow CD, Berner M, Egger M. St John's wort for depression. Cochrane Database Syst Rev. 2005(2):Cd000448.
69. Muller WE. Current St John's wort research from mode of action to clinical efficacy. Pharmacol Res. 2003;47(2):101–9.
70. Harrer G, Schmidt U, Kuhn U, Biller A. Comparison of equivalence between the St. John's wort extract LoHyp-57 and fluoxetine. Arzneimittelforschung. 1999;49(4):289–96.
71. Solomon D, Adams J, Graves N. Economic evaluation of St. John's wort (Hypericum perforatum) for the treatment of mild to moderate depression. J Affect Disord. 2013;148(2–3):228–34.
72. Kasper S, Gastpar M, Moller HJ, Muller WE, Volz HP, Dienel A, et al. Better tolerability of St. John's wort extract WS 5570 compared to treatment with SSRIs: a reanalysis of data from controlled clinical trials in acute major depression. Int Clin Psychopharmacol. 2010;25(4):204–13.
73. Moses EL, Mallinger AG. St. John's Wort: three cases of possible mania induction. J Clin Psychopharmacol. 2000;20(1):115–7.

74. Fahmi M, Huang C, Schweitzer I. A case of mania induced by hypericum. World J Biol Psychiatry. 2002;3(1):58–9.
75. Madhusoodanan S, Velama U, Parmar J, Goia D, Brenner R. A current review of cytochrome P450 interactions of psychotropic drugs. Ann Clin Psychiatry. 2014;26(2):120–38.
76. Henderson L, Yue QY, Bergquist C, Gerden B, Arlett P. St John's wort (*Hypericum perforatum*): drug interactions and clinical outcomes. Br J Clin Pharmacol. 2002;54(4):349–56.
77. Chiesa A, Serretti A. Mindfulness based cognitive therapy for psychiatric disorders: a systematic review and meta-analysis. Psychiatry Res. 2011;187(3):441–53.
78. Chiesa A, Serretti A. A systematic review of neurobiological and clinical features of mindfulness meditations. Psychol Med. 2010;40(8):1239–52.
79. Chiesa A, Serretti A. Mindfulness-based interventions for chronic pain: a systematic review of the evidence. J Altern Complement Med (New York, NY). 2011;17(1):83–93.
80. Chiesa A, Serretti A. Are mindfulness-based interventions effective for substance use disorders? A systematic review of the evidence. Subst Use Misuse. 2014;49(5):492–512.
81. Kabat-Zinn J. Wherever you go, there you are: mindfulness meditation in everyday life. New York: Hyperion; 2005. xxi, 280 p.
82. Kabat-Zinn J, Massion AO, Kristeller J, Peterson LG, Fletcher KE, Pbert L, et al. Effectiveness of a meditation-based stress reduction program in the treatment of anxiety disorders. Am J Psychiatry. 1992;149(7):936–43.
83. Kabat-Zinn J. An outpatient program in behavioral medicine for chronic pain patients based on the practice of mindfulness meditation: theoretical considerations and preliminary results. Gen Hosp Psychiatry. 1982;4(1):33–47.
84. Ma SH, Teasdale JD. Mindfulness-based cognitive therapy for depression: replication and exploration of differential relapse prevention effects. J Consult Clin Psychol. 2004;72(1):31–40.
85. Teasdale JD, Segal ZV, Williams JM, Ridgeway VA, Soulsby JM, Lau MA. Prevention of relapse/recurrence in major depression by mindfulness-based cognitive therapy. J Consult Clin Psychol. 2000;68(4):615–23.
86. Deckersbach T, Holzel BK, Eisner LR, Stange JP, Peckham AD, Dougherty DD, et al. Mindfulness-based cognitive therapy for nonremitted patients with bipolar disorder. CNS Neurosci Ther. 2012;18(2):133–41.
87. Williams JM, Alatiq Y, Crane C, Barnhofer T, Fennell MJ, Duggan DS, et al. Mindfulness-based Cognitive Therapy (MBCT) in bipolar disorder: preliminary evaluation of immediate effects on between-episode functioning. J Affect Disord. 2008;107(1–3):275–9.
88. Perich T, Manicavasagar V, Mitchell PB, Ball JR, Hadzi-Pavlovic D. A randomized controlled trial of mindfulness-based cognitive therapy for bipolar disorder. Acta Psychiatr Scand. 2013;127(5):333–43.
89. Segal ZV, Williams JMG, Teasdale JD. Mindfulness-based cognitive therapy for depression. 2nd ed. New York: Guilford Press; 2013. xix, 451 p.
90. Kuyken W, Byford S, Taylor RS, Watkins E, Holden E, White K, et al. Mindfulness-based cognitive therapy to prevent relapse in recurrent depression. J Consult Clin Psychol. 2008;76(6):966–78.
91. Eisendrath SJ, Gillung E, Delucchi K, Mathalon DH, Yang TT, Satre DD, et al. A preliminary study: efficacy of mindfulness-based cognitive therapy versus sertraline as first-line treatments for major depressive disorder. Mindfulness. 2015;6(3):475–82.
92. Stange JP, Eisner LR, Holzel BK, Peckham AD, Dougherty DD, Rauch SL, et al. Mindfulness-based cognitive therapy for bipolar disorder: effects on cognitive functioning. J Psychiatr Pract. 2011;17(6):410–9.

93. Lahera G, Bayon C, Fe Bravo-Ortiz M, Rodriguez-Vega B, Barbeito S, Saenz M, et al. Mindfulness-based cognitive therapy versus psychoeducational intervention in bipolar outpatients with sub-threshold depressive symptoms: a randomized controlled trial. BMC Psychiatry. 2014;14:215.
94. Townsend J, Bookheimer SY, Foland-Ross LC, Sugar CA, Altshuler LL. fMRI abnormalities in dorsolateral prefrontal cortex during a working memory task in manic, euthymic and depressed bipolar subjects. Psychiatry Res. 2010;182(1):22–9.
95. Burdick KE, Russo M, Frangou S, Mahon K, Braga RJ, Shanahan M, et al. Empirical evidence for discrete neurocognitive subgroups in bipolar disorder: clinical implications. Psychol Med. 2014;44(14):3083–96.
96. Malhi GS, Ivanovski B, Hadzi-Pavlovic D, Mitchell PB, Vieta E, Sachdev P. Neuropsychological deficits and functional impairment in bipolar depression, hypomania and euthymia. Bipolar Disord. 2007;9(1–2):114–25.
97. Robinson LJ, Ferrier IN. Evolution of cognitive impairment in bipolar disorder: a systematic review of cross-sectional evidence. Bipolar Disord. 2006;8(2):103–16.
98. Howells FM, Ives-Deliperi VL, Horn NR, Stein DJ. Mindfulness based cognitive therapy improves frontal control in bipolar disorder: a pilot EEG study. BMC Psychiatry. 2012;12:15.
99. Ives-Deliperi VL, Howells F, Stein DJ, Meintjes EM, Horn N. The effects of mindfulness-based cognitive therapy in patients with bipolar disorder: a controlled functional MRI investigation. J Affect Disord. 2013;150(3):1152–7.
100. Howells FM, Laurie Rauch HG, Ives-Deliperi VL, Horn NR, Stein DJ. Mindfulness based cognitive therapy may improve emotional processing in bipolar disorder: pilot ERP and HRV study. Metab Brain Dis. 2014;29(2):367–75.
101. Lopresti AL, Jacka FN. Diet and bipolar disorder: a review of its relationship and potential therapeutic mechanisms of action. J Altern Complement Med. 2015;21(12):733–9.
102. Thomson D, Turner A, Lauder S, Gigler ME, Berk L, Singh AB, et al. A brief review of exercise, bipolar disorder, and mechanistic pathways. Front Psychol. 2015;6:147.
103. Sylvia LG, Ametrano RM, Nierenberg AA. Exercise treatment for bipolar disorder: potential mechanisms of action mediated through increased neurogenesis and decreased allostatic load. Psychother Psychosom. 2010;79(2):87–96.
104. Fernandes BS, Berk M, Turck CW, Steiner J, Goncalves CA. Decreased peripheral brain-derived neurotrophic factor levels are a biomarker of disease activity in major psychiatric disorders: a comparative meta-analysis. Mol Psychiatry. 2014;19(7):750–1.
105. Fernandes BS, Gama CS, Cereser KM, Yatham LN, Fries GR, Colpo G, et al. Brain-derived neurotrophic factor as a state-marker of mood episodes in bipolar disorders: a systematic review and meta-regression analysis. J Psychiatr Res. 2011;45(8):995–1004.
106. de Sa Filho AS, de Souza Moura AM, Lamego MK, Rocha NB, Paes F, Oliveira AC, et al. Potential therapeutic effects of physical exercise for Bipolar Disorder. CNS Neurol Disord: Drug Targets. 2015;14(10):1255–9.
107. Goldstein BI, Kemp DE, Soczynska JK, McIntyre RS. Inflammation and the phenomenology, pathophysiology, comorbidity, and treatment of bipolar disorder: a systematic review of the literature. J Clin Psychiatry. 2009;70(8):1078–90.
108. Hamer M, Steptoe A. Association between physical fitness, parasympathetic control, and proinflammatory responses to mental stress. Psychosom Med. 2007;69(7):660–6.
109. Melo MC, Daher Ede F, Albuquerque SG, de Bruin VM. Exercise in bipolar patients: a systematic review. J Affect Disord. 2016;198:32–8.
110. Ng F, Dodd S, Berk M. The effects of physical activity in the acute treatment of bipolar disorder: a pilot study. J Affect Disord. 2007;101(1–3):259–62.
111. Knubben K, Reischies FM, Adli M, Schlattmann P, Bauer M, Dimeo F. A randomised, controlled study on the effects of a short-term endurance training programme in patients with major depression. Br J Sports Med. 2007;41(1):29–33.

112. Sylvia LG, Salcedo S, Bernstein EE, Baek JH, Nierenberg AA, Deckersbach T. Nutrition, exercise, and wellness treatment in bipolar disorder: proof of concept for a consolidated intervention. Int J Bipolar Disorders. 2013;1(1):24.
113. Van Citters AD, Pratt SI, Jue K, Williams G, Miller PT, Xie H, et al. A pilot evaluation of the In SHAPE individualized health promotion intervention for adults with mental illness. Commun Ment Health J. 2010;46(6):540–52.
114. Wright K, Armstrong T, Taylor A, Dean S. 'It's a double edged sword': a qualitative analysis of the experiences of exercise amongst people with Bipolar Disorder. J Affect Disord. 2012;136(3):634–42.
115. Crump C, Sundquist K, Winkleby MA, Sundquist J. Comorbidities and mortality in bipolar disorder: a Swedish national cohort study. JAMA Psychiatry. 2013;70(9):931–9.
116. Morriss R, Mohammed FA. Metabolism, lifestyle and bipolar affective disorder. J Psychopharmacol (Oxford, England). 2005;19(6 Suppl):94–101.
117. da Silva TL, Ravindran LN, Ravindran AV. Yoga in the treatment of mood and anxiety disorders: a review. Asian J Psychiatr. 2009;2(1):6–16.
118. Streeter CC, Gerbarg PL, Saper RB, Ciraulo DA, Brown RP. Effects of yoga on the autonomic nervous system, gamma-aminobutyric-acid, and allostasis in epilepsy, depression, and post-traumatic stress disorder. Med Hypotheses. 2012;78(5):571–9.
119. Brown RP, Gerbarg PL. Sudarshan Kriya Yogic breathing in the treatment of stress, anxiety, and depression. Part II–clinical applications and guidelines. J Altern Complement Med (New York, NY). 2005;11(4):711–7.
120. Uebelacker LA, Weinstock LM, Kraines MA. Self-reported benefits and risks of yoga in individuals with bipolar disorder. J Psychiatr Pract. 2014;20(5):345–52.
121. Abreu T, Braganca M. The bipolarity of light and dark: a review on bipolar disorder and circadian cycles. J Affect Disord. 2015;185:219–29.
122. Salvatore P, Ghidini S, Zita G, De Panfilis C, Lambertino S, Maggini C, et al. Circadian activity rhythm abnormalities in ill and recovered bipolar I disorder patients. Bipolar Disord. 2008;10(2):256–65.
123. Benedetti F, Colombo C, Pontiggia A, Bernasconi A, Florita M, Smeraldi E. Morning light treatment hastens the antidepressant effect of citalopram: a placebo-controlled trial. J Clin Psychiatry. 2003;64(6):648–53.
124. Lewy AJ, Wehr TA, Goodwin FK, Newsome DA, Markey SP. Light suppresses melatonin secretion in humans. Science (New York, NY). 1980;210(4475):1267–9.
125. Wu JC, Kelsoe JR, Schachat C, Bunney BG, DeModena A, Golshan S, et al. Rapid and sustained antidepressant response with sleep deprivation and chronotherapy in bipolar disorder. Biol Psychiatry. 2009;66(3):298–301.
126. Tseng PT, Chen YW, Tu KY, Chung W, Wang HY, Wu CK, et al. Light therapy in the treatment of patients with bipolar depression: a meta-analytic study. Eur Neuropsychopharmacol: J Eur College Neuropsychopharmacol. 2016;26(6):1037–47.
127. Sit D, Wisner KL, Hanusa BH, Stull S, Terman M. Light therapy for bipolar disorder: a case series in women. Bipolar Disord. 2007;9(8):918–27.

Treatment Settings for Older Age Bipolar Disorder: Inpatient, Partial Hospitalization, Outpatient, Models of Integrated Care

11

Colin Depp and Rachel C. Edelman

11.1 Introduction

Bipolar disorder is among the more challenging illnesses to treat across the life span, and research on the optimal service architecture for older adults with this illness is lacking. Nonetheless, innovations in reach and impact of mental health services will be critical in order to reduce the morbidity and excess mortality in bipolar disorder. As described elsewhere in this volume, the number of older adults with bipolar disorder is increasing at a rapid pace due to population aging and so virtually all mental health providers need to be prepared to provide services for older adults. In this chapter, we first briefly review the broader challenges in geriatric mental health care that have bearing on service access in older age bipolar disorder. We next review available data on service use in older age bipolar disorder across the care continuum, examine patient-level factors that pose challenges to access to care, and review findings on the population characteristics that differ across service settings. Finally, we discuss emerging service models, such as integrated and collaborative care, new technology, and practice-based networks in enhancing quality of care in older age bipolar disorder.

C. Depp (✉) · R.C. Edelman
Department of Psychiatry, University of California at San Diego,
9500 Gilman Drive, MC 0664, La Jolla, CA 92024, USA
e-mail: cdepp@ucsd.edu

R.C. Edelman
e-mail: rachelcedelman@gmail.com

R.C. Edelman
Los Angeles, CA 90403, USA

S.W. Lehmann and B.P. Forester (eds.), *Bipolar Disorder in Older Age Patients*,
DOI 10.1007/978-3-319-48912-4_11

11.2 Challenges Impacting Access to Mental Health Services in Older Age Bipolar Disorder

The threats to geriatric mental health services have been described for decades [1, 2]. Key concerns include a limited evidence base for effective treatment algorithms, an insufficient number of geriatrics-trained providers, caregiver burnout, care fragmentation, and suboptimal care of medical problems. These concerns are not specific to older age bipolar disorder. Yet, due to the typical complexity of bipolar disorder (e.g., high risk of comorbidities and high rates of service use in inpatient and other service sectors), older adults with this illness are especially vulnerable to shortcomings of the current geriatric mental healthcare system. A variety of approaches have begun to be undertaken to remedy these issues, but current practitioners working with older adults with bipolar disorder should be aware of the broader challenges in geriatric mental health services that are so often exemplified in older age bipolar disorder.

11.2.1 Impact of Paucity of Research on Treatment and Services

To date, there is very little in the way of empirical data on pharmacologic, non-pharmacologic, or service models specifically designed and adapted for older age bipolar disorder [3]. This is in contrast to late-life depression and to late-life schizophrenia, for which several randomized clinical trials of medications or psychotherapies have been conducted. This dearth of research leads to the necessity for clinicians to extrapolate evidence from younger people with bipolar disorder or from studies of older adults with other diagnoses, leading to what has been dubbed the practice of "evidence-free" medicine [4]. As Bartels and coworkers note, NIH-funded research applications require that investigators provide scientific justification for excluding children from research, which may increase the number of studies that incorporate children. However, no such justification is required for excluding older adults [2]. Similarly, services research in older age bipolar disorder has largely been descriptive and retrospective and only a handful of studies have employed prospective approaches such as clinical trials to systematically address which service models best accommodate the unique features of older age bipolar disorder.

11.2.2 Workforce Demand and Supply

In the USA, the number of geriatric psychiatrists and geriatric mental health specialized allied health professionals has remained largely static, while the number of older adults is expected to double between the years 2000 and 2030 [5]. There were approximately 1.5 geriatric psychiatrists per 10,000 people over the age of 75 in the year 2000, and projections for the year 2050 indicate that there will be only 0.3

geriatric psychiatrists per 10,000 older adults [6]. During the 2011–2012 academic year, there were only 58 geriatric psychiatry fellows in the country [7]. Despite geriatricians' higher job satisfaction than many other specialties, roughly 40 % of geriatric medicine fellowship slots are not filled. This dearth of providers is similar for allied health professions, with reports from psychology, nursing, and social work fields indicating severe gaps in developing the workforce for older adults with mental health problems. For example, only 4 % of psychologists specialize in geropsychology [8]. To date, remedies for addressing this shortage, including financial incentives for geriatricians, have not resulted in increases in participation in geriatrics specialty training over time. As a result, an alternative approach may be to promote the use of geriatric specialty providers to educate and support geriatric mental health services delivered by general adult practitioners. Even so, general adult mental health practitioners may not meet the needs of older adults with bipolar disorder. In 2010, only 54 % of outpatient psychiatrists accepted Medicare, which is generally attributed to the disadvantaged rate of reimbursement [9]. As such, limited availability of mental health care for older adults with bipolar disorder is evident in both general adult and specialty-trained geriatrics providers.

11.2.3 Diminished Access to and Quality of Care for Medical Comorbidities

Medical comorbidity accounts for a large proportion of the staggeringly high rate of years of life lost to bipolar disorder [10]. At least some of the excess morbidity from medical problems is due to diminished access to care, suboptimal quality of medical care, and primary care–mental healthcare fragmentation. People with bipolar disorder are less likely to receive care for diabetes or cardiovascular disease than are people without mental illnesses [11]. In the broader population of adults with serious mental illnesses, the prevalence of untreated chronic illnesses is staggering, estimated at 30 % for diabetes, 62 % for hypertension, and 88 % for hyperlipidemia [12]. In addition to undertreatment, individuals with serious mental illnesses also appear to experience worse outcomes following hospitalization for medical problems. In the Veterans Health System, patients with serious mental illnesses are less likely to receive preventative care [13].

Many factors likely contribute to higher rates of medical comorbidities in adults with serious mental illnesses. Patient-level factors include diminished care-seeking for chronic medical problems and lower rates of adherence to prescribed regimens or healthy lifestyles. Pragmatic patient-level barriers include poor access to transportation and poverty, which reduces access to some forms of care. Provider-level barriers include therapeutic nihilism (assumptions of limited potential to benefit from medical care given the patient-level barriers described above) and the often-limited participation of psychiatric providers in monitoring and treating medical comorbidities. System-level factors include fragmentation of medical and behavioral health services. Indeed, Bartels and colleagues demonstrated that one of the strongest predictors of engagement in mental *and* physical health services in a mixed-diagnosis sample of chronically mentally ill older adults was the physical distance between clinic settings. When medical and mental health clinics were located far apart from each other, the rate of successful referral to mental health services was lower [14].

11.2.4 Caregiver Burden

In addition to the burden on the health system, bipolar disorder is associated with substantial participation of informal caregivers in the day-to-day management of the illness. Tasks of caregiving in bipolar disorder are diverse and include assistance with managing medications and finances. In addition, caregivers must take an active role in care when the person with bipolar disorder is incapacitated by the illness. A small but compelling number of reports indicate that bipolar disorder is associated with substantial caregiver distress and experienced burden. The level of caregiver burden in bipolar disorder appears to be equivalent to that of caregivers of people with schizophrenia [15]. Indeed, caregivers themselves frequently require mental health services (29 % were current users of mental health services in one study) [16], and there is a strong association between caregiver burden and increased caregiver mental health service use among caregivers of people with bipolar disorder.

11.3 Mental Health Service Usage Patterns in Older Age Bipolar Disorder

11.3.1 Rates of Bipolar Disorder by Treatment Setting

Despite a prevalence of <1 % in community-based epidemiologic surveys of older adults, older age bipolar disorder is not an uncommon diagnosis in outpatient, inpatient, and residential treatment settings. Much of what is known about the prevalence of bipolar disorder in treatment settings is from chart reviews of selected sites and so exact estimates of proportions are not available. As reviewed previously, bipolar disorder accounts for approximately 8–10 % of inpatient geropsychiatry admissions, 6 % of outpatient geriatric psychiatry cases, and 14–17 % of older adults seen in psychiatric emergency settings [17]. In a handful of studies, about 3 % of patients in skilled nursing facilities have a diagnosis of bipolar disorder. It is clear that although bipolar disorder is relatively rare among community-dwelling older adults, it is commonly seen in treatment settings where psychiatric care is administered to older adults. At the same time, it is important to note that a sizable proportion of older adults with bipolar do not use any mental health services. Byers and coworkers evaluated the National Comorbidity Survey and found that 41 % of patients with bipolar disorder older than the age of 55 surveyed were not using any mental health services in the prior year [18].

11.3.2 Comparison with Other Diagnoses

Older adults with bipolar disorder, just as their younger counterparts, seem to consume more mental health services than patients with major depression. Bartels and coworkers compared service use patterns of older patients with bipolar disorder to those of older patients with major depression and found that the group with bipolar disorder used approximately four times the amount of mental health services than the group with major depression [19]. In particular, higher rates of mental health service utilization were observed for inpatient, partial hospitalization, and case management services, although the use of outpatient psychotherapy was comparatively lower for older adults with bipolar disorder. In comparison with older people with schizophrenia, the rate of hospitalization for older adults with bipolar disorder was slightly lower although the mean length of stay was longer.

11.3.3 Comparison with Younger Adults with Bipolar Disorder

Older adults with bipolar disorder have been reported to use a different array of mental health services compared to younger or middle-aged patients. Using administrative data from a sample of 40,000 patients who were clients of a large public mental health system, it seems that older adults (people over age 60) with bipolar disorder used substantially fewer crisis residential and emergency psychiatry services than did their younger counterparts [20]. However, older adults with bipolar disorder used more case management services. These data are consistent with the few studies of the long-term course of bipolar disorder, which suggest the severity of manic symptoms may decline with age [21], yet at the same time, cognitive and functional impairment becomes less distinguishable from that in schizophrenia, increasing the need for functional assistance such as case management [22].

11.4 Care Delivery in Common Treatment Settings

11.4.1 Inpatient Psychiatric Hospitalization

Inpatient hospitalization is a relatively frequent occurrence among older adults with bipolar disorder. In the current era of increased attention to rising healthcare costs, there has been substantial attention regarding the fiscal impact of inpatient psychiatric hospitalization. As of 2006, the average length of stay for adults with bipolar disorder was 9.4 days [23]. Examining inpatient treatment in community hospitals, the rate of hospitalization among older adults with bipolar disorder compared to younger adults with bipolar disorder was somewhat lower and the mean cost of hospitalization was approximately $8000 [23]. In a sample of 65,556 veterans with for bipolar disorder seen in the Veterans Health Administration setting, patients with bipolar disorder who were older than age 60 experienced psychiatric hospitalization approximately 6 times over a three-year period, which was equivalent to that of the middle-aged patients and slightly more than that of adults younger than age 30 [24]. However, adults over the age of 60 had average lengths of stay that were three times longer than that of younger adults, with the mean of 98 hospital days per patient compared to 30 days for younger adults. About 60 % of the inpatient hospitalizations in this sample were for mania and 40 % were for depression.

In attempting to contain costs associated with the "revolving door" of rehospitalization, attention has been paid to population factors that predict greater risk for hospitalization. In two separate retrospective chart review studies analyzing both diagnostic and non-diagnostic variation factors and risk of rehospitalization in separate geriatric inpatient psychiatric settings, bipolar disorder emerged as a strong predictor of risk of repeated hospitalization [25, 26]. Other factors that emerged in these studies in conjunction with bipolar disorder that predicted rehospitalization included male gender, living alone, and residing in supported housing. Within the population of older patients with bipolar disorder hospitalized for mania, Lehmann and Rabins [27] compared prehospitalization profiles of older adults with bipolar disorder in early-onset (onset <45 years) to late-onset (onset >45 years) subgroups and found that early-onset patients were (1) more likely to have had a recent dose change by a provider; (2) more likely to have been non-adherent to medications; and (3) more likely to have been exhibiting aggressive/agitated behavior. Other factors, such as the rate of comorbidities, and demographic variables were similar between early- and late-onset groups. Taken together, studies of the rate of inpatient hospitalization for bipolar disorder in later life are somewhat inconsistent as to whether risk of psychiatric hospitalization increases or decreases with age in older adults with bipolar disorder. There does appear to more consistent indication that older adults experience longer stays than their younger counterparts. Available data described above indicate that in geriatric inpatient psychiatry settings, bipolar disorder is a risk factor for rehospitalization compared to other diagnoses.

11.4.2 Skilled Nursing Facilities

As mentioned earlier, bipolar disorder is diagnosed in 2–3 % of patients in skilled nursing facilities. In a study conducted by the Department of Veterans Affairs, patients with bipolar disorder were approximately 28 % more likely to be admitted to skilled nursing facilities (SNFs) than people without mental illnesses [28]. Not surprisingly, patients with bipolar disorder in such facilities, compared to individuals with OABD in community settings, are more likely to have impairment in instrumental activities of daily living, greater cognitive impairment, fewer social supports, and more severe psychotic symptoms [29]. Within the population of residents of such facilities, people with serious mental illnesses are also more likely than individuals without serious mental illnesses to reside in skilled nursing facilities for greater than 90 days [30]. People with serious mental illnesses residing in skilled nursing faculties are also comparatively younger than residents without serious mental illnesses. Finally, patients with serious mental illnesses in SNFs are also more likely to be hospitalized than patients without serious mental illnesses, with high rates of hospitalizations for ambulatory care-sensitive conditions (i.e., ones that are seen as being likely to be treatable as an outpatient) [31].

The Olmstead Act (1999) required that "qualified" individuals with serious mental illnesses be placed in community settings rather than skilled nursing facilities whenever possible. Of note, while the general preference for consumers and for clinicians is for community placement, a study of older adults in New Hampshire residing in skilling nursing settings by Bartels et al. [32] revealed that there was a high degree of discordance between patients' preferred level of appropriateness for community placement and clinician-assigned level of appropriateness. In this study, the majority of clinicians believed that ideal transition settings were in community group homes, whereas patient consumers almost uniformly preferred apartment/independent living.

11.4.3 Partial Hospitalization

Partial hospitalization, according to Medicare's definition, is "a structured program of outpatient psychiatric services provided to patients as an alternative to inpatient psychiatric care." The term "partial hospitalization" is used interchangeably with day treatment. These services can be delivered in a community mental health or hospital setting and do not involve overnight stays. Medicare Part B provides coverage for partial hospitalization. Little is known about the prevalence of use or impact of partial hospitalization in bipolar disorder, although at least in one study older patients with bipolar disorder were more likely to use this service than were older patients with major depression [29]. Partial hospitalization programs vary in terms of structure and content, but typically sessions are held 2–4 times per week for 4–6 h per day, combining group and individual therapy as well as pharmacotherapy. Therapeutic targets include both symptom management and functional rehabilitation, with the involvement of multidisciplinary team care. One focus for partial hospitalization is for transitional care as a "step-down" from inpatient care. In light of recent attention to rapid rehospitalization in a variety of chronic medical illnesses, the case for partial hospitalization programs may build.

11.4.4 Outpatient Care

The National Comorbidity Survey [33] found that older adults with mental health diagnoses are less likely to participate in outpatient treatment than younger cohorts. The reasons for this lower rate of participation are unknown but generally attributed to patient-driven factors such as lower acceptance of mental health care among older adults and attendant stigmatization along with provider/system-driven factors such as diminished screening and recognition resulting in reduced referral to such services. As previously stated, 41 % of patients with OABD are not receiving mental health care, although this is a lower rate of non-participation than in older adults with other mood or anxiety diagnoses [18].

Additional national trends are for mental health services to be delivered by primary care providers rather than specialty mental health providers, although these trends are less prominent for bipolar disorder than other mood or anxiety disorders [34]. A recent study reported that older adults use a comparatively lower rate of psychotherapy than younger people, and only 25 % of older adults with mental health diagnoses use psychotherapy [35]. Older adults frequently report a preference to discuss mental health problems with family practitioners rather than specialty mental health providers [36]. In addition, a number of studies have reported that older adults with depressive symptoms prefer psychotherapy to antidepressant medication [37, 38], yet depression is typically managed in the family practice setting with medication treatment and not psychotherapy. As such, there is a disconnect between the site of preferred treatment and the preference for treatment modality in geriatric depression. The treatment preferences of older patients with bipolar disorder have received scant research attention. At least one study indicated that group psychotherapy was feasible and acceptable in a small sample of older patients with bipolar disorder [39].

11.5 Emerging Models of Mental Health Services

There are several emerging models of mental healthcare older adults that appear to be effective in addressing some of the many gaps in care outlined above. Broadly these interventions are aimed at improving access, cost, quality, coordination, and/or timeliness of care. We next describe these programs below and report data from older people with bipolar disorder where possible.

11.5.1 Collaborative Care

Recent research supports a collaborative model of chronic care for bipolar disorder, though there is a dearth of research investigating this model of care for older adults. One such model was implemented for three years across 11 Veteran Affairs Medical Centers resulting in positive outcomes including reductions in affective episode length and functional and quality-of-life improvements while remaining cost-neutral [40, 41]. The collaborative care intervention, termed the Bipolar Disorders Program, consisted of a specialty team of a nurse care coordinator and a psychiatrist, in an outpatient clinic. Care was provided during regularly scheduled appointments and phone contact as needed. The three key elements of the care included (1) psychoeducation to teach self-management skills; (2) a standardized, single algorithm and manual of practice guidelines in order to enhance evidence-based pharmacotherapy; and (3) a nurse care coordinator to ensure continuity of care, optimal access to care resources, and information flow between care providers and patients. Nurse care coordinators provided three types of contact including regularly scheduled appointments for patient monitoring, "demand-response services" for issues requiring same-day or next-business-day attention (i.e., alleviating side effects, addressing non-response to medication changes, and crisis management), and "outreach and inreach" for missed appointments and communication with other providers.

In a clinical trial [40, 41], the collaborative care and usual care conditions were relatively similar in terms of demographics and clinical characteristics, though patients in the intervention condition were slightly older, less likely to have prior suicide attempts, and more likely to have a lifetime substance-use disorder diagnosis. The average age of patients in this sample was 46 years. For the first six-month assessment, treatment satisfaction was higher for patients in the collaborative care group. In addition, the group of patients that received collaborative care saw a significant reduction in the number of weeks of manic episodes (although this was not seen for depressive episodes). By percentages, the intervention group reduced weeks spend in a manic episode by 23 %. Social function, including work, parental, and extended-family roles, as well as quality of mental life improved significantly for those who received collaborative care. Significant improvements in functioning and reduction in weeks in affective episodes began to emerge in the second year of intervention implementation, potentially suggesting a latency in time for the skills being taught to be learned, utilized, and effective. In terms of treatment costs, the intervention was less expensive than usual care, and while there was an insignificant increase in outpatient costs for the intervention, psychiatric and medical–surgical inpatients' costs were significantly reduced, which offset the outpatient increase. Overall, implementing collaborative care for bipolar disorder was essentially cost-neutral while boasting significant gains in several areas.

11.5.2 Primary Care Mental Healthcare Integration

Research shows that integrating mental health into primary care settings can improve screening and detection of mental illness [42]. The Veterans Health Administration (VHA) in 2010 implemented Patient-Aligned Care Team (PACT), a "proactive, personalized, team-based care oriented toward wellness and disease prevention" (www.va.gov). Essentially, PACT is a team of healthcare professionals that provide comprehensive primary care with mental health screenings and an emphasis on collaboration with mental health professionals for veterans who screen positive for mental health issues. The VA has thus far produced evaluation data that integrating primary care and mental health may be associated with lowering the risks of the poor outcomes associated with mental illness [42]. In a review of the 4,461,208 veterans who were seen in the first year of the PACT rollout nationwide, it was found that 1.15 million veterans were diagnosed with at least 1 mental illness, with depression being the most prevalent (13.5 %), followed by post-traumatic stress disorder (9.3 %), substance-use disorder (8.3 %), anxiety disorder (4.8), and serious mental illnesses including bipolar disorder (3.7 %). These rates are significantly higher when compared to the general population. All veterans with mental illness who were seen by primary care mental health integration (PCMHI) clinicians in that year lowered their risk of an emergency department visit compared to veterans not seen within the integrated care model. In addition, patients with depression, anxiety, serious mental illness, and substance-use disorder had lower risks of hospitalization and death compared to patients who were not seen in PCMHI. Because bipolar disorder was not among the top 5 most prevalent mental illnesses, data on the effectiveness of a PACT model of care for this disorder are limited. However, given the increased likelihood of hospitalization for patients with bipolar disorder, it is reasonable to assume that this model of care could be effective in lowering rates of hospitalization as well as lowering other poor mental health outcomes. In the Clinical Vignette below, primary care integrated behavioral health care is exemplified.

Clinical Vignette 11.1

Mr. L is a 66-year-old Caucasian male veteran who presented to the Veterans hospital for outpatient mental health treatment complaining of "fits of depression" and "hour long crying spells" that are difficult to control and are associated with thoughts of "putting a gun in my mouth and blowing my brains out." He adamantly denies having a specific plan or intent, citing his grandchildren in a neighboring state as his motivation to continue "living through the pain."

Mr. L described his 20s and 30s as the most exciting decades of life. He self-identified as "the life of the party," organized several spur of the moment extravagant trips with friends, went on spending sprees that accrued thousands of dollars of debt that he almost always narrowly managed to pay off with a high-paying, and exhilarating, job as an investment banker. He accrued some legal difficulties, mostly for speeding, but never faced serious consequences. At intake, he pined for the past and the discrete set of days that he had "miraculous levels of energy" that enabled him to start important projects around that house, though admitted that many of the projects would remain incomplete after he crashed from several days of little sleep. Currently, he reports that he will occasionally "get fired up" for 3 or 4 days and start art projects, read books, organize his house, and reach out to friends to provide financial help. During these times, people comment that his "sense of humor has returned" and he feels "happy and funny."

Mr. L has experienced a significant role transition and loss over the past two years. First, he retired from his job as a CFO from a bank. Initially, he was excited for the opportunity to travel with his wife and spend time with his grandchild. Three months after his retirement, his wife passed away from a sudden heart attack. Since then, he has found it difficult to motivate himself to do anything except sit on his porch all day and wait for his neighbor to come home around 5 o'clock so that they can drink scotch. In addition to crying spells and suicidal ideation, Mr. L is struggling with decreased motivation, difficulty concentrating, feelings of worthlessness and guilt, difficulty falling asleep and difficulty waking up in the morning.

While Mr. L was working, he used private health insurance. He chose providers in the community with separate offices around the city. His cardiologist, who he saw for atrial fibrillation, was located downtown, while his primary care physician, who prescribed medication for diabetes and opioids for chronic low back pain, was located uptown. After he retired, Mr. L decided to switch his medical care to the VA in order to "save money." It was during the veteran's initial primary care appointment that he was screened for depression and given a "warm handoff" to a patient-aligned care team psychologist, who diagnosed the patient with Bipolar II Disorder and set in motion his mental health treatment planning which included referral to specialty mental health care group psychotherapy with an emphasis on grief and loss. Through this program, the patient will have access to a variety of mental health treatment options, including psychiatry, individual and group therapy, access to a nurse care coordinator who can answer questions about medication over the phone and schedule follow-ups. All of his treatment, including specialty medical services, will be housed within the same facility and his team-based providers will be able to communicate on a regular basis to coordinate his ongoing care through a shared electronic record.

Mr. L's case exemplifies the potential for integrated care in which mental health services for OABD are first delivered in the primary care setting and a menu of treatment options are provided by a coordinated treatment team that communicates with one another via a shared electronic record.

Learning Points

- Many people with bipolar disorder take years to obtain the diagnosis, and a substantial proportion do not experience as pronounced behavioral disturbances in older age associated with mania when compared to their younger years.
- As many older adults access mental health care in the primary care setting, onsite mental health professional can aid in identifying patients who require speciality mental health services.
- Medical comorbidity, social isolation, and role transitions make for complex clinical management of older adults with bipolar disorder, frequently necessitating team-based services.

11.5.3 Technology-Facilitated Care

In light of the barriers to accessing services among older patients with bipolar disorder, as well as the complexities involved in managing multiple chronic medical and psychiatric conditions and their treatments, health technology may play an important role in managing older age bipolar disorder. The ongoing influx of information technology into medical services (e.g., electronic medical records and health registries) may have a broad impact on generating data to examine some of the fundamental knowledge gaps in OABD [43]. Additionally, interventions that directly leverage technology may support management of OABD outside of the clinic setting. Due to the fluctuating course of the illness and adherence to its treatment, bipolar disorder has often been the focus of mobile and home-based technologies that collect frequent data on behaviors and symptoms. Mobile devices such as smartphones have been used to assess mood symptoms on a frequent basis in bipolar disorder, similar to paper-and-pencil mood charting, and the data that emerge from mobile health devices appear to correspond better to clinician mood ratings than do paper-and-pencil ratings [44]. By leveraging real-time data on symptoms collected by mobile devices, it is possible to deliver interventions that respond to the symptoms [45]. For example, ratings of emergent suicidality may be linked with crisis services. Mobile or home-based technology could serve to extend the impact of brief psychosocial treatments, such as by prompting engagement in home practice, or by reducing the number of in-person sessions needed to mitigate against transportation barriers. Indeed, teletherapy models are particularly attractive for subgroups of older adults who have limited local access to mental health care. A recent randomized trial indicated that older adults with generalized anxiety found cognitive behavioral teletherapy acceptable and the outcomes for teletherapy were as good if not better than that in prior in-person treatments [46]. Of note, translating such interventions to the community is hampered by the low rate of insurance coverage for psychotherapy via medical supplemental insurance when it is not delivered in the clinic setting.

To date, research on such technology has been not directed at older people with bipolar disorder specifically, but home-based telehealth is a frequently used in the Veterans Health setting, in which a dedicated device is installed in the home and interactive algorithms elicit patient-reported data on medication adherence, vital signs, and symptoms [47, 48]. Data from these interactions are monitored remotely by care managers who then triage patient outreach based on thresholds or trends observed in patient reports. Reports from evaluations of public mental health users with mixed serious mental illness, including bipolar disorder, indicate that usage of such devices is associated with reduced rates of psychiatric hospitalization. It is doubtless that increasingly sophisticated home-based technologies, such as sensors or interactive devices, will become a more commonplace component of general outpatient care, transitional care from inpatient to outpatient settings, and integrated care models such as described above in older age bipolar disorder.

11.5.4 Home-Based Care

For older adults, being unable to leave the home unassisted or being homebound creates a significant barrier to accessing health services out in the community and, more specifically, detecting and treating mental health issues. Home-based models of care were created to address this issue and have been successfully implemented in communities around the USA. In 2007, the Veterans Health Administration initiated a mental health component to the existing Home-Based Primary Care (HBPC) program with the goal of promoting accessible and quality mental health services for homebound veterans who are at-risk or who have mental illness [49]. Given that 5 of the top 10 diagnoses among the HBPC population are mental illnesses (depression, anxiety, post-traumatic stress disorder, substance-use disorder, and schizophrenia), integrating a mental health provider on HBPC teams was a logical next step in providing comprehensive, interdisciplinary, and longitudinal care for veterans with chronic health needs. Essentially, Mental Health Home-Based Primary Care represents a model of care that integrates home-based mental health services into interdisciplinary primary care teams. Common features of home-based mental healthcare models reviewed by Reifler et al. [50] include serving adults age 60 and older, providing counseling and medication management delivered by bachelor-level case managers to psychiatrists, and treating either the full range of psychiatric disorders or limiting services to individuals with depression and anxiety. Overall, there is a paucity of research investigating the utility of such home-based programs for older adults with bipolar disorder, yet an evaluation of such models of care can be useful in developing care specific for older adults with bipolar disorder.

11.5.5 Practice-Based Networks and Registries

As discussed elsewhere in this volume, very few clinical trials have been conducted that specifically recruit and attempt to address questions about the treatment for older adults with bipolar disorder. Older adults with bipolar disorder are frequently not included in treatment trials of pharmacologic and non-pharmacologic interventions. In the absence of such evidence from prospective studies, comparative effectiveness approaches can be used to understand the impact of differing treatment strategies. Increasingly, administrative data culled from patient registries are used to address the benefits and risks of treatment strategies and could be used to fill gaps in understanding service models in late-life bipolar disorder. Practice-based research networks, which link data from diverse outpatient settings, could also be used to understand outpatient management of bipolar disorder. US Federal Agencies such as the Agency for Healthcare Research and Quality (AHRQ) have traditionally provided support for aiding in the infrastructure need to form such practice-based research collaborations. Outside of the USA, such networks are increasingly integrated with standardized outcome measurement to generate data for program planning, population characterization, and comparative effectiveness research [51].

11.6 Summary and Conclusions

Bipolar disorder is a common and challenging illness to treat at any age, and evidence suggests that older adults with this illness utilize a remarkably high rate of high-cost services. In addition to the use of high-cost services, bipolar disorder in older adults seems to predict greater risk for negative healthcare service outcomes that are currently targets of healthcare reform, such as hospitalization for ambulatory care-sensitive conditions or rapid rehospitalization. Although much needs to be known about how best to tailor mental health and medical services for older adults with bipolar disorder, there is hope that innovations in integrated medical and psychiatric treatment that uses technology to inform, monitor and deliver aspects of care could diminish morbidity and mortality in this population. Study of service utilization patterns of older people with bipolar disorder helps to shed light on the many gaps in geriatric mental health care and also how more emerging models of care might reduce the morbidity and mortality experienced by people with chronic complex conditions entering later life.

Clinical Pearls

- Despite low prevalence in community epidemiologic surveys of older adults, bipolar disorder is a common diagnosis in inpatient psychiatric, outpatient mental health, and skill nursing faculty settings.
- Challenges facing access to mental health services in late-life bipolar disorder include an insufficient workforce, caregiver burden, and poor integration between medical and mental health service sectors.
- Older adults with bipolar seem to have a longer length of stay in inpatient psychiatric settings are at significant risk for rehospitalization.
- Many older adults with bipolar disorder are not participating in any mental health service, and few are receiving non-pharmacologic treatments.
- Novel models for care include home-based care, collaborative care, primary care mental health integration, and technology-enabled care which appear to enhance outcomes in large population studies in geriatric mental health.

References

1. Kane R, Solomon D, Beck J, Keeler E, Kane R. The future need for geriatric manpower in the United States. N Engl J Med. 1980;302(24):1327–32.
2. Bartels SJ, Naslund JA. The underside of the silver tsunami—older adults and mental health care. N Engl J Med. 2013;368(6):493–6.

3. Sajatovic M. Treatment of bipolar disorder in older adults. Int J Geriatr Psychiatry. 2002;17:865–73.
4. Bartels SJ. Improving system of care for older adults with mental illness in the United States. Findings and recommendations for the President's New Freedom Commission on Mental Health. Am J Geriatr Psychiatry. 2003;11(5):486–97.
5. Jeste D, Alexopoulos GS, Bartels SJ, Cummings JL, Gallo JJ, Gottlieb GL, et al. Consensus statement on the upcoming crisis in geriatric mental health: research agenda for the next 2 decades. Arch Gen Psychiatry. 1999;56(9):848–53.
6. Bartels SJ. Improving the United States' system of care for older adults with mental illness: findings and recommendations for the President's New Freedom Commission on Mental Health. Am J Geriatr Psychiatry. 2003;11(5):486–97.
7. Eden J, Maslow K, Le M, Blazer D. The mental health and substance use workforce for older adults: in whose hands? Washington, DC: National Academies Press; 2012.
8. Hoge MA, Karel MJ, Zeiss AM, Alegria M, Moye J. Strengthening psychology's workforce for older adults: implications of the Institute of Medicine's report to Congress. Am Psychol. 2015;70(3):265.
9. Bishop TF, Press MJ, Keyhani S, Pincus H. Acceptance of insurance by psychiatrists and the implications for access to mental health care. JAMA Psychiatry. 2014;71(2):176–81.
10. Kupfer DJ. The increasing medical burden in bipolar disorder. JAMA. 2005;293(20):2528–30.
11. Kilbourne AM. The burden of general medical conditions in patients with bipolar disorder. Curr Psychiatry Rep. 2005;7(6):471–7.
12. Kilbourne AM, McCarthy JF, Welsh D, Blow F. Recognition of co-occurring medical conditions among patients with serious mental illness. J Nerv Ment Dis. 2006;194(8):598–602.
13. Kilbourne AM, Welsh D, McCarthy JF, Post EP, Blow FC. Quality of care for cardiovascular disease-related conditions in patients with and without mental disorders. J Gen Intern Med. 2008;23(10):1628–33.
14. Bartels SJ, Coakley EH, Zubritsky C, Ware JH, Miles KM, Arean PA, et al. Improving access to geriatric mental health services: a randomized trial comparing treatment engagement with integrated versus enhanced referral care for depression, anxiety, and at-risk alcohol use. Am J Psychiatry. 2004;161(8):1455–62.
15. Perlick DA, Rosenheck RA, Miklowitz DJ, Chessick C, Wolff N, Kaczynski R, et al. Prevalence and correlates of burden among caregivers of patients with bipolar disorder enrolled in the Systematic Treatment Enhancement Program for Bipolar Disorder. Bipolar Disord. 2007;9(3):262–73.
16. Perlick DA, Hohenstein JM, Clarkin JF, Kaczynski R, Rosenheck RA. Use of mental health and primary care services by caregivers of patients with bipolar disorder: a preliminary study. Bipolar Disord. 2005;7(2):126–35.
17. Depp C, Jeste DV. Bipolar disorder in older adults: a critical review. Bipolar Disord. 2004;6(5):343–67.
18. Byers AL, Arean PA, Yaffe K. Low use of mental health services among older Americans with mood and anxiety disorders. Psychiatr Serv. 2012;63(1):66–72.
19. Bartels SJ, Forester B, Miles KM, Joyce T. Mental health service use by elderly patients with bipolar disorder and unipolar major depression. Am J Geriatr Psychiatry. 2000;8(2):160–6.
20. Depp C, Lindamer L, Folsom D, Hough R, Gilmer T, Garcia P, et al. Differences in clinical features and mental health services use in bipolar disorder across the lifespan. Am J Geriatr Psychiatry. 2005;13(4):290–9.
21. Young RC, Falk J. Age, manic psychopathology, and treatment response. Int J Geriatr Psychiatry. 1989;4:73–8.
22. Depp CA, Moore DJ, Sitzer D, Palmer BW, Eyler LT, Roesch S, et al. Neurocognitive impairment in middle-aged and older adults with bipolar disorder: comparison to schizophrenia and normal comparison subjects. J Affect Disord. 2007;101(1–3):201–9.

23. Stensland M, Watson PR, Grazier KL. An examination of costs, charges, and payments for inpatient psychiatric treatment in community hospitals. Psychiatr Serv. 2012;63(7):666–71.
24. Sajatovic M, Blow FC, Ignacio R, Kales H. Age-related modifiers of clincial presentation and health service use among veterans with bipolar disorder. Psychiatr Serv. 2004;55(9):1014–21.
25. Yu C, Sylvestre JD, Segal M, Looper KJ, Rej S. Predictors of psychiatric re-hospitalization in older adults with severe mental illness. Int J Geriatr Psychiatry. 2015;30(11):1114–9.
26. Woo BK, Golshan S, Allen EC, Daly JW, Jeste DV, Sewell DD. Factors associated with frequent admissions to an acute geriatric psychiatric inpatient unit. J Geriatr Psychiatry Neurol. 2006;19(4):226–30.
27. Lehmann SW, Rabins PV. Factors related to hospitalization in elderly manic patients with early and late-onset bipolar disorder. Int J Geriatr Psychiatry. 2006;21(11):1060–4.
28. Miller EA, Rosenheck RA. Risk of nursing home admission in association with mental illness nationally in the department of veterans affairs. Med Care. 2006;44(4):343–51.
29. Bartels SJ, Mueser KT, Miles KM. A comparative study of elderly patients with schizophrenia and bipolar disorder in nursing homes and the community. Schizophr Res. 1997;27(2–3):181–90.
30. Grabowski DC, Aschbrenner KA, Feng Z, Mor V. Mental illness in nursing homes: variations across states. Health affairs (Project Hope). 2009;28(3):689–700.
31. Becker MA, Boaz TL, Andel R, Gum AM, Papadopoulos AS. Predictors of preventable nursing home hospitalizations: the role of mental disorders and dementia. Am J Geriatr Psychiatry. 2010;18(6):475–82.
32. Bartels SJ, Miles KM, Dums AR, Levine KJ. Are nursing homes appropriate for older adults with severe mental illness? Conflicting consumer and clinician views and implications for the Olmstead decision. J Am Geriatr Soc. 2003;51(11):1571–9.
33. Wang PS, Lane M, Olfson M, Pincus HA, Wells KB, Kessler RC. Twelve-month use of mental health services in the united states: results from the national comorbidity survey replication. Arch Gen Psychiatry. 2005;62(6):629–40.
34. Olfson M, Kroenke K, Wang S, Blanco C. Trends in office-based mental health care provided by psychiatrists and primary care physicians. J. Clin. Psychiatry 2014;75(3):247–53.
35. Karel MJ, Gatz M, Smyer MA. Aging and mental health in the decade ahead: what psychologists need to know. Am Psychol. 2012;67(3):184.
36. Klap R, Unroe KT, Unützer J. Caring for mental illness in the United States: a focus on older adults. Am J Geriatr Psychiatry. 2003;11(5):517–24.
37. McHugh RK, Whitton SW, Peckham AD, Welge JA, Otto MW. Patient preference for psychological vs. pharmacologic treatment of psychiatric disorders: a meta-analytic review. J Clin Psychiatry. 2013;74(6):1478–602.
38. Landreville P, Landry J, Baillargeon L, Guérette A, Matteau É. Older adults' acceptance of psychological and pharmacological treatments for depression. J Gerontol Ser B Psychol Sci Soc Sci. 2001;56(5):P285–91.
39. Depp C, Patterson TL, Lebowitz B, Lacro J, Jeste DV. Medication adherence skills training in middle aged and elderly adults with bipolar disorder: development and pilot study. Bipolar Disord. 2007;9(6):636–45.
40. Bauer MS, McBride L, Williford WO, Glick H, Kinosian B, Altshuler L, et al. Collaborative care for bipolar disorder: part II. Impact on clinical outcome, function, and costs. Psychiatr Serv. 2006;57(7):937–45.
41. Bauer MS, McBride L, Williford WO, Glick H, Kinosian B, Altshuler L, et al. Collaborative care for bipolar disorder: part I. Intervention and implementation in a randomized effectiveness trial. Psychiatr Serv. 2006;57(7):927–36.
42. Trivedi RB, Post EP, Sun H, Pomerantz A, Saxon AJ, Piette JD, et al. Prevalence, comorbidity, and prognosis of mental health among US veterans. Am J Public Health. 2015;105(12):2564–9.

43. Ben-Zeev D, Drake RE, Corrigan PW, Rotondi AJ, Nilsen W, Depp C. Using contemporary technologies in the assessment and treatment of serious mental illness. Am J Psychiatr Rehabil. 2012;15(4):357–76.
44. Depp CA, Kim DH, Vergel de Dios L, Wang V, Ceglowski JA. Pilot study of mood ratings captured by mobile phone versus paper-and-pencil mood charts in bipolar disorder. J Dual Diagn. 2012;8(4):326–32.
45. Depp CA, Ceglowski J, Wang VC, Yaghouti F, Mausbach BT, Thompson WK, et al. Augmenting psychoeducation with a mobile intervention for bipolar disorder: a randomized controlled trial. J Affect Disord. 2015;174:23–30.
46. Brenes GA, Danhauer SC, Lyles MF, Hogan PE, Miller ME. Telephone-delivered cognitive behavioral therapy and telephone-delivered nondirective supportive therapy for rural older adults with generalized anxiety disorder: a randomized clinical trial. JAMA Psychiatry. 2015;72(10):1012–20.
47. Pratt SI, Bartels SJ, Mueser KT, Naslund JA, Wolfe R, Pixley HS, et al. Feasibility and effectiveness of an automated telehealth intervention to improve illness self-management in people with serious psychiatric and medical disorders. Psychiatr Rehabil J. 2013;36(4):297.
48. Pratt SI, Naslund JA, Wolfe RS, Santos M, Bartels SJ. Automated telehealth for managing psychiatric instability in people with serious mental illness. J Mental Health. 2014;24:261–5.
49. Karlin BE, Karel MJ. National integration of mental health providers in VA home-based primary care: an innovative model for mental health care delivery with older adults. Gerontologist. 2014;54(5):868–79.
50. Reifler BV, Bruce ML. Home-based mental health services for older adults: a review of ten model programs. Am J Geriatr Psychiatry. 2014;22(3):241–7.
51. Veerbeek M, Oude Voshaar R, Depla M, Pot AM. Mental health care monitor older adults (MEMO): monitoring patient characteristics and outcome in Dutch mental health services for older adults. Int J Methods Psychiatr Res. 2013;22(2):100–9.

Index

Note: **Page numbers followed by *b*, *f*, *t* refer to boxes, figures, and tables, respectively**

S.W. Lehmann and B.P. Forester (eds.), *Bipolar Disorder in Older Age Patients*,
DOI 10.1007/978-3-319-48912-4

CPI Antony Rowe
Chippenham, UK
2017-06-14 01:03